PROGRESS IN
CLINICAL SURGERY

PROGRESS IN CLINICAL SURGERY

BY VARIOUS AUTHORS

Edited by

RODNEY SMITH
M.S., F.R.C.S.

Surgeon, St. George's Hospital, London

Series III

With 129 Illustrations

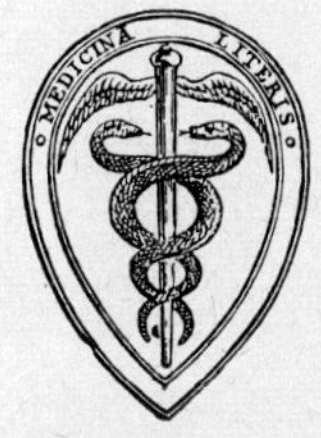

J. & A. CHURCHILL LTD.
104 Gloucester Place, London

1969

First Edition .   .   . 1954
Series II .   .   . 1961
Series III .   .   . 1969

Standard Book Number
7000 1395 4

Printed in Great Britain

PREFACE

The objectives in the preparation of Series III of progress in Clinical Surgery have been the same as in the preparation of Series I and II. Once again the main purpose has been to produce a volume of manageable length highlighting some of the surgical topics which have, for one reason or another, received special study during the last few years, and in particular those where recent work has led to some major re-appraisal.

This volume is intended primarily to help the postgraduate surgical student working for his final F.R.C.S. examination and the younger surgeon with a recent consultant appointment, and for this reason the emphasis has been placed upon practical general surgery rather than upon surgical research, though naturally it is through the application of surgical research to clinical surgery that progress is made. The distinction is a fine one but, to take an example, it has been considered that it will be of more help to the reader to include a detailed chapter upon "Advances in the management of major postoperative complications" than upon organ transplantation. The latter subject, though indeed the "growing edge" of surgery, has not yet become the province of the general surgeon and its study should probably at the moment begin by securing an appointment in one of the specialized units engaged in this work.

In arriving at the final selection of twenty surgical topics, the difficulty has been to decide what can be left out rather than what can be put in. Inevitably each reader will find some subject omitted which he would like to have seen included, and attempts to make this possible would have at least doubled the length of this book. In apologizing now for such omissions as may appear significant, I hope that the deeds of my contributors will compensate for the misdeeds of their editor, and take this opportunity of thanking them for all the care and trouble they have taken to cover so fully and concisely these selected subjects.

RODNEY SMITH

St. George's Hospital,
London. 1969.

v

CONTRIBUTORS

K. E. BARRETT, M.D.(Lond.), M.C.Path.
Head of the Department of Haematology, Ottawa Civic Hospital; Examiner to the Royal College of Physicians and Surgeons of Canada.

BRYAN BROOKE, M.D.(Birm.), M.Chir.(Camb.), F.R.C.S.(Eng.)
Professor of Surgery, University of London at St. George's Hospital Medical School.

D. CHURCHILL-DAVIDSON, M.A., M.B., B.Chir.(Camb.), F.R.C.S.(Eng.)
Consultant Orthopaedic Surgeon, Royal London Homoeopathic Hospital, London; Surgical Lt.-Cdr., R.N.R.

JOHN HAYWARD, M.B., B.S.(Lond.), F.R.C.S.(Eng.)
Member Scientific Staff, Imperial Cancer Research Fund; Research Fellow, Department of Surgery, Guy's Hospital, London.

A. H. HUNT, M.A., D.M., M.Ch., F.R.C.S.
Senior Surgeon and Surgeon in Charge, St. Bartholomew's Hospital; Surgeon, Royal Marsden Hospital, London.

A. W. KAY, M.D.(Glas.), Ch.M., F.R.C.S.(Ed. & Glas.)
Regius Professor of Surgery, University of Glasgow.

J. R. KENYON, B.Sc.(Glas.), Ch.M., F.R.C.S.(Ed. & Eng.)
Consultant Surgeon, St. Mary's Hospital, London and Paddington General Hospital.

LOUIS KREEL, M.B., B.Ch., M.R.C.P.(Lond.), F.F.R., D.M.R.D.(Eng.)
Consultant Radiologist, Royal Free Hospital and New End Hospital, London.

E. C. GRUEBEL LEE, M.B., B.Ch., F.R.C.S.(Ed.), F.R.C.S.(Eng.)
Senior Surgical Registrar, St. George's Hospital, London.

J. H. LOUW, Ch.M., F.R.C.S.
Professor of Surgery, University of Cape Town, Medical School.

ALLYN G. MAY, M.D.
University of Rochester, School of Medicine and Dentistry, Rochester, New York.

G. B. ONG, O.B.E., F.R.C.S.(Eng.), F.R.C.S., F.A.C.S.
Professor of Surgery, Hong Kong University.

ALAN PARKS, M.Ch.(Oxf.), F.R.C.S.(Eng.), M.R.C.P.(Lond.)
Consultant Surgeon, London Hospital and St. Mark's Hospital, London.

CHARLES G. ROB, M.C., M.A.(Camb.), M.D., M.Chir., F.R.C.S., M.R.C.S.
Chairman, Dept. of Surgery, University of Rochester School of Medicine and Dentistry, New York.

R. A. SELLWOOD, M.B., Ch.M.(Bristol), F.R.C.S.(Eng.)
Dept. of Surgery, Royal Postgraduate Medical School, London.

A. H. M. SIDDONS, M.R.C.P.(Lond.), M.Chir.(Camb.), F.R.C.S.(Eng.)
Consultant Surgeon, St. George's Hospital, London.

RODNEY SMITH, M.S.(Lond.), F.R.C.S.(Eng.)
Surgeon, St. George's Hospital, London.

R. B. WELBOURN, M.A.(Camb.), M.D., F.R.C.S.(Eng.)
Professor of Surgery, University of London; Director, Department of Surgery, Royal Postgraduate Medical School and Hammersmith Hospital.

A. W. WILKINSON, Ch.M.(Ed.), F.R.C.S.(Ed. & Eng.)
Nuffield Professor of Paediatric Surgery, Institute of Child Health, University of London; Surgeon, Hospital for Sick Children, Great Ormond Street.

E. D. WILLIAMS, M.A., M.B., B.Chir.(Camb.), M.C.Path.
Lecturer in Morbid Anatomy, Royal Postgraduate Medical School, London.

D. INNES WILLIAMS, M.A.(Camb.), M.D., M.Chir., F.R.C.S.(Eng.)
Surgeon, St. Peter's and St. Paul's Hospitals; Genito-Urinary Surgeon, Hospital for Sick Children, Great Ormond Street.

MICHAEL P. WRIGHT, B.M., B.Ch.(Oxon.), F.R.C.S.(Ed.)
Senior Registrar, Thoracic Surgery Unit, St. George's Hospital, London.

CONTENTS

CHAPTER 1

ADVANCES IN THE MANAGEMENT OF MAJOR POSTOPERATIVE COMPLICATIONS

E. C. GRUEBEL LEE

Introduction

A hundred years have passed since Lister. There has been a great increase of scientific knowledge, which has often resulted in changes being introduced rapidly into the practice of surgery. The last decade has shown a noticeable acceleration of the process. No surgeon doubts his ability to prepare, anaesthetize and carry out larger procedures for a widening range of pathology with better results than his predecessors. Until recently, however, British literature has failed to show an equal interest in the complications which all too often follow these operations.

Unwanted and unexpected sequelae may follow all surgical procedures. The training surgeon is expected to learn of these during his apprenticeship and is often unprepared by the written word for their extent and diversity. Inaccurate statistics result from a combination of lack of recognition of these complications, a dearth of reports from surgical units with trained staff, poor recording systems which prevent adequate retrospective analysis, and biased figures from surgical experts whose results (to which they devote a special interest) must be better than a busy general surgeon can hope to emulate. It is one of the greater failings of doctors in our unified Health Service, that we have not produced a unified clinical recording system allowing careful statistical analysis of our results throughout the country. Specialized training of junior staff and students is urgently required to use the complicated computer technology being introduced into hospitals. Clinical practice will otherwise mirror the antiquated hospitals in which we are forced to work. With the increase of knowledge, hard work and careful planning is required just to maintain high clinical standards.

The problem of complications remains a challenge. In the face of falling morbidity and mortality, patients still have the chance of dying from the most trivial operation. In the elderly, even the most major surgery may be tolerated with surprising equanimity, but like modern war the onset of a minor complication may be followed by a series of increasingly overwhelming incidents, which could be called an escalating complication syndrome. In one series of patients over 75, 45·8 per cent of emergency cases, and 20·3 per cent of cold cases died after operation (Luccioni *et al.*).

The Changing Nature of Disease

The Hippocratic maxim "The progress of a disease should be so guided, where guidance is needed, that it develops in the most favourable manner according to its natural tendency" has unfortunately become clouded. It is difficult to demonstrate to students the natural history of a pathological process. Not only have modern drugs changed the character of tissue reaction, but multiple pathologies occurring in an older age group of patients, and the altered physiological process resulting from chemical and surgical treatment produce an increasingly complicated picture of disease. Many surgical patients carry pathology previously lethal, but now held in check by modern medicine.

Metabolic Changes during Surgery

The effect of surgery is to produce a complex biochemical change of the whole organism against which background local healing or complications must be assessed. Ignoring the changes may lead to severe metabolic derangements, particularly when they occur in the very young, the elderly, severely diseased, or when the pathological process is extensive or sustained. Since 1932 (Cuthbertson, 1932; Kinney, 1960) it has been known that retention of water, sodium ion, increased K^+ ion excretion and excretion of an acid urine resulting in mild alkalosis, is the natural result of trauma or surgery in a healthy patient. Isotopic dilution studies have yielded accurate information of electrolyte changes in cells and other fluid compartments in the body (Moore, 1967). Careful nitrogen, fat, and carbohydrate studies are recorded in various pathological states (Moore *et al.*, 1963). Cell mass is rapidly lost and extracellular fluid accumulation may occur leading to a state of oedematous wasting. Haemorrhage further deranges the constituents of fluid compartments. Multiple hormone response has been demonstrated to bring about these changes involving renin, angiotension, aldosterone and vaso-pressin (Skillman, 1967). Adrenal cortical hormones (Sandberg, 1954), thyroid hormones (Clark & Horn, 1965; Blomstedt, 1965) and insulin (Evans & Butterfield, 1951) also play a part (Johnson, 1967) in the complex response.

GENERAL COMPLICATIONS

Balanced Chemical Requirement Problems

FLUIDS AND ELECTROLYTES (Marcus, 1962; Reitermeier, 1962)

Since the war, surgeons have taken great interest in careful balance of fluid and electrolytes in the pre-operative preparation and post-

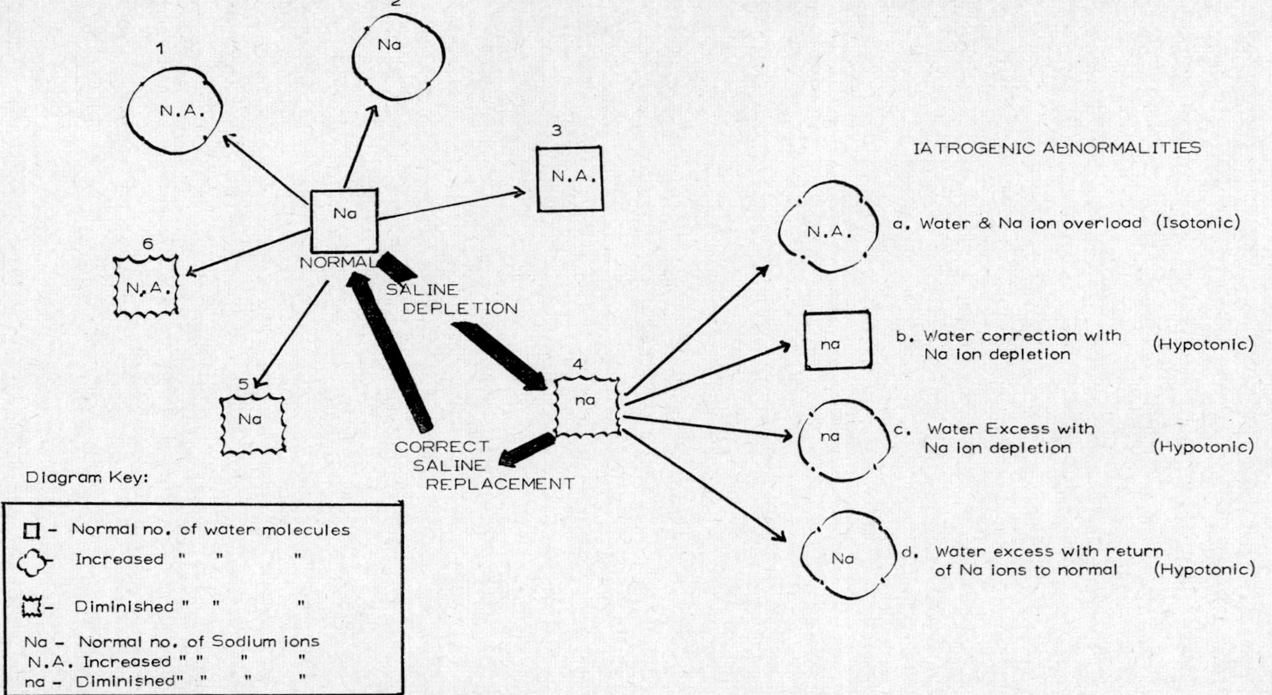

Fig. 1.1. The possible altered relationships of water molecules and Na ions. Pathway 4 demonstrates the common surgical abnormality of loss of water molecules and Na ions in isotonic concentrations.

operative management. Too often major defects result from iatrogenic deficiency (Le Quesney, 1967). Alterations occur in three ways. Firstly, an abnormal intake, deficiency being more common than excess; secondly, abnormal loss inadequately replaced; and thirdly, endogenous alterations of body fluid and constituents normally occurring in association with primary renal or cardiac disease.

The condition occurs with vomiting, aspiration of bowel contents, fistula, haemorrhage, serum loss or diarrhoea. If the saline is not replaced correctly, hypotonic dilution results either from excess water or insufficient Na ion replacement. The usual fluid balance chart helps to make this possible by not differentiating between saline loss and plain water replacement (5 per cent dextrose). Potassium ion loss must be replaced, but oral administration of enteric-coated capsules may produce ulceration in the small bowel leading to haemorrhage, perforation or stenosis (Campbell and Knapp, 1966; Alexander and Schwartz, 1966).

DERANGEMENT OF ACID BASE BALANCE (Walker, 1967; Van Slyke, 1966; Anderson, 1965)

Acidosis is clinically regarded as an increase, or a tendency to increase, in the hydrogen ions in the blood with an inverse change in the pH. Alkalosis is the converse (Morgan *et al.*, 1963). These changes result from respiratory or metabolic causes defined by changes in carbon-dioxide tension (PCO_2) and buffer base respectively.

Acidosis produces cardiovascular changes which may result in decreased cardiac output and eventual ventricular fibrillation and death (Clowes *et al.*, 1961; Ebert *et al.*, 1962). It is the more common major acid-base defect in surgery, and results from poor tissue diffusion of blood, excess loss of base or excess CO_2 retention (Lyons and Moore, 1966). Recently Moore has drawn attention to the dangers of alkalosis which may kill by producing tetany and convulsions. Combined derangements may occur. The normal mild alkalosis may be made worse by anaesthetic hyperventilation. More lactic acid is produced to buffer the respiratory alkalosis. Post-operatively blood loss may increase the metabolic acidosis and if hypoventilation is allowed to occur after the anaesthetic, respiratory acidosis is superimposed to produce a severe, or even fatal derangement.

Other Requirements

Deficient intake of protein (Rhoads, 1952), carbohydrate and vitamins (Rice *et al.*, 1950) occurs when the clinician ignores the increased requirements of the post-operative patient and may lead to states of gross hypoproteinaemia and wound healing deficiency. High calorie parenteral or alimentary feeding reduces post-operative negative nitrogen balance (Johnston *et al.*, 1966). Positive balance begins in the second week after high calorie intake.

Shock (Shoemaker and Baker, 1967)

Shock has been defined as a disparity in volume or distribution between the blood and its vascular bed, resulting in peripheral circulatory failure. Usually a reduction of venous return (low central venous pressure) results in diminution of the ventricular stroke volume, and the arterial blood pressure falls. Reflex homeostasis is mediated by the sympathetic system to produce peripheral constriction and tachycardia, which raised the blood pressure (compensated shock). If this mechanism is insufficient to bring the arterial pressure back to normal the patient is said to be in a state of decompensated shock and requires urgent replacement of circulating volume. Recent literature elucidates (Robins, 1966) the secondary changes produced by deficient capillary perfusion, with ischaemic anoxia resulting in severe metabolic acidosis. Finally, extensive intravascular coagulation occurs in the microcirculation throughout the body potentiating the biochemical changes, increasing the permeability of cells lining the capillary bed and allowing further loss of blood constituents to the extracellular compartment (Hardway, 1966).

Evidence of cellular ischaemia is seen with the widespread mucosal necrosis throughout the bowel and renal tubular necrosis. The term irreversible shock has been applied when the condition fails to improve because cellular damage has been overwhelming, therapy has been inadequate or slow, or as the result of major biochemical defects, as yet unrecognized.

It will be seen that combinations of factors produce increasing complexity of the clinical situation if therapy does not immediately return the circulation to normal. In cardiogenic shock attempts to expand the circulating volume by transfusion are dangerous and may overload an already strained myocardium. This patchy distribution of volumes, and poor mixing prevents the blood volume estimation, predicting the volume of fluid which requires to be replaced. Direct central venous pressure measurements are much more useful in assessing the functional requirements of volume replacement. It can be readily carried out by retrograde catheterization of veins in the arm or by direct subclavian puncture (Aubaniac, 1952; Davidson *et al.*, 1963), and has proved important in the management of severely shocked patients.

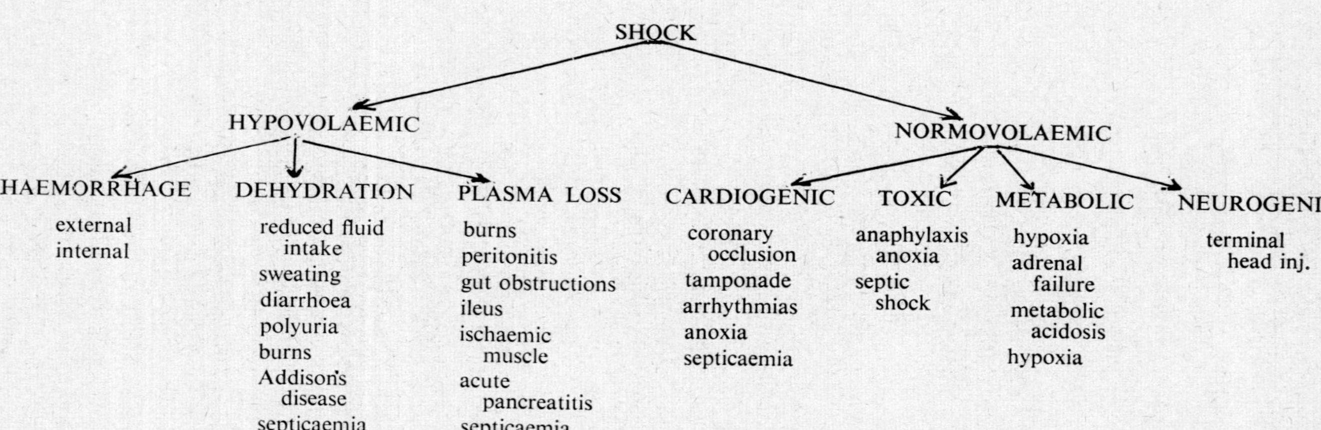

Fig. 1.2. Common causes of shock (Brooks, 1967; Gitlitz and Hurwitt, 1964).

Septic Shock

Recent interest centres on septic shock which used to have a high mortality. Etiology is complex and illustrates some of the factors involved in all types of shock. It results from the action of bacterial toxins on the myocardium (Seigel, 1965) and the blood vessels, and causes severe biochemical changes. It may follow severe infection (Lansing, 1963) trauma, surgery, haemorrhage (Ravin *et al.*, 1960) instrumentation or blood transfusion. Four clinical types have been described (Brooks, 1967).

TYPE I, with predominant myocardial damage. There is poor response to transfusion in spite of a rising venous pressure. Bradycardia may occur.

TYPE II. Dilatation of the capillary bed is masked and the patient often has warm dilated extremities. Adequate quantities of urine with a low osmolarity are excreted. Metabolic acidosis may occur in severe cases resulting in a change in the clinical picture to one of worsening hypotension, a rise in the central venous pressure and peripheral constriction.

TYPE III is characterized by loss of large quantities of protein rich fluid into an "abnormal body cavity" (e.g. gut, peritoneum) or through a damaged capillary endothelium into the extracellular space.

TYPE IV. Irreversible shock.

Treatment. Changes in the modern treatment of shock are based upon the following points:

(i) Careful monitoring of vital signs by a trained team in an intensive care unit has been used extensively, particularly in the U.S.A. Peripheral blood pressure and central venous pressure readings provide the best guide to progress (Sykes, 1963; McLean, 1964).

(ii) Expansion of circulating volume by intravenous administration of blood, plasma (particularly when protein leakage is high) in synthetic plasma expanders. Low molecular weight dextran solutions seem useful because of their function to prevent microcirculation sludging and allow better tissue perfusion (Yeo, 1966; Rousell, 1966).

(iii) With cardiogenic shock, great care must be taken not to overload the circulation. Digitalis administration and isoprenaline infusion may help because of a direct stimulation of cardiac output (Du Toit *et al.*, 1966; Brooks, 1967).

(iv) The use of Na bicarbonate infusions is required in sufficient quantities to counteract developing metabolic acidosis.

(v) Broad spectrum antibiotics (e.g. chloramphenicol) and hydro-cortisone are required in septic shock. The latter must be given in large doses for its pharmacological effect on the reduction of capillary permeability.

(vi) Drugs affecting the tone of peripheral arterioles. Controversy rages about the beneficial effect of the peripheral constriction of nor-adrenalin. In many cases its use results in a transient rise in blood pressure with subsequent deterioration. It seems sensible that some cases with obviously dilated, warm periphery may benefit, but in these, as in the hypotensive anaesthesia, tissue perfusion of blood is probably adequate. Recently it has been shown that certain cases do not respond to fluid replacement in spite of normal central venous pressure measurements. This capacitance defect of peripheral vessels probably indicates maximal arteriolar constriction with capillary bed dilatation or capillary lining defects allowing extracellular leakage of blood constituents. Steroids may be helpful but must be used in pharmacological rather than physiological doses (i.e. 5–8 g. of hydrocortisone), and adrenergic blocker drugs have been used to overcome maximal sympathomimetic activity on the terminal arteriole combined with very rapid expansion of plasma volume (Arbulu and Thal, 1966; Thal and Wilson, 1965; Keddie *et al.*, 1966). The technique is dangerous and requires careful preparation of adequate size intravenous canulation to allow the fluid to be infused as fast as possible. Two or more drips may be set up as a necessary precaution.

Haemorrhage

Paucity of reports of post-operative haemorrhage is not mirrored by practical experience. Most cases occur within the first 24 hours after surgery and the term reactionary haemorrhage has been applied. All surgeons have experienced cases which bleed after careful haemostasis, and all cases becoming shocked soon after the operation should be considered to have bled until proven otherwise. Bleeding may occur from the wound, into the wound, into dead space, intraperitoneally, into the substance of a viscus or into its lumen. Intraluminar bleeding is not confined to the gut; bleeding into the urinary tract is not uncommon. Jaundice may result from haemobilia following exploration of the common bile duct (MacVaugh *et al.*, 1966). Exsanguinating haemorrhage is, of course, more common from the sites of major abdominal, thoracic or vascular surgery, but bleeding from sites unrelated to the operation is not uncommon. Loss may occur from oesophageal varices or an old or acute peptic ulcer. Beil *et al.*, (1964) analysed 35 cases of massive post-operative haemorrhage from acute peptic ulceration of stomach and duodenum. Although most were seen within one week of surgery, a few occurred as late as the 42nd post-operative day. Fifty per cent of cases had associated intraperitoneal infections and a further 24 per cent infection at other sites. The bleeding site may not be immediately obvious. Unexplained shock warrants the passage of a nasogastric tube. Treatment is by immediate blood replacement. Early exploration and haemostasis lowers the subsequent morbidity and mortality. Causes of death include continued haemorrhage, infection, pulmonary complications and renal tubular necrosis. Osmolar diuresis may help prevent renal failure when used with plasma expanders (Stremple, Ellison and Carey, 1966). A septic intraperitoneal haematoma is particularly lethal. Gross biochemical changes may occur including uraemia and severe metabolic acidosis.

Disorders of the Clotting Mechanism

Clotting defects fall into two main categories.

The Tendency to Bleed

Recent work has classified the defects which can occur after operations. Transfusion of a large volume of blood results in excess administration of citrate (used to prevent coagulation within the bottle), and calcium gluconate should be given with each bottle to replace bonded calcium ions. Secondary deficiency of items in the normal clotting mechanism may occur when bleeding continues and has to be replaced by large quantities of blood.

Thrombocytopaenia may require transfusion of freshly drawn blood. Vascular and cardiac surgeons realize that in spite of adequate volume replacement, the more severe the loss, the more likely is the bleeding to continue. Some of the causes of this clotting defect are as yet unknown but centre on pathological fibrinolytic states (McNichol, 1966).

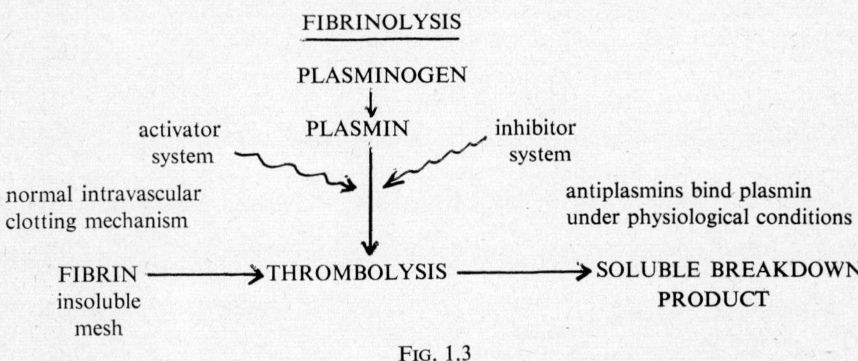

Fig. 1.3

The enzyme plasmin has a fibrinolytic role to clear insoluble plasmin from the vascular tree. Under physiological conditions antiplasmins bind and block any plasmins produced. When intramuscular thrombosis occurs the balance shifts towards thrombolytic activity. Under abnormal conditions a state of excess fibrinolytic activity may occur when vast quantities of plasminogen activator are released. Hyperplasminaemia allows digestion of fibrinogen, prothrombin and certain factors involved in the generation of thromboplastin, as well as fibrin itself. A true clotting defect is thus imposed on excess fibrinolysis.

The diagnosis is made when a patient with a predisposing lesion develops incoagulable blood, prolonged clotting and prothrombin time and a low or zero level of plasma plasminogen. Predisposing causes occur in obstetrics, prostatic carcinoma, malignant metastases, pancreatic neoplasms, leukaemia and hepatic cirrhosis. Hypothermia, hypotension, massive tissue damage or dissection, and anoxia are associated with massive release of plasminogen activator. Episolaminocaproic acid (EACA), a synthetic amino acid, is a potent inhibitor of the fibrinolytic system. It has been used when bleeding is serious in spite of the theoretical hazard of intravascular thrombosis (McNicol, 1964).

Tendency to Form Excess Thrombin

Venous Thrombosis (Poole, 1967)

In 1947 Homan (Homan, 1947) reported 2 per cent incidence of intravascular thrombosis. Of his series 50 per cent developed pulmonary embolus with a 20 per cent mortality. In the older age groups the incidence is probably much higher (15 per cent in cases over 50 years of age). Again statistical evidence of the complication is not adequately recorded in the U.K.

Virchows triad of alteration in the vessel wall, stasis and blood composition changes have received modern confirmation (Gibbs, 1967; Quick, 1958). Two periods of increased coaguability exist (a) during surgery and (b) after a latent period during the first five days. Clotting may occur in the venous or arterial tree (e.g. coronary thrombosis). Massive thrombosis may result in venous gangrene (Young *et al.*, 1966). Special risk of thrombosis has been described in the early post-operative period, during pregnancy, infections, heart disease, malignancy, the elderly, large fractures, polycythaemia, paralysed limbs, varicose veins and obesity. The last two are particularly important in young people. Recent suggestion has been made that women on oral contraceptives may have a predisposition to thrombose. Even gentle exercise has been shown to increase fibrinolysis and prevent thrombosis (Menton *et al.*, 1967). Most surgeons anticoagulate their patients for 10 days when venous thrombosis is diagnosed. Intravenous Dextran solutions have been used in the treatment (Bryant, Bloom and Brewer, 1966).
Diagnosis. The old problem of early diagnosis of venous thrombosis

before it has become fixed to the vessel wall by inflammation, has not been solved. Signs are unusual in the early dangerous stage when embolism is likely to occur. Coon and Willis (1959) reported no previous evidence of venous thrombosis in 80 per cent of a series of fatal pulmonary emboli. Phlebography has been tried but seems a major procedure in a dangerous situation.

[131]I-labelled fibrinogen has been administered and scintillation counter activity used to localize thrombi in animals. Plasmin and fibrinolytic enzymes have been similarly labelled in experimental situations. Clinically a method has been described where ^{131}I-labelled antibody to fibrinogen localizes and concentrates on preformed thrombi (Reich, 1966). In the future it may be possible to screen patients with suspicious tachycardia or pyrexia which often precedes the local signs of inflammation. Some surgeons advocate thrombectomy for massive venous thrombosis (Homans, 1947; Mahorner, 1966).

Pulmonary Embolism (Sasahara and Stein, 1965)

(Acute Pulmonary Embolism, Editorial, *Lancet*, 1965, **2,** 70–71.) Incidence of embolization after venous thrombosis is uncertain because:

(a) Many cases are not recorded.
(b) Difficulty to diagnose minor embolic phenomena.
(c) Difficulty of diagnosing occult thrombosis.

Incidence has been estimated as 0·5 per cent of hospital admissions and 10 per cent of autopsies.

Gibbs (1967) recorded 33 per cent embolic rate in post-operative cases developing a deep vein thrombosis, but recent studies using radioactive intravascular macro-molecules and pulmonary angiography have shown that minor vascular occusions can occur with minor systemic changes. Alternatively, vascular constriction of the pulmonary tree may convert a relatively minor block into a major clinical syndrome. Isotopic follow-up of the blocked vascular tree in those who survive has shown the expected clearing of the block by lysis or recanilization. Multiple minor embolism may be the cause of idiopathic pulmonary hypertension.

The mean time from operation to embolization in a large series was stated by Meyerowitz (1966) to be 21 days. Spring and autumn months seem to have a higher incidence.

Of 67 fatal cases, 37 presented as sudden unexpected fatalities. Fifteen collapsed whilst straining on the toilet or bedpan. In only five of these cases was death delayed for up to 30 minutes. Only eight cases had previous signs of deep vein thrombosis. These had been treated with anticoagulants. Most writers agree about the brief interval between acute episode shock and death. Diagnosis is made in the less severe case by the sudden onset of shock, respiratory distress and chest pain in a patient at risk. E.C.G. changes of acute (R) heart strain or recent (R) bundle branch block may be helpful. The X-ray changes of wedge opacity are not usually seen at an early stage. It is suspected that many more incidents of less severe embolization occur and escape detection unless repeated episodes manifest themselves. Major importance is attached to the prevention of venous thrombosis. Strict pre-operative care to prevent calf pressure during the operation and early mobilization are important factors (Gibbs, 1967). Anticoagulation as soon as venous thrombosis is diagnosed seems of value. Many authors prefer Heparin to the use of the newer oral anticoagulants.

Treatment. Much recent work centres on the early diagnosis because development of new cardiac by-pass procedures allows removal of the embolic obstruction in a carefully prepared clinical situation with the chance to save a number of lives each year.

Heroic surgery as suggested by Trendelenburg may still have a place in the rapidly fatal case but the presence of a disposable oxygenator with cardiac by-pass pump could allow oxygenation until the patient could be taken to theatre for embolectomy.

Prevention of further embolization has been tried by various operations on the inferior vena cava. Mozes *et al.* suggest the following criteria as indications when anticoagulation fails to prevent embolization:

   (i) Single P.E. with dramatic deterioration of the patient's condition.

  (ii) Single P.E. from thrombosis in the known drainage area of the vena cava.

 (iii) Repeated P.E.'s when the source of embolization is unknown.

 (iv) Cases of respiratory insufficiency when microemboli are suspected.

OPERATIONS ON THE VENA CAVA (Mozes *et al.*, 1966)

Caval ligation is the operation most commonly employed. Mortality may be as high as 41 per cent in ill patients. Plication operations and simple obliteration by clip have been tried.

Major Infections in the Post-operative Period (Maitland, 1965)

In spite of the introduction of antibiotics, infection continues to be a major problem of surgery (Dineen, 1964). In a review of 15,000 major surgical procedures (Howe and Mozden, 1963) infection was demonstrated in 40 per cent of cases. Pulmonary and wound sepsis continue to be the common sites. Peritonitis, intraperitoneal abscesses, septicaemia and genito-urinary infections are still hazardous, especially in combination with other complications such as fluid abnormalities.

General Predisposing Factors

THE ORGANISMS

Pneumococci and haemolytic streptococci play a diminishing role in surgical infection (Finland, Jones and Barnes, 1959) but a great increase in staphylococcal infections has occurred particularly in hospital practice where antibiotics have produced a resistant population of organisms. Great care has to be taken to keep these organisms in check (Nahmias and Elkhoff, 1961). Infection with staphylococcus does not usually occur from the patient's own skin. Of 27 per cent of nasal carriers undergoing operations, 1·43 per cent developed wound infections compared with 1·39 per cent of the remaining 72 per cent of non-carriers (Rogers and Duffy, 1965). Recently the introduction of another generation of Penicillins and other antibiotics has reduced the hazard. The problem remains a constant threat on the surgical horizon.

SUSCEPTIBLE HOSTS

Experimental alteration of host defences in normal animals pre-disposes to infection (Miles and Burke, 1957; Elek & Conen, 1957). Clinical correlation of this theory of "Primary Lodgement" suggests that recent increase of infection may be due to a change in the age, general health and nutrition of the patient, and the severity of the technical procedure carried out (Barnes *et al.*, 1959, 1961).

HOSPITAL ENVIRONMENT

No surgeon doubts that "Asepsis" is one of the main supporting pillars on which modern surgery rests. A voluminous literature exists, describing modern concepts of hospital, ward and theatre design, sterilization, surgical and nursing technique, and the isolation and reduction of infection which does occur. How far British practice falls short of the ideal in most hospitals is too well known to describe. No statistical analysis exists which shows the cost to the Health Service of infective complications (which may be as high as 40 per cent). The inefficiency of old hospitals would not be tolerated in an industry in which capital investment in new plant and the cost of running old plants were correlated. However, the medical practitioner must take more responsibility to prevent infection.

Treatment of Infection

Prevention is more important than cure. Once infection is established, the old maxims have not been altered by antibiotic therapy. When pus is present, early drainage is imperative. Antibiotics should be administered in short, high-dose courses. In most cases it is better to prescribe the drug when the sensitivity of the organism has been found by culture.

Combinations of suitable antibiotics may prevent the development of resistance.

The prophylactic use of antibiotics is a vexed question. In non-infected cases it has been shown to predispose to wound and pulmonary infection (Meyers, 1959; Petersdorf *et al.*, 1957). However, antibiotic cover has been shown to be useful in operations on contaminated fields, such as the drainage of deep abscesses, for operations to relieve chronic obstruction of the bowel, urinary tract or common bile duct. As a cover for operations on patients with specific infections, its use is undoubted, e.g. tuberculosis. Antibiotics may be very useful in eliminating sources of infection such as medical staff who are nasal carriers of pathogenic organisms (Williams *et al.*, 1959).

Surgical technique is as important as ever to obliterate dead space, carry out careful haemostasis, to dissect with the least possible trauma to surrounding tissues, and suture with minimal tension. Allergic tissue reactions to the suture materials themselves, may play a part in the localization of organisms. Catgut gives the most, monofilament nylon and wire the least reaction.

Sites of Infection

WOUND INFECTION (Dineen, 1964; Howe and Mozden, 1963)

In the best hands, the level of wound sepsis still remains at about 4 per cent, but must be much higher in units with less interest in their results (Barnes *et al.*, 1959). Staphylococci, organisms of the enteric group, or combinations of organisms are the usual cause of infection. Haemolytic streptococci are now rare in surgical wounds and easily overcome with penicillin.

SUBPHRENIC ABSCESSES (Ozeran, 1967)

Localization of pus under the diaphragm is less common as a complication of abdominal surgery than formally, but it continues to occur. Since the introduction of antibiotics the diagnosis is seldom made in the early stages, and the obscure symptomatology may cause many weeks' delay. More commonly, after major peritoneal sepsis, a number of intraperitoneal localizations occurs, one of which may occupy a subphrenic space. Long continued use of antibiotics leads to a static (often sterile) collection of pus surrounded by hard granulation tissue undergoing fibrosis. Subacute bad health, weight loss, recurrent pyrexia and bursts of diarrhoea, should suggest the diagnosis. Occasionally these hidden abscesses declare themselves by pulmonary symptoms. Delayed diagnosis has been reported as late as seven years after operation (Dineen and McSherry, 1962). Diagnosis is made by X-ray changes of elevation and restricted movement of the leaf of the diaphragm associated with a minor pleural effusion. In difficult cases radio-isotope scan of the liver may show the mass displacing it from the diaphragm above (Bodon and Holzwasser, 1964). Extension into the pleural space may occur (Adams, 1961).

Detailed anatomical division of the subphrenic spaces into six seems excessive and to bear little relation to clinical findings (Boyd, 1958). Four spaces are of clinical importance. Right and left subphrenic, subhepatic and the lesser sac. Infection of the right subphrenic and subhepatic spaces usually follows operations on the stomach and biliary tree. The left has, in addition, to contend with pancreatic and splenic procedures. Colonic operations are an occasional source of abscesses.

Treatment is by operation (Bondi and Erikson, 1964). Left to themselves some abscesses will penetrate into the thoracic cavity and even discharge spontaneously into a main bronchus. The retroperitoneal approach (Nather and Oschner, 1923) through the bed of the 12th rib is used less commonly today. Antibiotics have reduced the chance of fulminating generalized peritonitis and most cases are better drained through an anterior transperitoneal approach. Recently a transpleural operation has been advocated (Moore, 1963) but it seems to have many practical and theoretical disadvantages.

ABSCESSES IN OTHER INTRAPERITONEAL SITES

Localization of collections of pus may occur throughout the abdomen after peritonitis or anastomotic leaks. The commonest site is still the pelvis. Diagnosis is often obvious and drainage is increasingly undertaken through the peritoneal cavity rather than the rectum. In the early days after operation, the abscess walls may give a combined clinical picture of ileus, organic obstruction and generalized infection. Diarrhoea is a common symptom.

Other Important Infections

Genito-urinary infections are not uncommon after surgery, particularly in older patients, especially if inadequate fluid replacement results in oliguria. Most cases respond rapidly to fluids and to appropriate antibiotics (Kass, 1957).

Peritonitis is usually localized to the section of the peritoneal cavity in which it has arisen. Even today, however, a rapidly fatal generalized peritonitis may occur, as in the days before antibiotics. Bacteraemia, pyaemia and septicaemia are still serious infections and result in multiple abscesses, bacterial endocarditis and septic shock.

Pseudomembranous enterocolitis is the result of a staphylococcal infection of the bowel and usually follows abdominal surgery combined with unsuitable antibiotic administration (Altemeier, Hummel and Hill, 1963).

Post-operative Respiratory Complications

Pulmonary complications are so common following upper abdominal surgery today that many surgeons accept them as part of the healing process (Kurzweg, 1953; Anscombe, 1957). This is particularly true in Britain where an ageing population, air pollution and cigarette smoking result in a high incidence of chronic bronchitis. They may occur at any age, however, and one series reports that more than half the patients undergoing upper abdominal surgery developed a productive cough, fever and X-ray abnormalities (Dudley, Baker and Anderson, 1962). Nor are these complications trivial. Chest infections were the main cause of death in as many as one third of such cases (Walters *et al.*, 1952; Modell and Moya, 1966). Onset is usually within 48 hours of surgery.

Complications most frequently encountered are hypoventilation, atelectasis and collapse, infection (Palmer 1967; Karlson, 1964). Pneumothorax results from damage to the pleura. It may pass unrecognized during operations on the kidney or neck. Effusion, haemothorax and empyema usually occur after the chest has been opened or with a subphrenic abscess.

Prevention of these Complications (Anderson *et al.*, 1963; Fomon, 1957)

Pre-operative investigation of pulmonary function assists the surgeon in choosing those patients who require special care. A history of dyspnoea warrants expert lung function tests (Badger, 1957; Veith *et al.*, 1959; Meneely *et al.*, 1961). Of these, timed vital capacity and maximum breathing capacity are probably the most useful clinical tests (Comroe *et al.*, 1962). Studies of the blood gases help confirm pulmonary inadequacy.

Culture of sputum before the operation allows the eradication of pathogenic organisms and helps the clinician in his choice of antibiotic should post-operative infection occur. Careful training by a physiotherapist may strengthen the power of respiratory muscles and help clear the bronchial tree of excess or thick, retained sputum. Bronchodilators help the asthmatics. Infection should be cleared from the mouth and the upper and lower respiratory tract. Postural drainage clears the retention of copious sputum.

Hypoventilation (Nunn and Payne, 1962; Kinney, 1963). Arterial desaturation and carbon dioxide retention results from hypoventilation and is more common after anaesthesia than usually supposed. Anxiety, restlessness, mental confusion, sweating, peripheral constriction and hypotension are suggestive. Cyanosis is much less common and only occurs when O_2 saturation falls below 70 per cent in arterial blood (Knowles, 1959). Previous airway obstruction, bronchospasm, chronic bronchitis, defects of pulmonary parenchyma and restrictions of expansion, predispose to its development. Pain from high abdominal wounds, distension and respiratory depressant drugs add a further load. Mechanical assistance may be required (Woolmer, 1958).

Aspiration of gastric contents is an anaesthetic hazard of bowel obstruction, but may be a terminal event in severely shocked or unconscious patients, particularly if acute dilation of the stomach develops. Immediate tracheobronchial aspiration may be life saving. Airway obstruction is an uncommon hazard after abdominal operations, but may occur after surgery on the neck. Bleeding after thyroidectomy causing dyspnoea, warrants immediate opening of the wound.

Collapse of alveolae. Collapse of a lung, lobe or bronchopulmonary segment follows blockage of the bronchial tree by retained secretions. Major collapse may shock or kill with great rapidity (Collins, 1960). Unless the airway is cleared, bacterial contamination leads to pneumonia.

Infection. Tracheitis, bronchitis, infected collapsed segments and bronchopneumonia are all common complications and require antibiotics and vigorous physiotherapy.

Treatment of Complications

Many patients develop a mixture of hypoventilation, collapse and infection. These must be treated by a combination of respiratory assistance analgesia, aspiration of distended gut, removal of retained secretions by nasotracheal aspiration, bronchoscopy or tracheostomy, bronchodilators and antibiotics as required. Unless the patients are treated correctly at an early stage, the mortality is high, other complications may arise, or they may survive as chronic pulmonary cripples (Palmer, 1961).

Dehiscence or Disruption of Abdominal Wounds
(Guiney *et al.*, 1966; Efron, 1965)

Dehiscence is often taken to mean separation of all layers of the abdominal incision after intra-abdominal surgery. All types of wounds have been known to separate including chest incisions. Partial disruption, without separation of skin and subcutaneous tissue, but deep muscle separation resulting in ventral herniation, is much more common than usually suspected. This would account for variation of reported incidence from less than 0·5 to 3 per cent or more.

Predisposing factors (Alexander and Prudden, 1966). Disruption occurs most commonly in the elderly males, with upper abdominal wounds. It is often associated with other major disease—30 per cent have hypoproteinaemia, or low haemoglobin. Experimentally vitamin C lack has proved important and may be a clinical factor. Steroid administration may delay healing. Disseminated carcinomatosis and jaundice may be implicated. Associated post-operative complications are common. Dehiscence is often one of the major events in a multi-complication syndrome. Tracheo-pulmonary complications, ileus and abdominal distension are the most frequent concomitants (87 per cent in one series). The combination of delayed wound healing and increased intra-abdominal pressure sets the stage for the final insult, usually straining to cough, vomit, hiccough or pass urine or stool. Experiments designed to test the strength of healing wounds demonstrate three main stages, the lag phase, accelerated healing phase and plateau phase.

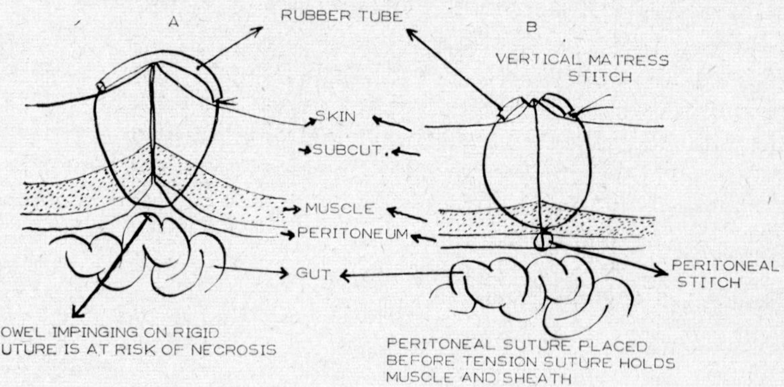

Fig. 1.4. Technique of Tension Suture.

Treatment should aim at prevention by holding the wound together with widely placed strong sutures through all layers except peritoneum, until the plateau stage is reached. Monofilament nylon or wire proves adequate and should be left in situ for two weeks or more in cases predisposed to delayed healing. When disruption has occurred most cases require to be resutured. Multiple interrupted sutures are best, but probably should not be placed through the peritoneum as they may damage underlying bowel by pressure necrosis.

Secondary or even tertiary disruptions are not unknown. Since standardization of statistics is not adequate mortality figures cannot be computed but probably lie in the neighbourhood of 10 per cent.

The Problem Abdomen

Shock in the immediate post-operative period usually means haemorrhage but the onset of trouble at a later stage (usually between the fifth and fourteenth day) may present the surgeons with a diagnosis of great difficulty. Not only may the patient be suffering from multiple complications outside the abdominal cavity, such as fluid and electrolyte abnormalities and chest infection, but it is often extremely difficult to elucidate the nature of the underlying pathological process. The very fact that a healing wound is present makes abdominal examination difficult. It is not uncommon to find a combination of signs of peritonitis, abscess formation and distension due to a mixture of paralytic ileus and organic obstruction.

Leakage from Suture Lines

Intraperitoneal leak of bowel contents or associated secretions is the most important potential hazard of surgery to any hollow viscus. It is wise to consider the possibility when the post-operative course is not entirely uneventful. The leak is usually secondary to rupture of an intramural haematoma or area of infarction. Total avascular infarction of the gastric remnant after gastrectomy has been recorded (Rodgers, 1966). In other cases leakage of secretions such as urine or bile may occur soon after operation and lead to a severe and fatal peritonitis. The later the leak occurs, the more likely it is to be localized to the immediate site of the operation by adhesions.

Distal obstruction of the viscus retains its importance as a potent cause of leakage and many surgeons use decompression procedures when viability of the anastomosis is in doubt (e.g. gastrostomy, jejunostomy or proximal colostomy).

The clinical presentation varies from the sudden onset of shock and peritonitis to a mild syndrome of pyrexia and tachycardia in which the leak becomes obvious when the wound or drain, discharges serous fluid or recognizable food. Faecal peritonitis rapidly progresses to shock and septicaemia unless it discharges on to the skin. Biliary peritonitis following unrecognized injury to the bile duct or liver bed, or missed distal obstruction after cholecystectomy or common bile duct exploration, is a major hazard. Means (1964) noted a 20 per cent mortality in localized, and an 80 per cent mortality in generalized bile peritonitis. Culture of the bile often grows *E. coli* or paracolibacterium organisms. These cases occurred in spite of routine drainage with soft Penrose drains.

Treatment of the shock and toxaemia and early drainage of a major leak is life saving.

Fistula (Chapman *et al.*, 1964)

Drainage of anastomotic leaks produces a fistula which will close spontaneously unless distal obstruction exists. Secondary complications of the fistula include chronic intraperitoneal abscess, skin digestion, fluid and electrolyte imbalance and malnutrition. General peritonitis and septicaemia occur in the early stages. Mortality depends upon the anatomical level of the fistula; Welch and Edmunds (1966) report

> 87 per cent mortality—gastric and duodenal fistulae
> 71 per cent mortality—jejunal or ileal fistulae
> 29 per cent mortality—colonic fistulae.

Prevention of fistulae is of great importance. Prevention of afferent loop obstruction in Polya-type gastrectomies has markedly reduced the rate of leakage from the duodenal stump. Tube duodenostomy of a hard, scarred stump allows external drainage without intraperitoneal leakage. Technical errors of anastomosis predisposing to leakage include unrecognized distal obstruction, unrecognized damage to bowel wall and its blood supply, tension of the anastomosis, and transfixion of intestine during closure of the peritoneum. The use of through and through all layer sutures may allow sloughing of an adjacent piece of bowel against a tense suture.

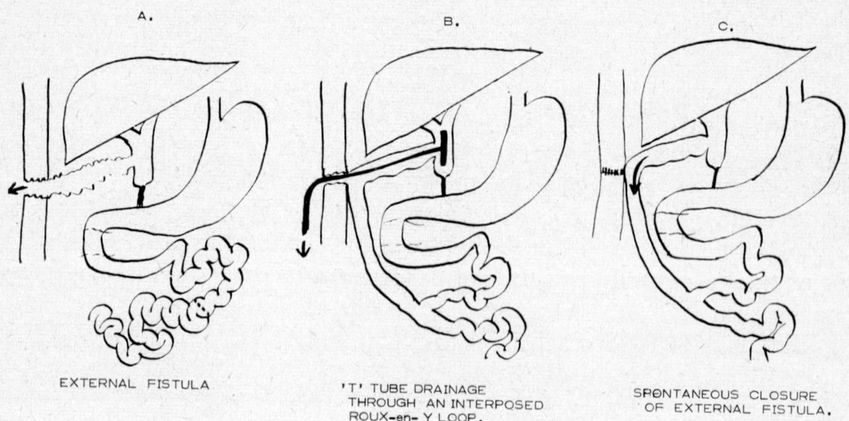

FIG. 1.5. The use of a Roux-en-Y loop to convert an external biliary fistula into an internal fistula into the small bowel segment. The tube allows the development of a second "external fistula" of the bowel, and drains the original site, in this case the common bile duct. When the tube is removed distal obstruction to the bile duct keeps the internal fistula open. The external fistula will close since the distal bowel is not obstructed. Variations of this procedure may be tailored to the patient's requirements (Rodney Smith, 1967).

Treatment. More active approach to fistulae has been advocated during the last few years. Defunctioning of high fistulae by nasogastric and duodenal intubation, or diverting ileostomy or colostomy may help. Barium or soluble dye studies should always be carried out to exclude distal obstruction.

Specific treatment. Early suture of the perforation at the laparotomy to drain a leak may be successful. Small bowel fistulae tend to do poorly on conservative management because of the electrolyte imbalance, poor nutrition and skin damage.

Pancreatic fistulae are particularly difficult to manage. Prone nursing helps the skin but promotes increased fluid leakage. Pancreatectomy distal to a pancreatic duct stricture may be required.

The Problem of Intestinal Obstruction after Abdominal Surgery

The concept that post-operative ileus or absent intestinal peristalsis is the usual result of manipulation of the bowel during intraperitoneal procedure has undergone a change during recent years. It has been shown that duodenal peristalsis begins as early as 24 hours after vagotomy and pyloroplasty. This has led to earlier removal of gastric aspiration tubes and recently to "tubeless" upper abdominal surgery. There seems to be no difference between pre- and post-operative small bowel absorption (Glicksman *et al.*, 1966). However, some cases require more prolonged aspiration of intestinal contents and replacement of fluid and electrolytes. The problem case is often a secondary phenomenon occurring within the first or second week, when a patient's condition deteriorates. Vomiting and abdominal distension occurs. Does the patient have an ileus or is there an organic intestinal obstruction? Further difficulty is the masking of signs of strangulation. Tenderness, pyrexia and leucocytosis are more likely to be due to infection causing the ileus, than to a strangulating loop of bowel.

The differentiation is no mere diagnostic exercise. All agree that correct treatment of ileus is expectant with supportive measures, whilst a true obstruction which is strangulating requires urgent operation to save the patient's life. Further difficulties arise about the nature of the ileus. The concept of total bowel paralysis has been changed by the use of X-rays which often demonstrate dilation of segments of bowel adjoining pathological regions, with normal bowel movement (and bowel sounds) in the rest of the gut. These regionalized segments have been called sentinal loops and may serve to pin-point the site of pathology. Even with generalized peritonitis following infection or anastomotic leaks, bowel sounds may be present.

Parts of the gastro-intestinal tract regain motility at different times after abdominal surgery and ileus, the duodenum and small bowel being most active and the distal colon most sluggish (Well *et al.*, 1961). Gaseous distension is often the cause rather than the result of ileus and severe cases may be prevented by constant nasogastric or duodenal suction. Absorption has been shown to be surprisingly good and hydration may be maintained by intravenous or jejunal feeding although the latter is rarely used today.

Exploration of the abdomen has often demonstrated areas of gross dilatation due to ileus in association with partial obstruction of gut lumen by abscess walls. Functional and organic obstruction may certainly co-exist. It is generally agreed that these cases should be treated conservatively except to drain collections of pus, bile or leaking bowel contents.

The diagnosis of a "problem abdomen" has been helped during recent years by modern X-ray techniques. In the past it was impossible to outline the bowel lumen safely with insoluble barium salts because

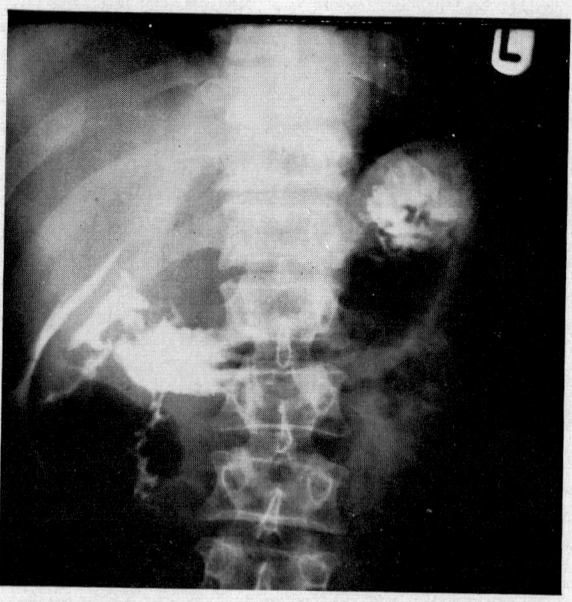

FIG. 1.6. Free duodenal perforation in a patient with minimal evidence of peritonitis using the plane film technique.

the thick residue may complete a partial obstruction, or severe toxicity may result from peritoneal absorption. Since 1955 (Moore, 1955; Canada, 1955) water soluble dyes have been used with little toxicity from absorption. The addition of an emulsifying agent, Tween 80, reduces surface tension and allows rapid diffusion through the fluid content of the lumen. The fact that opacification is much less than with barium is compensated by electronic intensification of the image (Samuel, 1961).

In the severely ill patient the author has investigated the use of the dye as an adjunct to plane film technique since manipulations necessary for screening may further damage his condition. 40–80 ml. of dye are swallowed or injected down a nasogastric tube. The patient is turned in his bed from the left to the right side, whilst sitting at 45°. Palpation of the abdomen at intervals allows dyed content to spill from one dilated loop to the next.

A single film is taken after 30 minutes and in most cases the dye can be shown to have entered the colon in spite of what appears to be severe ileus.

The technique is also of use in the patient where anastomotic leak or duodenal perforation is suspected. Barium peritonitis is hazardous

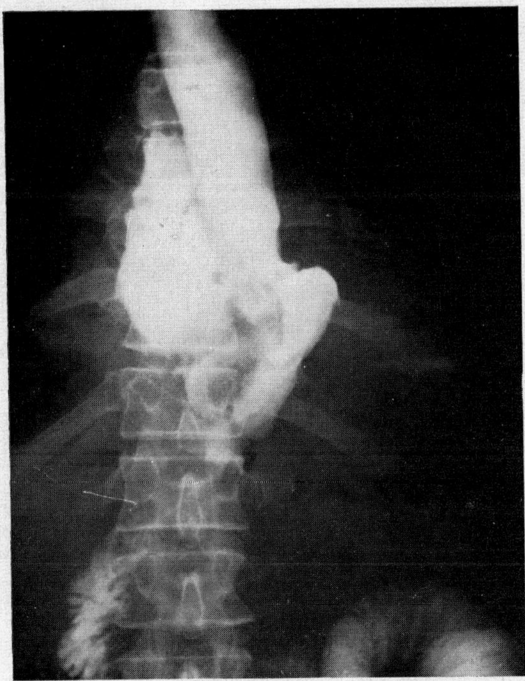

Fig. 1.7. Intrathoracic leak from the anastomosis after oesophago-gastrectomy heralded by shock. The plane films indicated which cavity required to be drained.

(Westfall and Nelson, 1966). Chronic granulomata may result from intraperitoneal leakage (Herrington, 1966).

It is possible to exclude total organic obstruction in many cases. Difficulties are found in the main in those cases with severe distension. There is a danger in saline depleted patients that the hypertonic solution may reduce circulating volume further.

Mortality in intestinal obstruction (Sauer, 1965) is higher in the older age group particularly when bowel gangrene occurs or even when the bowel has been opened by the surgeon.

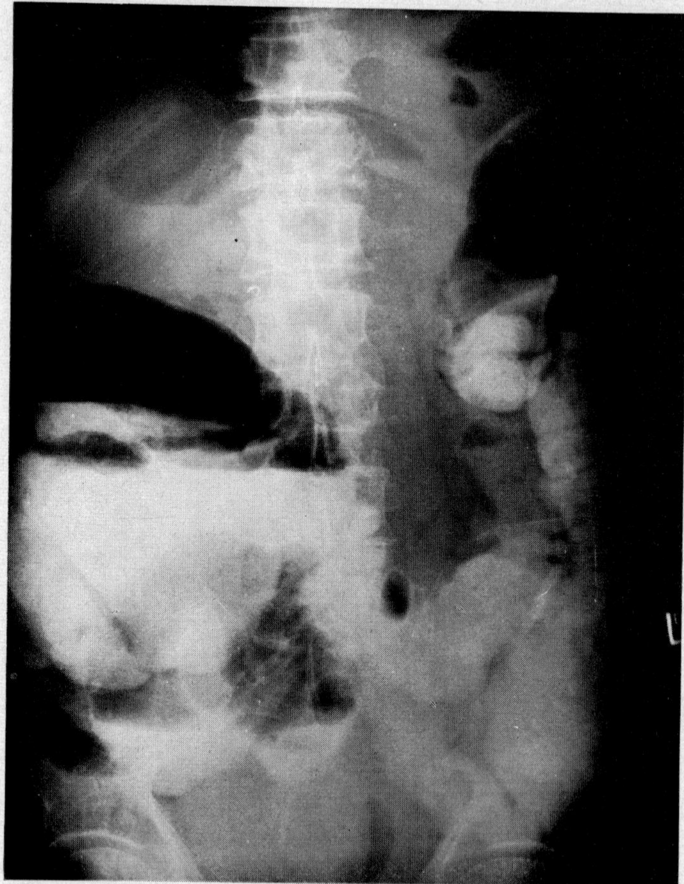

FIG. 1.8. In spite of massive distension of the right colon suspiciously like an organic obstruction, gastrografin passed through to the rectum within three hours of oral administration.

Conclusion

There has been marked change in the practice of surgery in recent years and it has brought with it complications of an increasing range and complexity. With limited space, it is only possible to touch on some of the important developments. In the future surgeons will have to read widely to be aware of unwanted sequelae of their surgery.

References

Introduction

LUCCIONI, F., *et al.* (1965). *Marseille Chir.*, **17**, 414–419.

Metabolic changes during surgery

BLOMSTEDT, D. (1965). *Acta Chir., Scand.*, **130**, 424.
EVANS, E. I. and BUTTERFIELD, W. J. H. (1951). *Ann. Surg.*, **134**, 588.
CLERK, F. and HORN, D. B. (1965). *J. Clin. Endocr. Metab.*, **25**, 39.
CUTHBERTSON, D. P. (1932). *Q. Jl. Med.*, **1**, 233.
JOHNSTON, I. D. A. (1967). *Brit. J. Surg.*, **54** (Suppl. No.), 438–441.
KINNEY, J. M. (1966). *Bull. N.Y. Acad. Med.*, **36**, 617.
MOORE, F. D., *et al.*, (1963). "The Body Cell Mass and its Supporting Environment".
    Saunders, Philadelphia.
MOORE, F. D. (1967). *Brit. J. Surg.*, **54** (8p. No.), 431–435.
SANDBERG, A. A., *et al.* (1954). *J. Clin. Invest.*, **33**, 1509.

Fluids and electrolytes

ALEXANDER, H. C. and SCHWARTZ, G. F. (1966). *Gastroenterology*, **50**, 224.
CAMPBELL, J. R. and KNAPP, R. W. (1966). *Ann. Surg.*, **163**, 291.
LE QUESNE, L. P. (1967). *Brit. J. Surg.*, **54**, 449–451.
MARCUS, E. (1962). *Surg. Clin. N. Amer.*, **42**, 35–54.
REITERMEIER, R. J. (1962). *M. Clin. N. Amer.*, **46**, 1001–12.

Derangements of acid-base balance

ANDERSON, O. S., ASTRUP, CAMPELL, E., CHINARD, F. and NAHAS, G. (1965). *Lancet*, **2**,
    1010.
CLOWES, G. H. A., *et al.* (1961). *Ann. Surg.*, **154**, 524.
EBERT, P. A., GREENFIELD, L. J., AUSTEN, W. G. and MORRON, A. G. (1962). *Surg. Gynec.*
    & Obstets., **114**, 357–67.
LYONS, J. H. and MOORE, F. D. (1966). *Surgery*, **60**, 93–106.
MORGAN, H. G., OGILVIE, R. R. and WALKER, W. F. (1963). *J. Clin. Path.* **16**, 545.
VAN SLYKE, D. D. (1966). *Ann. N.Y. Acad. Sci.*, **133**, 5–14.
WALKER, W. F. (1967). *Brit. J. Surg.*, **54**, 452–54.

Other requirements

JOHNSTON, I. D. A., MARINO, J. D. and STEVENS, J. Z. (1966). *Brit. J. Surg.*, **53**, 885–89.
RHOADS, J. E. (1952). *Surg. Gynec. & Obstets.*, **94**, 417.
RICE, C. O., *et al.* (1950). *Ann. Surg.*, **131**, 289.

Shock

AUBANIAC, R. (1952). *Pr. méd.*, **60**, 1456.
BROOKS, D. K. (1957). "Resuscitation". Arnold, London.
DAVIDSON, J. J., *et al.* (Nov. 1963). *Lancet*, **3**, 1139.
GITLITZ, G. F. and HURWITZ, E. (1964). *Surg. Clin. N. Amer.*, **44**, 505–33.
HARDAWAY, R. M. (1966). "Syndromes of Dissemmated Intravascular Coagulation".
    Thomas, Illinois.
ROBINS, J. (1966). *Obstets. Gynec.*, **28**, 130–38.
SHOEMAKER, W. C. and BAKER, R. J. (1967). *Surg. Clin. N. Amer.*, **47**, 3–16.

Septic shock

BROOKS, D. K. (1967). "Resuscitation". Arnold, London.
LANSING, A. M. (1963). *Canad. Med. Ass. J.*, **89**, 583–88.
RAVIN, H. A., *et al.* (1960). *J. exp. Med.*, **112**, 782–92.
SIEGEL, J. H. (1965). *Clin. Res.*, **13**, 220.

Treatment of shock

ARBULU and THAL (1966). *Surg.*, **60**, 60–68.
BROOKS, D. K. (1967). *Brit. J. Surg.*, **54**, 441–446.
DU TOIT, H. J., DU PLESSIS, J. M. and DOMMISSE, J., *et al.* (1966). *Lancet*, **2**, 143–46.
KEDDIE, N. C., *et al.* (1966). *Surg.*, **60**, 427–33.
MCLEAN, L. D. (1964). *Surg. Gynec. & Obstets.*, **118**, 594.

ROUSELL, R. H. (1966). *Brit. Med. J.*, **2**, 691.
SYKES, M. K. (1963). *Ann. Roy. Coll. of Surg. Eng.*, **33**, 185.
THAL, A. P. and WILSON, R. F. (1965). *Current Problems Surg.* (Sept.), 1–62.
YEO, R. (1966). *Lancet*, **1**, 817.
YEO, R. (1966). *Lancet*, **2**, 497.

Haemorrhage

BEIL, A. R., MANNIX, H. and BEAL, J. M. (1964). *Amer. J. Surg.*, **108**, 324–30.
MacVAUGH, H., *et al.* (1966). *Surgery*, **60**, 547–553.
STREMPLE, ELLISON and CAREY (1966). *Surgery*, **60**, 924–937.

The tendency to bleed

McNICOL, G. P. and DOUGLAS, A. S. (1964). *Brit. med. Bull.*, **20**, 233–39.
McNICOL, G. P., *et al.* (1966). *Brit. J. Surg.*, **53**, 26–29.

Venous thrombosis

BRYANT, M. F., BLOOM, W. L. and BREWER, S. S. (1966). *Amer. Surg.*, **32**, 13–16.
GIBBS, N. M. (1967). *Brit. J. Surg.*, **40**, 209.
HOMANS, J. (1947). *Amer. J. Med.*, **3**, 345–54.
QUICK, A. J. (1958). *Surg. Clin. N. Amer.*, **38**, 1031–43.
MENTON, *et al.* (1967). *Lancet*, **1**, 700.
POOLE, J. C. F. (1967). *Brit. J. Surg.*, **54**, 463–65.
YOUNG, T. W., *et al.* (1966). *Brit. J. Surg.*, **53**, 387–89.

Diagnosis of venous thrombosis

COON, W. W. and WILLIS, P. W. (1959). *Amer. J. Cardiol.*, **4**, 611–621.
HOMANS, J. (1947). *Amer. J. Med.*, **3**, 345.
MAHORNER, H. (1966). *Surg.*, **60**, 773–77.
REICH, T., *et al.* (1966). *Surg.*, **60**, 1211–15.

Pulmonary embolism

GIBBS, N. M. (1967). *Brit. J. Surg.*, **40**, 209.
EDITORIAL (1965). *Lancet*, **2**, 70–71.
MEYEROWITZ, B. (1966). *Surg.*, **60**, 521–535.
MOZES, M., *et al.* (1966). *Surg.*, **60**, 790–94.
SASAHARA, A. A. and STEIN, M. (Editors) (1965). "Pulmonary Embolic Disease". Stephen
    Green Press, New York.

Major infections in the post-operative period

DINEEN, P. (1964). *Surg. Clin. N. Amer.*, **44**, 553–64.
HOWE, C. W. & MOZDEN, P. J. (1963). *Surg. Clin. N. Amer.*, **43**, 859–82.
MAITLAND, A. I. L. (1965). *Brit. J. Surg.*, **52**, 931–40.

The organisms

FINLAND, M., JONES, W. F., JR. and BARNES, M. W. (1959). *J. Amer. Med. Ass.*, **170**
    2188–97.
NAHMIAS, A. J. & EICKHOFF, T. C. (1961). *New Eng. J. Med.*, **265**, 177–82.
ROGERS, L. S., DUFFY, J. P. and MOLL, T. W. (1965). *Arch. Surg.* (*Chicago*), **90**, 294.

Susceptible hosts

BARNES, B. A., *et al.* (1959). *Surgery*, **46**, 247–60.
BARNES, B. A., *et al.* (1961). *Ann. Surg.*, **154**, 585–98.
ELEK, S. D. and CONEN, P. E. (1957). *Brit. J. exp. Path.*, **38**, 573–86.
MILES, A. A., MILES, E. M. and BURKE, J. (1957). *Brit. J. exp. Path.* **38**, 79–96.

Treatment of infection

MYERS, R. S. (1959). *Surg. Gynec. & Obstets.*, **108**, 721–25.
PETERSDORF, R. G., *et al.* (1957). *New Eng. J. Med.*, **257**, 1001–9.
WILLIAMS, R. E. O., *et al.* (1959). *Brit. med. J.*, **II**, 658–62.

Wound infection

DINEEN, P. (1964). *Surg. Clin. N. Amer.*, **44**, 553–64.
HOWE, C. W. and MOZDEN, P. J. (1963). *Surg. Clin. N. Amer.*, **34**, 859–82.
BARNES, B. A., *et al.* (1959). *Surgery*, **46**, 247–60.

Subphrenic abscesses

ADAMS, H. P. (1961). *Surg. Clin. N. Amer.*, **41**, 847–52.
BODON, G. R. and HOLZWASSER, G. R. (1964). *Surg. Gynec. & Obstets.*, **119**, 601–602.
BONDI, F. R. and ERICKSON, E. W. (1964). *Amer. J. Surg.*, **107**, 614–19.
BOYD, D. P. (1958). *Surg. Clin. N. Amer.*, **38**, 619–26.
DINEEN, P. and MCSHERRY, C. K. (1962). *Ann. Surg.*, **155**, 506–17.
MOORE, H. D. (1963). *Ann. Surg.*, **158**, 240–48.
NATHER, C. and OCHSNER, E. W. A. (1923). *Surg. Gynec. & Obstets.*, **37**, 665–673.
OZERAN, R. S. (1967). *Amer. Surg.*, **33**, 64–67.

Other important infections

ALTEMEIER, W. A., *et al.* (1963). *Ann. Surg.*, **157**, 847–58.
KASS, E. H. (1957). *Arch. Int. Med.*, **100**, 709–14.

Post-operative respiratory complications

ANSCOME, A. R. (1957). "Pulmonary Complications of Abdominal Surgery". Year Book
    Publishers, Chicago.
DUDLEY, H. A. F., BAKER, L. W. and ANDERSON, W. A. (1962). *J. Roy. Coll. Surg. Ed.*, **7**,
    121–27.
KARLSON, K. E. (1964). *Surg. Clin. N. Amer.*, **44**, 537–52.
KURZWEG, F. T. (1953). *Amer. Surg.* **19**, 967–74.
MODELL, J. H. and MOYA, F. (1966). *Anesth. Analg. (Cleveland)*, **45**, 432–39.
PALMER, K. N. V. (1967). *Brit. J. Surg.* **54**, 479–481.
WALTERS, W., *et al.* (1952). *Proc. Staff Meeting, Mayo Clin.*, **27**, 39.

Prevention of pulmonary complications

ANDERSON, W. H., *et al.* (1963). *J. Amer. Med. Ass.*, **186**, 763–66.
BADGER, T. L. (1957). *Calif. Med.*, **86**, 207–16.
COMROE, J. H., *et al.* (1962). "The Lung: Clinical Physiology and Pulmonary Function
    Tests". Year Book Publishers, Chicago.
FOMON, J. J. (1957). *Amer. J. Surg.*, **94**, 611–14.
MENEELY, G. R. and FERGUSON, J. L. (1961). *J. Amer. Med. Ass.*, **175**, 1074–80.
VEITH, F. J. and ROCCO, A. G. (1959). *Surgery*, **45**, 905–11.

Hypoventilation

KINNEY, J. M. (1963). *Surg. Clin. N. Amer.*, **43**, 619–36.
KNOWLES, J. H. C. (1959). "Respiratory Physiology and its Clinical Application". Harvard
    University Press, Cambridge, Mass.
NUNN, J. F. and PAYNE, J. P. (1962). *Lancet*, **2**, 631–32.
WOOLMER, R. (1958). *Brit. Med. Bull.*, **14**, 54–57.

Collapse of alvaeolae

COLLINS, V. J. (1960). *J. Amer. Med. Ass.*, **172**, 549–55.

Treatment of complications

PALMER, K. N. U. (1961). *Lancet*, **1**, 191–92.

Dehiscence of abdominal wounds

ALEXANDER, H. C. and PRUDDEN, J. F. (1966). *Surg. Gynec. Obstet.*, **122**, 1223–29.
EFRON, G. (1965). *Lancet*, **1**, 1287–90.
GUINEY, E. J., MORRIS, P. J. and DONALDSON, G. A. (1966). *Arch. Surg.*, **92**, 47–51.

Leakage from suture lines

RODGERS, J. B. (1966). *Arch. Surgery*, **92**, 917–21.

Fistula

CHAPMAN, R., FORAN, R. and ENGELBERT-DUNPHY, J. (1964). *Amer. J. Surg.*, **108**, 157.
SMITH, RODNEY (1967). Personal communication.
WELCH, C. E. and EDMUNDS, L. H. (1962). *Surg. Clin. N. Amer.*, **42**, 1311–20.

Intestinal obstruction

GLUCKSMAN, *et al.* (1966). *Surg.*, **60**, 1020–25.
CANADA, W. J. (1955). *Radiology*, **64**, 867–73.
HERRINGTON, J. L. (1966). *Ann. Surg.*, **164**, 162–66.
MOORE, H. D. (1955). *Lancet*, **1**, 163–69.
SAMUEL, E. (1960). *Brit. J. Radiol.*, **33**, 82–91.
WELLS, C., *et al.* (1961). *Lancet*, **2**, 136–37.
WESTFALL, R. H., NELSON, R. H. and MUSSELMAN, M. M. (1966). *Amer. J. Surg.*, **112**, 760–63.
SAUER, H. (1965). *Klin. Med. (Wein)*, **20**, 509–516.

Chapter 2

SURGERY IN HAEMOPHILIA AND OTHER BLEEDING STATES

K. E. Barrett

Haemophilia is a rare hereditary disease characterized by abnormal coagulation of blood resulting in excessive bleeding from or into tissues. This bleeding commonly arises from trauma which may be trivial but haematomas frequently occur spontaneously.

The disease was thought to affect males exclusively but a few well substantiated reports have appeared describing women who are true haemophiliacs. This situation results from the union of a carrier of the disease with a male haemophiliac. Experience has shown that a significant number of carriers themselves suffer from abnormal bleeding which is usually mild in degree but may assume serious proportions after surgery.

Mechanism of Coagulation

Much new knowledge has accumulated about the apparently simple function of blood coagulation. It is now clear that the mechanism is highly involved and still far from settled. There is little point in general clinicians attempting to keep abreast of the minutiae in this field. It is, however, helpful to know of the major advances in the theory of coagulation. The original Classical theory (Schmidt, 1892; Morawitz, 1905) provided a useful framework upon which so much subsequent work has been based. It propounded that Prothrombin was converted to Thrombin and that the latter acted upon Fibrinogen to translate it to Fibrin. It was not until 1947 that this theory was significantly expanded first by Owren (1947) and then by Biggs and Douglas (1953) of the theory that a substance was generated which acted as a precursor to prothrombin. This was then alluded to as plasma thromboplastin but is now referred to as prothrombin activator. Further modifications have led to the current concept of Macfarlane's Cascade Theory. This postulates the interaction of a relatively few factors forming products which act on others and these in turn develop later products until the end point—fibrin—is generated. A schematic illustration is provided in Fig. 2.1.

Haemophilia A is caused by a deficiency in the plasma of a protein termed anti-haemophilic globulin (Factor VIII) and results in a life long liability to a variety of clinical manifestations, some common, others rather rare. Haemophilia B (Christmas disease) is associated with a deficiency of Factor IX.

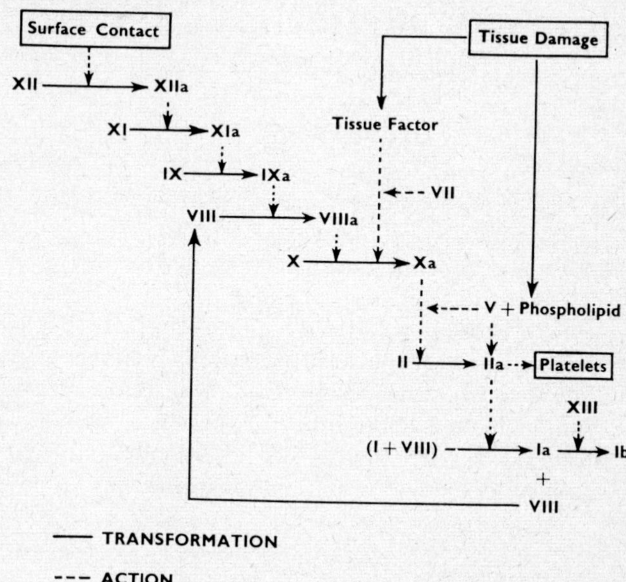

Fig. 2.1. A schematic representation of coagulation of blood
(Cascade Theory of Macfarlane, 1964).

Clinical Presentation

In a survey of 267 patients with haemophilia including classical haemophilia A or haemophilia B, (Christmas disease) (Wilkinson, Nour-Eldin, Israëls and Barrett, 1961) the frequencies of haemorrhagic manifestations were as given in Table I.

This shows that traumatic bleeding, haemarthroses, spontaneous bruising and haematomas together with bleeding from dental causes are the most common presentations. Other manifestations less likely to present in surgical practice include haematuria, alimentary tract bleeding, retro-peritoneal haematoma and bleeding after circumcision. In addition non-haemophilic disease may develop and be influenced by the haemorrhagic diathesis.

A history of male bleeders in the patient's relatives provides useful confirmatory evidence but its absence by no means excludes the probability. Not infrequently it becomes clear from genaelogical study that the disease has arisen apparently *de novo* and this happens as a result of mutation in the patient's mother.

Examination of the patient, particularly if he is seriously affected, may reveal some of the stigmata. With improved methods of treatment however these are becoming less common. The most frequent are orthopaedic disabilities, notably flexion deformities of the knees and elbows, muscular wasting round haemophilic arthropathic joints, anaemia, bruises, cut-down scars, and occasionally nerve palsies.

TABLE I. *Haemorrhagic Symptoms in Haemophilia Syndromes (Haemophilia and Christmas Disease Combined, 267 cases)*

	Patients affected	
	No.	%
Traumatic bleeding, excessive	246	93·0
Haemarthrosis	177	66·4
Spontaneous bruises and haematoma	174	65·2
Bleeding from gums	167	62·5
Epistaxis	101	38·8
Haematuria	63	23·6
Alimentary-tract bleeding	51	19·0
Retroperitoneal haemorrhage	33	12·3
Throat and sublingual haemorrhage	33	12·3
Circumcision	21	7·8
Central-nervous system haemorrhage	13	4·8
Peripheral-nerve haemorrhage	12	4·5
Tonsillar haemorrhage	11	4·2
Haemothorax	4	1·5
Purpura	2	0·8
Others	9	—

It is thus seen that most haemophiliacs can be diagnosed as being bleeders from a careful history and examination. Mildly affected patients may not fit into the above description. It may be useful to ask about bleeding after dental extraction. Experience shows that even the most mildly affected haemophiliac bleeds persistently, i.e., for more than 24 hr. after extraction. The final assessment however in determining the type and the severity of the coagulation defect rests upon tests of the haemostatic mechanism.

Special Investigations

In all patients suffering from Haemophilia A or B special tests will reveal the disease. These investigations are such as could reasonably be expected to be available in a good general hospital. Deficiencies of other coagulation factors which may lead to presentations similar to haemophilia, also occur although special measures are required for their identification.

It is not appropriate at present to embark on a description of the complete investigation of a patient with a bleeding diathesis since there are other causes of this than the haemophilia syndromes. Certain cardinal screening tests must be mentioned.

The *whole blood clotting time* has for many years occupied a hallowed position in the diagnosis of bleeding disorders. Reliance on this test to exclude the diagnosis of haemophilia is not recommended. It was carried out on 225 patients with haemophilia and 94 (41·7%) had normal clotting times. Of 38 with haemophilia B, 20 (52·6%) also gave normal results. (Wilkinson, *et al.*, 1961). Thus, approximately half of such patients may not be diagnosed if this test is the sole laboratory criterion used. This point is particularly applicable to the mildly affected patient who may have little clinical evidence of the disease but who nevertheless may run into severe trouble if surgery is carried out.

The *bleeding time* is normal in this disease but the test should always be carried out as a screening measure in a suspected bleeder. In a study of 51 patients with Von Willebrand's disease approximately one third have deficiencies of anti-haemophilic factor (personal observation). It is not uncommon for the two conditions to be confused as there is superficial similarity. The matter may be settled by the result of the bleeding time which is prolonged in Von Willebrand's disease but not in haemophilia.

In addition to the bleeding time a full blood and platelet count is essential together with a prothrombin determination. One of the most valuable diagnostic tests for the diagnosis of coagulation deficiencies is the thromboplastin generation test (T.G.T.) (Biggs and Douglas, 1953). This, together with the prothrombin determination will detect not only the type of coagulation abnormality but also by modification reveal even the mildest of deficiencies. It is adaptable also to allow correction tests which form the ultimate means of typing the abnormality and finally by further modification to permit assay of coagulation factors. Other simpler tests are now available which are very valuable for crude screening purposes but these are no substitute for accurate diagnosis or for haemostatic control of a patient. A number of tests based on the partial thromboplastin time (P.P.T.) are in vogue. Probably the most sensitive is the *Kaolin cephalin time* but this group will only inform on the presence and not on the type of deficiency. This is a practical consideration since these tests are inappropriate for haemostatic control of a haemophiliac undergoing surgery and only the thromboplastin generation test or assay techniques based on this are allowable for the purpose.

Assessment for Proposed Surgery

Criteria for Operation

Patients with haemophilia may fall into one of three categories.

1. Extremely grave conditions, usually traumatic such as road accident and fire-arm injuries requiring immediate operative procedures. It may not be possible immediately to institute the programme to be described and this should be commenced as soon as possible after surgery and in any case within a few hours.

2. Essential surgery of a nature that allows time to prepare a safe programme. Such conditions as intra-cranial bleeding, associated with fractured skull, acute abdominal emergencies, orthopaedic procedures for fractures, fall into this group.

3. Non-urgent surgical conditions.

The results of surgery in a haemophiliac are significantly better if there is close co-operation between the surgeon and a haematologist experienced in dealing with these patients, (McIntyre, Barrett and Israëls, 1964). This is particularly apparent when dealing with non-urgent surgery. An example is peptic ulceration complicated by frequent dangerous haemorrhages. In such a situation we have relied on vigorous and repeated courses of medical treatment and plasma transfusion, proceeding where this has failed to gastrectomy.

In haemophiliacs a retro-peritoneal haematoma on the right side of the abdomen may convincingly mimic acute appendicitis. The presence or absence of polymorphonuclear leucocytosis does not help in distinguishing the lesion.

For clear cut appendicitis, the patient is submitted to surgery. If doubt arises a medical regime is instituted for the treatment both of acute appendicitis and retro-peritoneal haematoma. This relies on gastric aspiration, the administration of anti-haemophilic globulin fraction and broad spectrum antibiotic therapy. It will be realised that oral and intra-muscular antibiotics are out of the question. Experience has confirmed the value of methicillin or erythromycin administered by intravenous route.

The value of relying on a conservative approach is provided by a problem recently posed. A man of 45 years, a known haemophiliac, presented with profound iron deficiency anaemia due to intractable haemoptysis, a symptom virtually never met in this disease unless there is underlying lung pathology. Bronchography revealed a left lower lobe bronchiectasis of a type which was considered suitable for lobectomy. Instead of operation, however, he was given massive continuous antibiotic therapy and the bleeding stopped. In spite of this treatment if the bleeding recurs he will be reconsidered for operation.

Venous Status

In addition to assessment of the need for operative surgery, a very careful evaluation of the venous status has to be made. In a normal patient this is not usually a serious consideration. By contrast a haemophiliac may, during his life time, have many hundreds of transfusions so that continuing access to veins is essential. Unfortunately it has been found particularly in children that they have had repeated "cut downs" robbing one of their subsequent and possibly equally vital use. The programme to be described requires administration of a number of agents, including anti-haemophilic globulin fraction, plasma, blood, electrolytes and anti-biotics. This may go on for as long as three weeks. Assuming that one vein lasts four days, the patient should have at least five good accessible veins. The administration of the substances mentioned is best not carried out by repeated venepunctures. Experience shows that catheters inserted through a needle are valuable, but they should be big enough to take packed red cells.

The Correction of the Haemostatic Defect

This has to be achieved immediately before, during and for a varying period after operation. It may be partially effected by fresh plasma, fresh blood or more completely by anti-haemophilic globulin concentrates. It has been mentioned that it may be necessary for concentrates to be given for up to three weeks. Usually it is considerably less than this, around ten to fourteen days. It is essential that at least seven days supply of anti-haemophilic globulin be available or reserved before operation commences. The danger period is not usually at operation but during the period of five to ten days afterwards. Fresh blood and plasma are not adequate for safe cover of operations. Reports appear of surgery carried out under this cover, but it is now generally accepted that there is too little margin of safety for it to be recommended. In the relatively minor trauma of dental extractions carried out under such cover it may sometimes be necessary to resort to administration of AHG fraction as an emergency measure and if this is not available large quantities of blood may have to be given. The reason for the relatively unsatisfactory results after plasma lies in the degree of haemostatic correction one may achieve.

Normal A.H.G. levels in humans vary between 65–150 per cent (Pitney, 1956). In haemophilia the concentration is commonly nil but occasionally may be as high as 10 per cent. The administration of 750–1,000 mls. of fresh plasma will raise the plasma A.H.G. level in a haemophiliac from nil to around 10–15 per cent (Biggs and Macfarlane, 1962). Larger volumes of plasma lead to the risk of overloading of the circulation. Adequate haemostasis occurs at levels higher than 25 per cent (Biggs and Macfarlane, 1962). Thus it is seen that using fresh plasma there is still a deficit of about 20 per cent before a satisfactory haemostatic level prevails.

For operative surgery this problem is overcome by using A.H.G. concentrates instead of fresh blood or plasma. Plasma concentrations well in excess of haemostatic levels are easily obtained. Fraction is available in three forms: 1. Human A.H.G. 2. Pig A.H.G. 3. Bovine A.H.G.

Human A.H.G. is scarce, highly expensive and is reserved for medical emergencies or essential surgery. Its advantage lies in non-antigenicity and thus it may be used on more than one occasion. Its use sometimes initiates the formation of circulating anti-coagulants usually to Factor VIII, clearly a dangerous complication which is an indication for stopping this treatment.

Animal A.H.G. (Bidwell, 1955) is used almost exclusively in the United Kingdom. It is highly effective, fairly readily available through commercial sources, and although not cheap, costs considerably less than human fraction. There are disadvantages. It is anti-genic although anti-body concentrations do not usually assume significant proportions until 10–14 days after its initial use, a period which would permit most types of operation to be carried out safely. Its continued administration confers the extra risk of anaphylactoid reactions. Clearly only one course of such treatment is advisable in a patient's lifetime. Cross immunological reactions between pig and bovine A.H.G. do not occur, and the use of pig fraction will not detract from the subsequent value of bovine fraction. The latter has a propensity for causing thrombocytopenia.

A recent observation (Pool, 1965) notes that a precipitate rich in A.H.G. and fibrinogen is obtained by exposing fresh plasma to very low temperatures. It is termed cryoprecipitate and exploratory clinical investigation (personal observation) has confirmed that from a technical and medical view point this material shows considerable promise. There are at present administrative problems relating to methods of collection of blood by Regional Transfusion Centres which will have to be surmounted before it can be accepted as a routine method for use in surgery.

All liquid A.H.G. is highly labile both in vitro and in vivo so that the concentrate is best given every six to eight hours depending on its strength and on clinical indications. It is given rapidly and with no delay between its preparation and administration.

Haemostatic Programme

Pre-operative

The disease varies in severity from a severe form which requires frequent medical attention and hospital admissions to the mildest involving perhaps only prolonged bleeding after dental extraction. The amount of A.H.G. required to cover operation is thus modified accordingly. Reliance on blood tests to determine the degree of severity is not recommended in preference to evaluation of the previous haemorrhagic history. Nevertheless it is useful to have available the plasma A.H.G. assay result before fraction has been given so that the rise which occurs afterwards is accurately assessed.

(*a*) Pre-infusion A.H.G. assay. The technique is unfortunately highly involved and executed only in a few centres.

(*b*) Insertion of intravenous catheter.

(*c*) Four pints of blood are crossmatched two of which should be suitable for red cell packing. They need not be fresh blood. The blood group of registered haemophiliacs is included on the green card that they should always carry.

(*d*) One hour before operation A.H.G. fraction is administered into the catheter. If human fraction is selected the amount is two bottles (= 450–650 mls. of fresh plasma per bottle). If animal fraction is chosen 400–600 units (1 porcine A.H.G. vial = 200 Oxford units) is given.

(*e*) If possible plasma A.H.G. levels are assayed 1 hr. after fraction has been given to determine whether a haemostatic level has been reached. This need only be done once in each 24 hr. Similar assays are also necessary once each day in the post-operative period.

Post-operative

(*f*) Further fraction is required at regular intervals usually every 6 to 8 hrs. If human A.H.G. is being used one bottle is required but if animal fraction has been chosen 400 units is the amount necessary.

(*g*) Daily haemoglobin estimations are carried out to assess blood loss and blood transfusion requirements. Also platelet counts are particularly necessary if animal fraction is used as this has a propensity for inducing thrombocytopenia sometimes to a marked degree, this complication being an indication to stop its administration and change to human A.H.G.

A further complication which may occur with all forms of fraction is the development of circulating anti-coagulants acting against clotting factors. It will be seen that this is a highly dangerous event since continued replacement therapy is not only useless but incurs the risk of potentiating the circulating anti-coagulant. This complication most commonly occurs after human fraction is used and unlike the reactions following administration of animal fraction are not antigen/antibody in nature, do not respond to treatment with steroids and are commonly transient.

Usually the measures described control bleeding and the first few days after operation are uneventful. The unwary may be tempted to relax the haemostatic measures but to do so is unwise. Haemophilic tissues heal badly and wounds tend to break down easily particularly if adequate haemostasis is not maintained. The latter is continued until firm healing has definitely occurred and all bleeding stopped. Sutures are left in for a day or two longer than in non-haemophilic patients. Confinement to bed for between one and two weeks is advisable since ambulation involves increased utilization of plasma A.H.G. and this is undesirable. Active exercises to leg muscles will reduce the chance of haemarthroses of knees and ankles when weight bearing commences.

Surgery in Christmas Disease: (Haemophilia B)

This condition has a natural history, genetic transmission, and symptomatology similar to that of Haemophilia A. It differs in two main respects. The coagulation abnormality arises as a result of deficiency of Factor IX, a characteristic identified by using the thromboplastin generation test, and also by certain limitations in treatment which do not apply in Haemophilia A. So far as treatment of Christmas disease with fresh blood or plasma is concerned, the principles are also similar but unlike Haemophilia A, concentrates are not generally available and it is unlikely that they will become so. Therefore indications for surgery in this condition must be even more stringently sought and are confined virtually to life threatening situations.

Orthopaedic Conditions in Haemophilia Syndromes

Unfortunately orthopaedic complications are frequent in haemophilia even with improved initial management and from many points of view surgical correction of such deformities would be desirable. At present such measures are not usually practicable, not only because of limitations imposed by paucity of A.H.G. fraction but also because of poor healing of haemophilic tissues.

Many major orthopaedic abnormalities would not arise if the present imperfect methods of treatment could be improved. Treatment of haemarthroses and haematomas of muscle form a high proportion of the work undertaken by haemophilia centres, both as in-and out-patients and are also responsible for much disability leading to interference with schooling and employment.

Easy access to transfusions of fresh plasma and to physiotherapy by staff experienced in this field significantly reduces the incidence of major deformities. It does not, unfortunately eliminate them. It is probable that improvement in the materials available for transfusions in these patients, such as cryoprecipitate, will lead to a corresponding reduction in orthopaedic disabilities.

Acute or recurrent haemarthroses are treated by transfusions of fresh plasma daily until signs of subsidence occur. This usually happens in about three to four days. As soon as the range of movement of the joint shows even slight improvement, physiotherapy is started, paying particular attention to maintaining power of the muscles around the joint. Wasting is a common feature and predisposes, because of the joint instability which follows, to further bleeding. Thus a vicious circle may be established. Certain caveats have been found to apply. The aspiration of blood from joints into which bleeding has occurred is inadvisable. Bleeding virtually always recurs and to this is added a needle track which provides a further possible source of bleeding and of infection. Immobilization in plaster casts has two disadvantages. It encourages muscle wasting, a complication to be avoided and also it may mask swelling arising from continued bleeding into the joint. It has been found to cause dangerous pressure features.

Judicious manipulation of flexion deformities of joints under cover of fresh plasma transfusions may sometimes be effective in increasing function, but of course there is the risk of initiating fresh bleeding.

Finally, the introduction of concentrates together with easy access to fresh blood has during the last decade made surgery in haemophilia a practicable proposition so long as certain safeguards are applied. Further improvements are possible and much material is available for elective surgery but this is unlikely to come about until present facilities for manufacture of A.H.G. fraction are considerably supplemented. The outlook for surgery in Christmas disease has remained practically unchanged.

References

BIDWELL, E. (1955). Purification of Bovine anti-haemophilic globulin. *Brit. J. Haemat.*, **1**, 35.
BIGGS, R. and DOUGLAS, A. S. (1953). The Thromboplastin Generation Test. *J. Clin. Path.*, **6**, 23.
BIGGS, R. and MACFARLANE, R. (1962). Human Blood Coagulation. Blackwell, Oxford.
MACFARLANE, R. (1964). Cascade Theory. *Nature*, **202**, 498.
MCINTYRE, H., BARRETT, K. E. and ISRAËLS, M. C. G. (1964). Dental treatment in the haemophilia syndromes. *Lancet*, **1**, 584.
MORAWITZ, P. (1905). Die Chemie der Bluterinung. *Ergebn Physiol.*, **4**, 307.

OWREN, P. A. (1947). The Coagulation of blood; investigations on a new clotting factor. *Acta. med. Scand. Supp.*, 194.

PITNEY, W. R. (1956). The assay of anti-haemophilic globulin in plasma. *Brit. J. Haemat.*, **2**, 250.

POOL, J. G. (1965). Preparation and testing of anti-haemophilic globulin. Sources for transfusion therapy in Haemophilia. *Scand. J. Clin. Lab. Invest. Supp.*, **84**, 70.

SCHMIDT, A. (1892). Quoted by Morawitz (1905). *zur Blutlehre*, Leipzig.

WILKINSON, J. F., NOUR-ELDIN, F., ISRAËLS, M. C. G. and BARRETT, K. E. (1961). Haemophilia Syndromes; a Survey of 267 patients. *Lancet*, **2**, 947.

CHAPTER 3

CIRCULATING CANCER CELLS

R. A. SELLWOOD

When tumours invade blood vessels cells become detached very easily and are swept away to other parts of the body in the circulation. This way in which cancer spreads to regions distant from the primary tumour has been recognized since the careful histological studies of Schmidt (1903) who found emboli of tumour cells in the lungs of patients who had died from abdominal cancer. Until recently, however, there have been few convincing demonstrations of malignant cells in samples of blood from living patients. Engell (1955) examined 274 samples of blood from 140 patients with cancer and reported that cancer cells were present in 59 per cent of patients. His findings suggested a way of studying directly some of the mechanisms involved in the vascular dissemination of cancer, and investigators from several centres designed new methods for extracting cancer cells from blood.

Methods for Isolating Circulating Cancer Cells

Each of the major groups of investigators has developed a new method or modified an existing one. Goldblatt and Nadel (1965), in a review, found that at least 20 different methods had been used. This suggests that none is completely satisfactory. Three main problems are involved. (1) It is necessary to remove all or a major proportion of the relatively enormous numbers of normal cells in blood so that a few abnormal cells may be concentrated for study. (2) The final preparation must provide a clear field with cells which are intact morphologically and which have been stained appropriately. (3) Firm criteria must be defined for the positive identification of malignant cells. These requirements should be satisfied by a method which is simple, cheap and quick. If possible, it should be quantitative.

Removal of Normal Cells

Red cells may be removed by lysis or by sedimentation.

Early workers used water or acetic acid to haemolyse the red cells but water damages cancer cells and acetic acid coagulates protein making preparations unsuitable for microscopic study. Many have preferred to use Saponin which lyses red cells rapidly and completely, without damaging cancer cells. Streptolysin O destroys both red cells and polymorphs but the enzyme is expensive and unstable and deteriorates rapidly, even if refrigerated. In these circumstances destruction of the polymorphs, in particular, may be incomplete and the final preparation obscured by debris and partially lysed cells. Cancer cells are not damaged by the enzyme and several workers have reported good preparations with this method.

When blood is allowed to stand and prevented from clotting the erythrocytes settle slowly to the bottom of the container. Sedimentation may be accelerated by adding agents which cause red cells to agglutinate and this provides a means for rapid separation of red cells from other elements of the blood. Bovine fibrinogen has been used for this purpose by several workers but strings of fibrin may form and interfere with the clarity of the final preparation. For this reason others have preferred to use dextran or phytohaemagglutinin. Sedimentation is simple, cheap and quick but cannot give quantitative results as some cancer cells are carried down with the erythrocytes.

Several investigators have been content to remove the erythrocytes only to make preparations containing all the remaining cells. The large numbers of white cells in such preparations make it necessary for many slides to be screened and this process is tedious and time-consuming. Most workers use methods in which some, at least, of the leucocytes are removed also.

Polymorphs have a higher specific gravity than cancer cells and may be separated from them by special methods of centrifugation. After removal of erythrocytes, the remaining cells and plasma may be layered over a solution of albumin with a specific gravity of 1·065. The two solutions, which remain separate with a clear interface, are centrifuged; polymorphs, having a specific gravity greater than 1·065, are deposited at the bottom of the centrifuge tube. Cancer cells and lymphocytes, being less dense, remain at the interface and may be aspirated with a pipette and smeared on slides. In a similar method, a mixture of silicone oils may be used instead of albumin.

A simple and ingenious method for removing polymorphs depends on their ability to phagocytose small particles. Samples of blood are incubated with finely divided carbonyl iron powder. The particles of iron are ingested by the polymorphs which are then removed with a magnet.

Preparation for Microscopy

The cells recovered may be embedded in paraffin wax and sectioned serially, or may be smeared on slides and prepared in the ways usual for examining smears of blood. These methods provide excellent cytological detail but cells are inevitably lost during preparation and in an attempt to provide quantitative results, many workers have preferred to use membrane filters. These are thin plastic membranes with fine pores, approximately 5 microns in diameter. Fluids may be drawn through a filter using a small negative pressure and any cells present are retained on the surface of the membrane. Membranes can be treated with fixatives and stains and become completely transparent when "cleared" with xylene. They are then mounted on slides and examined microscopically.

Most cancer cells are bigger than the other cells found in blood. Recently, attempts have been made to design a sieve through which blood can be strained to catch cancer cells and on which cells can be examined directly under the microscope. Some success has been claimed with strips of thin perforated plastic tape and with membrane filters with large pores.

Methods of staining depend largely on the preference and experience of individual observers. They include haematoxylin and eosin, the Papanicolaou method and Romanowsky stains. Particular success has been reported with Acridine orange, a fluorescent stain, but the appearances are difficult to interpret and several workers have found it of no more value than conventional methods.

Recognition of Malignant Cells

Malignant cells are usually larger than normal ones and the nuclei are large in relation to the cytoplasm. The nuclear chromatin may stain more deeply than normal and is arranged in coarse clumps. Nuclei are often irregular in outline and unusual in shape. Among a group of cells there is considerable variation in size, shape and distribution of chromatin. Nucleoli may be large, multiple and irregular.

These are changes of degree rather than of kind and occur to a greater or lesser extent in any actively dividing colony of cells. They may all be seen in smears from normal bone marrow which has been stained suitably. In these circumstances it is doubtful whether any given single cell from blood may be regarded as malignant. Clumps of cells are required in which the typical changes are present.

New methods for concentrating leucocytes have revealed a remarkable variety of non-malignant cells which may occur singly or in small numbers in circulating blood. (Alexander and Spriggs, 1960). The large and irregular nuclei of megakaryocytes have been implicated particularly as a source of false positive results. Primitive cells from bone marrow are found more often in patients with cancer than in normal individuals, and are particularly common in the leucoerythroblastic anaemia of advanced malignant disease. Other cells which may cause confusion include endothelial cells, plasma cells, osteoblasts and cells from tissues traversed by the aspirating needle.

The Incidence of Circulating Cancer Cells

The first results obtained from application of the new methods suggested that the incidence of circulating cancer cells was high (Moore *et al.*, 1957; Malmgren *et al.*, 1958; Roberts *et al.*, 1958). By 1959 cells had been found on average in 38 per cent of patients with cancer and this raised hopes for a diagnostic test for cancer, a means of assessing the prognosis of individual patients and an experimental method for studying the spread of cancer. During the next three years, however, workers from several centres reported their inability to reproduce these results and by 1962 the incidence reported varied from 0 to 100 per cent of patients.

Several factors might have been responsible for this situation. The numbers and volumes of the samples of blood studied by different investigators varied and were not always recorded. Some samples were taken from local veins and some from peripheral veins. Patients were studied with tumours of different organs and at different stages of the disease. Preparations were made by different methods, stained in different ways and assessed by observers who varied considerably in skill and experience. It seems clear, however, that the main reason for the considerable differences in the results from various centres is the difficulty of cytological identification.

The diagnostic research branch of the National Cancer Institute sponsored a series of meetings of senior investigators to discuss the problem, and in 1962 they published a *Cautionary note to those concerned with cancer cells in the blood*. Malignant cells had unquestionably been demonstrated in some patients with cancer but the clinical significance of this finding was not clear. More extensive well controlled studies, improved techniques and sharper criteria for recognition of cancer cells were required. An Expert Committee of the World Health Organisation (1963) made a similar statement. They concluded that the identification of cancer cells in the peripheral blood should not be regarded as a routine method of diagnosis. Much research was needed to determine whether the finding had any clinical application.

As members of the various investigative teams have become more experienced the reported incidence of cancer cells in blood has fallen, and the most recent reports suggest that cells are found in peripheral blood from less than 10 per cent of patients (Moore and Sandberg, 1965).

Cells are found more often in blood from local veins, which drain regions involved by tumour, than in blood from peripheral veins. They are found more often in patients with advanced disease than in those with relatively early disease. In patients with some prospect of surgical cure the incidence of cells is negligible. The site of the primary tumour and the degree of differentiation appear to have no effect on the incidence of cells.

The Effect of Surgical Trauma and Manipulation

Patients with previously slow-growing malignant tumours may deteriorate rapidly and die of widespread metastases shortly after surgical intervention, possibly as a result of dissemination of tumour cells by the trauma of operation. There is no doubt that, in certain circumstances, operative manipulation can release emboli of tumour cells into the circulation. Fatal pulmonary emboli of tumour fragments have been detached during mobilization of hypernephromas, and massive systemic emboli have arisen during resections for pulmonary carcinomas. Various experiments with animals seem to confirm that trauma and manipulation of tumours play a part in dissemination. This suggests that tumours should be handled with care and that the main veins draining regions involved by tumour should be ligated early in the course of the operation.

Biopsy of tumours might be dangerous if trauma causes dissemination and it has been described as "a criminal act". This view is based largely on observations of individual patients, and in a controlled study of patients with squamous carcinoma the incidence of metastases was not increased by biopsy (Paterson and Nuttall, 1939). Biopsy does not alter significantly the incidence of metastases nor the average survival period in experimental rats (Maun and Dunning, 1946) and there is no significant difference in the prognosis of patients submitted to aspiration biopsy for carcinoma of the breast and those who are not (Robbins *et al.*, 1954). In a series of patients with carcinoma of the breast reported from the Mayo Clinic it was found that a previous biopsy did not affect survival adversely. (Pierce *et al.*, 1956.)

The development of techniques for isolating circulating cancer cells has made it possible to examine this problem by more direct methods. Observations by several workers suggest that, in some patients, cancer cells may appear in the bloodstream only during surgical operations and in some cases showers of cells may be liberated at the time of operation. (Roberts *et al.*, 1960; Fleming, 1963; Griffiths and Salsbury, 1965). Others, however, have been unable to confirm these results (Sellwood *et al.*, 1965) and the effect of surgical trauma may be no greater than that of a modern brassiere and of the movements of peristalsis and respiration.

The Prognostic Significance of Circulating Cancer Cells

Some circulating cancer cells are presumably potential metastases and their presence might be expected to imply a grave prognosis. There is no doubt that some patients in whom cells are found can survive for many years with apparent freedom from disease. On the other hand when groups of patients are considered collectively those with cells fare worse than those without. This difference appears to be due to the advanced stage of the disease in many of those with cells.

The Fate of Circulating Cancer Cells

The presence of cancer cells in the circulation does not necessarily imply that metastases will develop. When emboli of cells arrest in small vessels they become surrounded by thrombus and most cells perish as organization takes place. Paradoxically, thrombosis seems necessary for the development of secondary deposits. The early stages of this process have been studied in the capillaries of rabbits' ear-chamber preparations (Wood, 1958). Initially there is adhesion of cancer cells to the endothelium and after a few minutes they become surrounded by thrombus. Within hours there is loss of definition in the adjacent endothelium and leucocytes accumulate and pass through the injured wall leaving defects through which cancer cells emigrate into the surrounding tissues.

Arrest in capillaries is not inevitable. Cells injected into the circulation of animals can pass freely through the lungs, liver and kidneys (Griffiths and Salsbury, 1963). Some may pass through arterio-venous shunts, and others, when impacted in capillaries, may elongate and become wormlike in order to traverse the vessels (Zeidman, 1961).

The factors which determine the arrest and growth of circulating cancer cells are presumably similar to those which decide whether or not bacterial contamination becomes infection. They are (1) the viability, virulence or invasiveness of the cells, (2) the number of cells present and (3) the resistance of the host.

Viability, Virulence and Invasiveness

Cancer cells in the blood can be of little importance if they are not alive and able to form metastases. In animals these properties can be demonstrated by the transmission of transplantable tumours when blood from affected animals is inoculated in the circulation of normal ones. In patients the numbers of cells found are usually small and viability is difficult to demonstrate. Attempts have been made to grow cancer cells from human blood in tissue cultures but the results are difficult to interpret as cells of epithelioid appearance can be grown from normal blood and bone marrow. Some cultured cells, however, have resembled closely those of the primary tumour.

Evidence of active mitosis suggests that cells are capable of forming metastases. For division to take place it is necessary for cells to synthesize deoxyribonucleic acid (D.N.A.). The amino acid thymidine is a precursor of D.N.A. and is taken up avidly by cells which are about to divide. Dividing cells may be recognized by making autoradiographs after allowing them to take up thymidine which has been labelled with tritium to make it radioactive. In this way clear autoradiographs have been obtained from circulating cancer cells in patients with carcinoma of the bronchus (Kuper and Bignall, 1964).

The Numbers of Cells

Experiments with animals suggest that many viable cells are necessary for the development of metastases. When cells from transplantable tumours are inoculated intravenously in isologous animals the numbers of tumours which develop appear to be roughly proportional to the numbers of cells injected. The number of cells required to produce any tumours at all varies in different experimental systems from 50 to 750,000, and it may vary in the same system when studied at different times. It has been suggested that only certain mutant cells have the ability to metastasize (Zeidman, 1965).

The Resistance of the Host

As large numbers of viable cells are required to produce tumours in animals, many must be destroyed by the defences of the host. The nature of host resistance to cancer is not understood but certain factors may inhibit or augment it and thus increase or decrease the development of metastases.

Surgical trauma—There is increasing evidence from experiments with animals that the stress of major operations may decrease the resistance of the host to cancer cells. Laparotomy increases the incidence and rate of growth of tumours when small numbers of transplantable cells are inoculated subcutaneously in rats (Creath *et al.*, 1959) and accelerates the appearance and growth of chemically-induced tumours in mice (Gottfried and Molomut, 1961). A second laparotomy increases the incidence of hepatic tumours when cells are injected into the portal veins of rats. This effect is enhanced when the liver is manipulated at operation, or when partial hepatectomy is done (Fisher and Fisher, 1965). In some transplantable tumours in mice, the numbers of spontaneous metastases are increased by surgery (Romsdahl, 1964). Other forms of stress reported to augment the production of metastases include chronic bleeding, excessive heat or cold and auditory stress.

Adrenal steroids—In animals, treatment with steroids may increase the number of spontaneous metastases and of those induced artificially by intravenous injection of cells. The effect is proportional to the gluco-corticoid activity of the steroids and does not occur with those having solely mineralo-corticoid properties. (Albert and Zeidman, 1962).

Anticoagulants—Heparin and dicoumarol, which impede the clotting of blood, inhibit significantly the development of tumours when transplantable cells are injected into the circulation of animals (Koike, 1964).

Fibrinolysins behave in a similar way and substances which inhibit fibrinolytic enzymes have an opposite effect (Cliffton and Agostino, 1964). Presumably the effect of anti-coagulants is due to the prevention of thrombosis around emboli of cancer cells in small vessels. Treatment with anti-coagulants is the only known means of consistently decreasing metastases in animals and a clinical trial in human patients with cancer seems desirable.

Summary

If samples of blood from patients with cancer are studied in special ways it is possible sometimes to find cancer cells in them. Such cells are seldom found in patients with any prospect of surgical cure. There is evidence to suggest that cells may be disseminated by surgical trauma and manipulation, but few circulating cells survive to form metastases. In experimental animals the incidence of metastases may be increased by surgical trauma or by treatment with corticosteroids and decreased by treatment with anti-coagulants.

References

ALBERT, D., ZEIDMAN, I. (1962). *Cancer Res.*, **22**, 1297.
ALEXANDER, R. F., SPRIGGS, A. I. (1960). *J. Clin. Path.*, **13**, 414.
Cautionary note to those concerned with cancer cells in the blood. (1962). *J. Lab. Cancer Inst.*, **29**, 1023.
CLIFFTON, E. E., AGOSTINO, D. (1964). *J. Lab. Cancer Inst.*, **33**, 753.
CREATH, J. R., McDONALD, G. D., COLE, W. H. (1959). *Surg. Forum*, **10**, 45.
ENGELL, H. C. (1955). *Acta. Chir. Scand. Suppl. No.* 201.
FISHER, E. R., FISHER, B. (1965). *Acta. Cytol.*, **9**, 146.
FLEMING, J. A. (1963). *Proc. Roy. Soc. Med.*, **56**, 497.
GOLDBLATT, S. A., NADEL, E. M. (1965). *Acta. Cytol.*, **9**, 6.
GOTTFRIED, B., MOLUMUT, N. (1961). *J. Int. Coll. Surg.*, **36**, 596.
GRIFFITHS, J. D., SALSBURY, A. J. (1963). *Brit. J. Cancer.*, **17**, 546.
GRIFFITHS, J. D., SALSBURY, A. J. (1965). Circulating Cancer Cells. Ch. 3, p. 53. Thomas, Springfield, Illinois.
KOIKE, A. (1964). *Cancer*, **17**, 450.
KUPER, S. W. A., BIGNALL, J. R. (1964). *Lancet*, **1**, 1412.
MALMGREN, R. A., PRITT, J. C., DEL VECCHIO, P. R., POTTER, J. F. (1958). *J. Nat. Cancer Inst.*, **20**, 1203.
MAUN, M. E., DUNNING, W. F. (1946). *Surg. Gynec. Obstet.*, **82**, 567.
MOORE, G. E., SANDBERG, A. (1965). *Acta. Cytol.*, **9**, 175.

MOORE, G. E., SANDBERG, A., SCHUBARG, J. R. (1957). *Ann. Surg.*, **146**, 580.

PATERSON, R., NUTTALL, J. R. (1939). *Amer. J. Cancer.*, **37**, 64.

PIERCE, E. H., CLAGETT, O. T., MCDONALD, J, R., CAGE, R. P. (1956). *Surg. Gynec. Obstet.*, **103**, 559.

ROBBINS, G. F., BROTHERS, J. H., EBERHART, W. F., QUAN, S. (1954). *Cancer* **7**, 774.

ROBERTS, S., LONG, L., JONASSON, O., MCGRATH, R., MCGREN, E., COLE, W. H. (1960). *Surg. Gynec. Obstet.*, **111**, 3.

ROBERTS, S., WATNE, A., MCGRATH, R., MCGREW, E., COLE, W. H. (1958). *A.M.A. Arch. Surg.*, **76**, 334.

ROMSDAHL, M. M. (1964). *J. Surg. Research*, **4**, 363.

SCHMIDT, M. B. (1903). Die Verbreitungswege der Karzinome und die Begiehung Generalisierter Sarkome zie den Leukamischen Neubildungen. *Jena.*

SELLWOOD, R. A., KUPER, S. W. A., WALLACE, E. N., BURN, J. I. (1965). *Brit. J. Surg.*, **52**, 770.

WOOD, S. (1958). *A.M.A. Arch. Path.*, **66**, 550.

World Health Organization (1963). Technical Report. Series No. 251. Cancer Control 1st report of expert committee, p. 23.

ZEIDMAN, I. (1961). *Cancer Research*, **21**, 38.

ZEIDMAN, I. (1965). *Acta. Cytol.*, **9**, 136.

CHAPTER 4

SURGICAL TREATMENT OF ANEURYSM

ALLYN G. MAY and CHARLES G. ROB

Aneurysms develop in segments of arterial wall weakened by disease. Thus, aneurysms may arise from incomplete development of arterial musculature (congenital aneurysms), defective development (Marfan's syndrome), destruction of arterial wall by infection (mycotic and syphilitic aneurysms), degeneration (atherosclerosis), and injury of the arterial wall (traumatic aneurysms). By far the most common aneurysms encountered today are atherosclerotic in origin. The lesion occurs in two anatomical forms, the fusiform and the saccular, or in a combination of these. In the fusiform aneurysm, the entire circumference of the arterial wall expands in all directions along the arterial axis; whereas in the saccular, only a fraction of the circumference of the arterial wall is involved and enlargement occurs in one direction.

Indications for Surgical Treatment

If allowed to evolve without interference, an aneurysm will produce symptoms by compression of adjacent structures, by thrombosis and ischemia, or by rupture and haemorrhage. Ideally, all aneurysms should be treated surgically. Practically, the indications for surgery must be balanced against the risks in the individual patient. Rupture is an absolute indication for surgery. Pain, large size (greater than 7 cm. in diameter for abdominal aortic aneurysms), and noticeable enlargement are strong relative indications. These conditions suggest the imminence of rupture and argue for early operation in order to achieve the low mortality rate associated with elective resection and to avoid the higher mortality rate associated with emergency resection.

Special Contra-Indications

Diffuse aneurysmal dilatation of the aorta and multiple aneurysms of the major arteries are contra-indications to surgical treatment. Similarly, lower abdominal aortic aneurysms in patients without patent distal arteries to provide satisfactory "runoff" should not be excised. Although severe ischemic heart disease is a contra-indication to elective resection of aortic aneurysms, a healed myocardial infarction is not. Patients with evidence of pre-existing coronary artery disease suffer a higher incidence of cardiac complications after elective aneurysmectomy in comparison to patients who do not show such evidence. However, the overall mortality rate for elective resection is low and the fraction of patients having fatal post-operative myocardial infarctions is vanishingly small. Indeed, 65 per cent of our patients with documented pre-existing coronary artery disease experience no cardiac complication with elective resection. In patients with ruptured aneurysm there is no increase in mortality associated with pre-existing coronary artery disease. The consequences of rupture exert more influence in deciding the outcome of resection than does the state of the coronary circulation.

Pre-Operative Preparation

Elective Resection of Aortic Aneurysms

Because most aneurysms occur in patients with generalized atherosclerosis, preparation for resection of intact aneurysms should include a search for historical evidence of other atherosclerotic disease, such as intermittent claudication and cerebral or coronary insufficiency. A knowledge of the significance of atherosclerosis at other sites puts the aneurysm disease in the correct perspective for intelligent management. Attention should be paid to the presence or absence of peripheral pulses and vascular bruits. These physical findings may prove of service in detecting operative thrombo-embolism, should such a complication occur. Nonatherosclerotic aneurysms, such as the mycotic or syphilitic, should be recognized because specific treatment in addition to surgery may be necessary for cure.

A history of previous colon surgery should be noted, as the marginal artery of Drummond may have been interrupted and the collateral blood supply of the descending colon made inadequate. In such a patient, ligation of a patent inferior mesenteric artery during the resection may result in ischemic necrosis of the colon. The bowel should, then, be prepared pre-operatively with enemas and anti-biotics in case a colon resection proves necessary.

Base-line determinations of renal function (blood urea nitrogen, serum creatinine, an intravenous pyelogram, and isotopic renogram), serum electrolytes, and an electrocardiogram and chest film should be obtained before surgery. Aortography is rarely indicated for evaluation of the aneurysm because most aneurysms are lined with thrombus and the lumen as seen by aortography may be of normal dimensions.

The day before surgery broad spectrum anti-biotic coverage is started in view of the prosthetic material to be implanted. Two hours before surgery on intravenous infusion of 5 per cent Dextrose and water places the kidneys in a favourable state of diuresis. Insertion of an indwelling urinary catheter decompresses the bladder just before surgery and allows monitoring of urine production during and after operation.

Emergency Resection of Aortic Aneurysms

Speed is essential in the successful treatment of ruptured abdominal aortic aneurysm. The diagnosis must be considered immediately for any patient with severe abdominal pain of sudden onset, and it must be confirmed promptly by demonstration of a pulsatile mass. Preparation for surgery must often begin on the way to the operating room. One or two large bore intravenous needles are placed in veins of the upper extremities to allow blood replacement. Blood is made ready for transfusion, but, if necessary, unmatched O-negative blood, plasma, or physiological saline may be given to combat shock. Transfusion should be limited to maintenance of adequate vital signs, not designed to restore perfect blood volume, until the aorta is clamped and further haemorrhage prevented.

Although shock may not be present when the patient is first examined, it may develop with induction of anesthesia, presumably from relaxation of the abdominal musculature, reduction of intra-abdominal pressure, and release of its tamponading effect. This phenomenon can many times be prevented by a certain anesthesia tactic. An endotracheal tube is passed with the aid of a topical anesthetic agent and an intravenously administered hypnotic. Muscular relaxation is not allowed until the incision has been carried down to the peritoneum. Then a relaxant is given, the peritoneal cavity opened, and rapid control of the aorta achieved.

Operations for Aneurysm

Arterial Ligation

Simple ligature of the arteries entering and leaving an aneurysm will prevent embolization and rupture. The operation suffers, however, from the disadvantage of interfering with blood flow. In main arteries, this may produce intolerable distal ischemia. Aneurysms of certain arteries, such as the splenic artery, may be treated in this manner because a very adequate collateral circulation is present. Occasionally ruptured intracranial aneurysms must be handled with this technique.

Reinforcing Procedures

Wrapping with fascia or plastic materials has little to offer in the surgical treatment of most aneurysms. However, the principle has been profitably applied to intact intracranial aneurysms which can be reinforced with a coating of rapidly setting plastic. This avoids arterial ligation and thus minimizes the danger of stroke.

Aneurysmorrhaphy

In this operation the aneurysm is only partially excised and the arterial lumen reconstructed with the remnant of remaining vessel. This procedure is most satisfactory with small-mouthed, saccular aneurysms in which the diseased sac can be totally excised and the defect closed by lateral suture of healthy arterial wall. Traumatic aneurysms, such as result from arterial lacerations, are particularly amenable to this technique. Fusiform aneurysms, however, tend to recur when treated in this manner because diseased aneurysm wall must be used for reconstruction of the artery.

Wiring

This operation is useful in poor risk patients with difficult aneurysms. Its purpose is to introduce into the aneurysm random coils of stainless steel wire. The wire causes clotting of blood within the aneurysm, except for a central channel which remains open. The wire and thrombus provide a strengthening frame work for the weak aneurysm wall.

Wiring of an abdominal aortic aneurysm may be performed through a small abdominal incision which exposes only the anterior surface of the lesion. A No. 18 hypodermic needle is introduced through the aneurysm wall and 200 to 1,000 ft. of No. 36 stainless steel wire from a spool is fed through the needle into the lesion. Care and patience is necessary to introduce enough wire to be effective. When sufficient wire has been introduced, the needle is withdrawn, the wire cut, and the end of the wire pushed into the aneurysm.

Excision and Reconstruction of Aneurysms of the Lower Abdominal Aorta

Elective Resection of Intact Aneurysms—The patient is placed supine on an operating table designed to allow operative arteriography of the lower extremities. The skin of the abdomen, lower chest, flanks, groins, and upper thighs is scrubbed. Sterile drapes are applied so as to expose the abdomen and groins in continuity. This allows access to the femoral arteries through separate incisions in case the prosthesis must be brought to that level or in case the peripheral arterial tree must be exposed for thrombo-embolism.

The peritoneal cavity is opened through a midline or left paramedian incision from the costal margin to the pubis. The aneurysm is exposed by incising the posterior peritoneum to the right of the midline and dissecting it, together with the peri-aortic fibroadipose tissue, from the aneurysm. The inferior mesenteric artery is ligated and divided near its origin.

With large aneurysms, it is sometimes necessary to mobilize the third portion of the duodenum and the left renal vein in order to expose the aorta sufficiently for application of the proximal clamp. The vena cava at this level is usually not closely applied to the aorta and presents no obstacle in dissecting a space posterior to the aorta for the clamp. A pair of lumbar arteries is ligated and divided to provide hemostasis in an aortic cuff of adequate length.

Distal control of the aneurysm is usually obtained at the common iliac

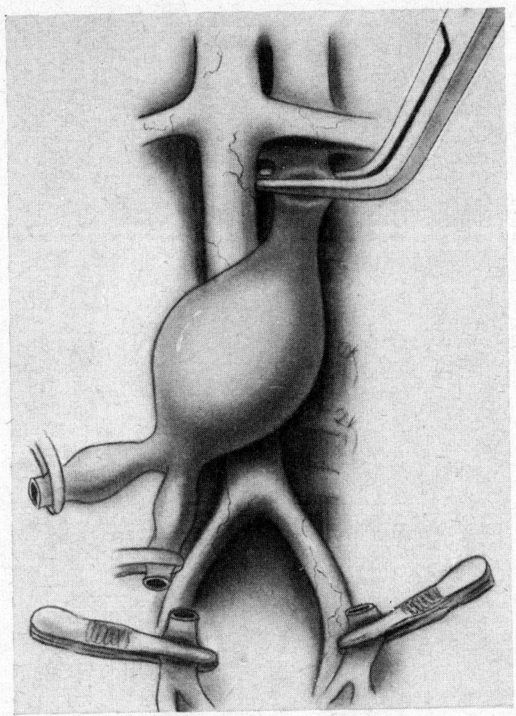

FIG. 4.1. When total excision of the aneurysm is performed, the lumbar arteries are clamped and ligated as the aneurysm is dissected from the vertebrae and inferior vena cava.

artery level, for most lower abdominal aortic aneurysms involve the aortic bifurcation. Occasionally the aneurysm and the adjacent common iliac arteries may be densely adherent to the vena cava and iliac veins. In this case it is safer to develop a plane of dissection between the iliac arteries and veins at a lower level where these vessels normally begin to diverge.

The aortic clamp should be applied first. A relatively healthy segment of aorta, as free of calcification as possible, should be chosen for clamping. Occasionally, the clamp can be oriented to minimize stressing of calcified portions of the aortic wall. Vascular clamps are then applied to the iliac arteries and, proximal to these, Kelly clamps.

The iliac arteries are transected between these clamps leaving adequate cuffs of distal artery for construction of the anastomoses (Fig. 4.1). The aneurysm is then opened longitudinally. All clot and debris

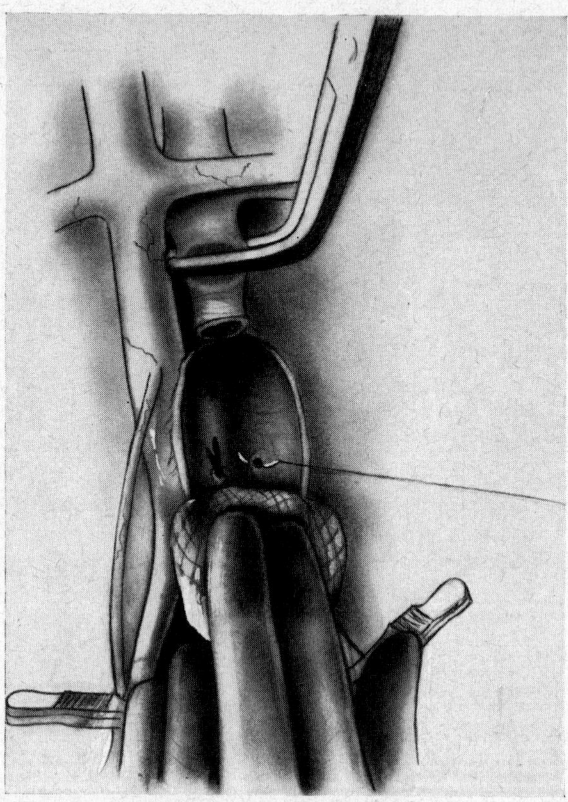

Fig. 4.2. Large aneurysms, which tend to be densely adherent to the inferior vena cava, may more safely be partially excised. After application of proximal and distal clamps for control of bleeding the aneurysm is opened and the lumbar arterial orifices are sutured from within the aneurysm. Then the anterior portions of the aneurysm are excised.

are removed, the lumbar and middle sacral arteries are controlled by sutures from within the aneurysm (Fig. 4.2). The portion of the aneurysm adherent to the iliac arteries and inferior vena cava is left *in situ* and its unattached margins are excised. The aorta is transected below the proximal aortic clamp leaving a cuff of proximal aorta sufficient for the anastomosis. (An alternative technique is to remove the entire aneurysm. However, in the case of large aneurysms this

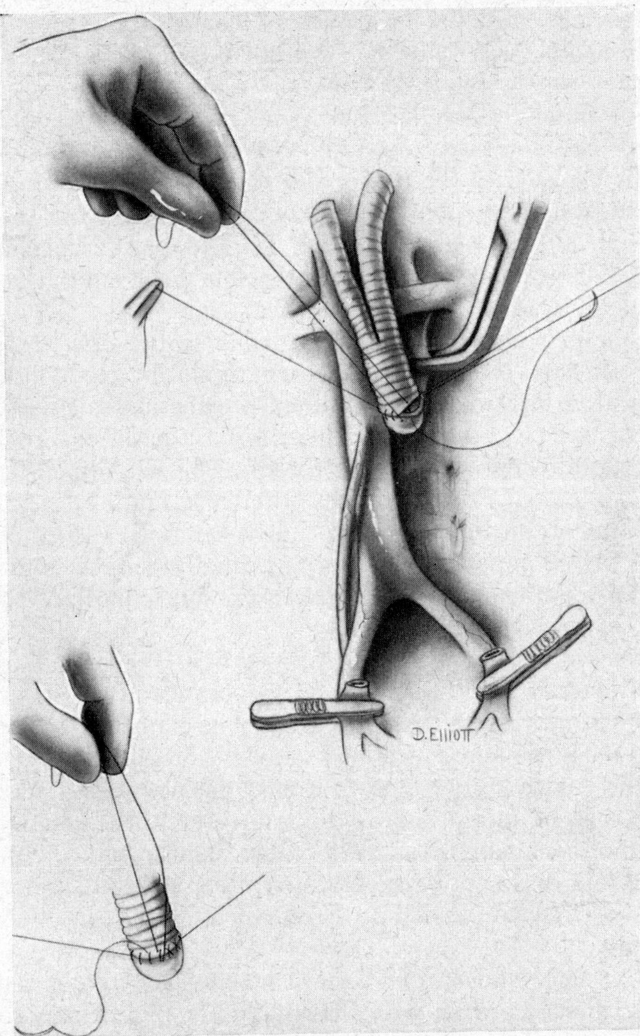

FIG. 4.3. The proximal aortic anastomosis is constructed first, using two interlocking rows of continuous arterial silk sutures.

technique is associated with an increased incidence of venous haemorrhage.)

Should venous bleeding occur during removal of the aneurysm, it
should be controlled by local pressure with the finger or a swab. If the
bleeding is from a torn lumbar vein, simple ligation will control it.
If it is from a small tear in the vena cava, then local pressure for a full
10 mins. may control it. A large tear will require careful application
of a vascular clamp and suture repair with fine silk. Should these

manoeuvres fail, then the cava must be ligated above and below the tear while haemorrhage is being controlled by local pressure.

The aneurysm is delivered from the abdomen by transecting the aorta immediately above the aneurysm's neck. The adventitia on the aortic cuff should not be trimmed for it adds considerable strength and hemostatic capacity to the proximal anastomosis. Loose fragments of intima and atheroma should, however, be removed from the interior of the aortic cuff. It is occasionally necessary to remove calcified intimal plaques to enable passage of the suture needle. Each arterial cuff should be thoroughly washed with physiological saline.

A prosthesis is chosen to fit the proximal aorta. The porosity of a woven prosthesis is low enough to prevent significant blood loss through the fabric after implantation. A knitted prosthesis is relatively porous and should be "preclotted" by immersion in a basin containing 20 to 30 ml. of clottable blood from the patient. This will diminish bleeding through the interstices of the fabric after restoration of aortic blood flow. It is important that all blood clot be carefully washed out of the prosthesis before implantation. If a bifurcated prosthesis is to be used, the proximal limb may be kept relatively short, most of the defect being bridged by its two iliac limbs.

The proximal anastomosis is performed first (Fig. 4.3). Two double ended 0–0 dacron arterial sutures fix the prosthesis to the aorta and act as stays at the extremities of the transverse diameter. The prosthesis is held up for sewing the posterior part of the anastomosis. One end of each double ended suture is sewn across the posterior suture line to make two rows of interlocking continuous sutures. The anterior part of the anastomosis is completed in the same manner with the prosthesis lying in its bed. In the presence of a very diseased aorta, a more secure anastomosis is achieved when rather large bites of aorta are included in the suture.

Each iliac anastomosis is performed with single rows of continuous 0000 arterial suture (Fig. 4.4). The stays are placed anteriorly and posteriorly to facilitate twisting the vessel from side to side for better exposure of the suture line during sewing. With one iliac anastomosis completed, bleeding is allowed into the prosthesis from below and above by momentary release of the iliac and aortic clamps in succession. This flushes any clot or atheroma from these vessels. The prosthesis is irrigated and aspirated through its unanastomosed iliac limb which is then clamped at its origin. The prosthesis is allowed to fill with blood by removal of the iliac clamp. Finally, removal of the aortic clamp restores blood flow to one limb.

A fall in systemic blood pressure is frequently encountered with restoration of blood flow. This results from loss of circulating blood volume into the previously ischemic limb. Haemorrhage from the suture lines and through the fabric of the prosthesis will contribute to this phenomenon. The hypotension should be anticipated and blood made ready for transfusion before the aortic clamp is removed. The surgeon initially should limit the flow of blood through the prosthesis for a few minutes after removal of clamps by compression of the proximal aorta between his fingers. At first, only one pulse beat in five may be allowed to pass, then one in three, alternate beats, and finally each beat when the blood pressure remains stable at a satisfactory level.

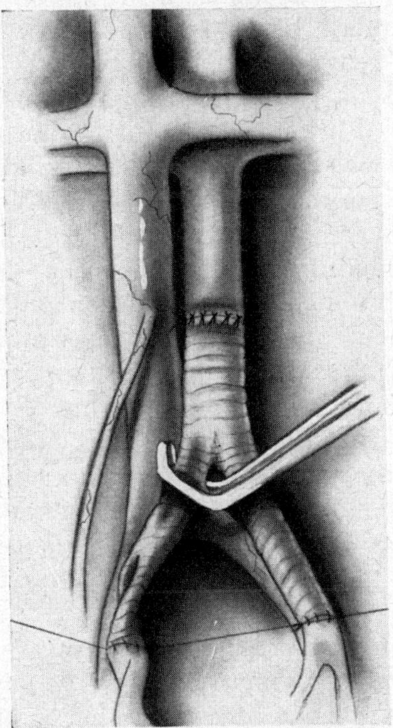

FIG. 4.4. Blood flow may be re-established through one limb of a bifurcated prosthesis whilst the final distal anastomosis is being completed.

Some anastomotic bleeding always occurs. Usually it is brief, ceases spontaneously, and involves only a small blood loss. Such bleeding can be stopped by packing dry gauze about the anastomosis and application of gentle pressure for a full ten-minute period. If haemorrhage should persist in spite of this measure, then additional sutures may be required. The exact site of bleeding should be established, then the proximal aorta is reoccluded and the suture inserted and tied without delay. The proximal clamp should be reapplied for only as short a time as possible to avoid thrombosis of the prosthesis.

The second iliac anastomosis is carried out with the same technique. Before placing the last few sutures, the distal clamp is momentarily opened to flush the adjacent vessel. The unfinished limb of the prosthesis is irrigated and aspirated, then the anastomosis is completed and the remaining prosthetic limb opened by removal first of the distal clamp, to expel air from the prosthesis lumen, and then the proximal clamp.

The peri-aortic fibroadipose tissue and posterior peritoneum is closed over the prosthesis and its anastomoses with continuous 0–0 chromic catgut suture. It is important to interpose sufficient tissue between the prosthesis and duodenum to prevent development of an aorticoduodenal fistula. Reconstruction of the anterior abdominal wall should include heavy retention sutures inserted at frequent intervals. The fascia and anterior peritoneum are closed as one layer with 0–0 silk in the case of a midline incision. In the paramedian incision the peritoneum and posterior rectus fascia are repaired as one layer and the anterior rectus fascia as a second layer. The skin edges are approximated with interrupted fine silk sutures.

Emergency Resection of Ruptured Aneurysm—Initial control of the proximal aorta is absolutely necessary when rupture has occurred. If the rupture has occurred into the retroperitoneal space, then the bleeding may be tamponaded for several hours. Nevertheless, success of the operation still depends upon acquiring control of the proximal aorta without incurring haemorrhage. This necessitates approaching the aorta well above the aneurysm. The aorta may be approached and clamped in the upper abdomen or in the chest through a separate thoracotomy incision. The haematoma is seldom so extensive as to preclude control of the upper abdominal aorta through the midline laparotomy incision.

A midline incision from the xiphoid process to pubis opens the peritoneal cavity (Fig. 4.5). The stomach is retracted inferiorly and an opening is made in the lesser omentum large enough to admit several fingers. With the right hand, a straight aortic clamp is inserted through the opening and its jaws, guided by the fingers of the left hand, are closed on the aorta well above the hematoma. It is occasionally necessary to open the posterior peritoneum for proper application of the clamp. The aorta is clamped at this level to avoid entering the large haematoma which surrounds the rupture and tamponades further haemorrhage. This life-saving manoeuvre should take only seconds to perform. After control of the proximal aorta has been acquired, the patient may be transfused with less danger of causing massive haemorrhage by restoration of blood pressure.

Next, the transverse colon and small intestine are swung superiorly and the posterior peritoneum is incised vertically over the aneurysm.

If the field had been dry up to this time, it may now be momentarily obscured by blood released from the retroperitoneal haematoma. Frequently, infiltration of blood in the retroperitoneal space has already accomplished much of the dissection necessary for application

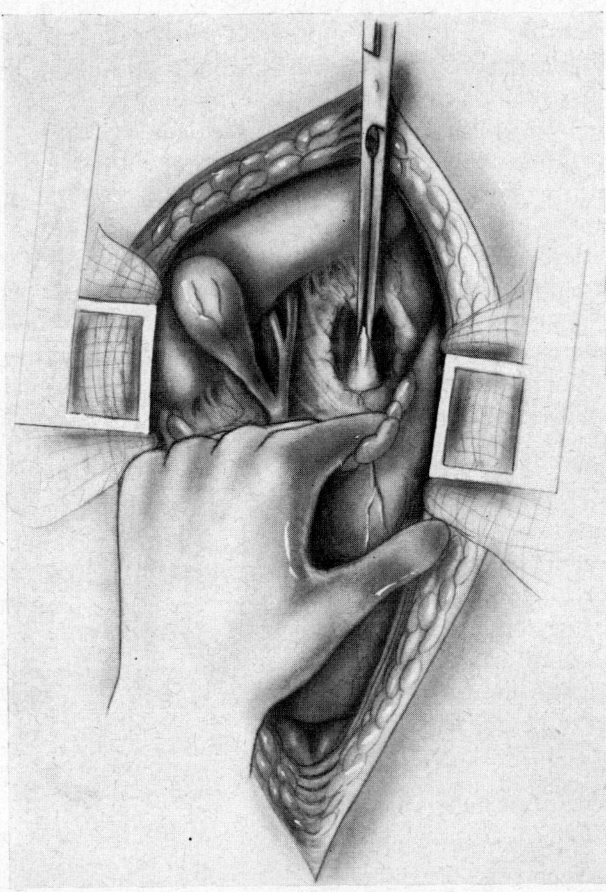

FIG. 4.5. In ruptures abdominal aortic aneurysm control of the aorta proximal to the lesion must precede dissection about the aneurysm. Decompression of a retroperitoneal haematoma without control of the proximal aorta will lead to fatal haemorrhage.

of the second aortic clamp just above the aneurysm and below the renal arteries. Using blunt dissection, the finger is passed posterior to the aorta at the upper extremity of the aneurysm. As soon as the aorta has been clamped at this level, the clamp above the renal arteries is removed. Total interference with renal blood flow should seldom be more than five or ten minutes. From this point on, the technique of resecting the ruptured aneurysm is essentially the same as that for the intact aneurysm.

Partial Aneurysmectomy—Some aneurysms of the lower abdominal aorta are densely adherent to the vena cava. There is a high incidence of dangerous venous bleeding associated with complete removal of such an aneurysm. In this situation the technique of partial excision is useful. The exposure of the aneurysm and application of proximal and distal vascular clamps is the same as previously described. As much of the aneurysm is dissected from the vena cava as is compatible with safety. Then the aneurysm is opened widely by a longitudinal incision on its anterior surface. The thrombus and atheromatous material in the aneurysm are scooped out. Back bleeding from the lumbar arteries, which arise from the aneurysm, is controlled by packing and pressure until each is ligated with a figure of 8 suture placed from within the aneurysmal sac (Fig. 4.2). The aneurysm wall is then trimmed to its attachment to the vena cava and this portion is left *in situ*. The area is thoroughly irrigated free of debris. The aneurysmal remnant becomes a part of the prosthetic bed.

The Extraperitoneal approach to the Abdominal Aorta—This approach has the following advantages:

1. Less post-operative ileus.
2. Reduced incidence of wound dehiscence.
3. Less post-operative atelectasis.
4. Easier anesthesia.
5. Less discomfort.
6. Shorter stay in bed.
7. Earlier discharge from the hospital.
8. Faster return to work.

But it has the following disadvantages:

1. Large aneurysms difficult.
2. High aneurysms very difficult.
3. Exposure requires more vigorous retraction.
4. The collateral circulation of the aorta suffers more interference.

The patient is placed supine with 5° elevation of the left hip. The abdomen, groins, and left flank are prepared in the usual manner and drapes are applied. The incision begins slightly to the right of the midline and passes obliquely about 1 in. below the umbilicus arcing upward and across the left flank to end just below the tip of the eleventh rib (Fig. 4.6). The external oblique muscle and its aponeurosis are split and the underlying internal oblique muscle is divided in the direction of the incision. The transversus abdominis muscle and transversal is

fascia are incised carefully to avoid cutting the peritoneum. The trans-
versalis fascia is dissected from the underlying peritoneum over a wide
area for the length of the incision. It is easy to tear the peritoneum
inadvertently where it is closely applied to the posterior rectus sheath.
If this should happen, the rent must be closed with fine interrupted silk
sutures. The posterior peritoneal space is developed by blunt dissection.

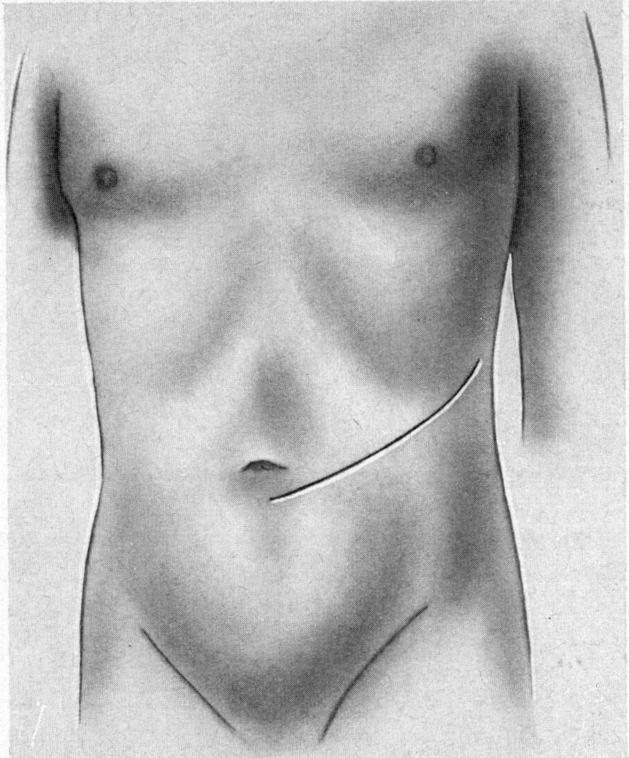

Fig. 4.6. The extra-peritoneal approach to the abdominal aorta.

The contents of the abdominal cavity, enveloped by the peritoneum,
are retracted anteriorly and medially until first the psoas muscle and
then the aorta are exposed (Fig. 4.7). The left ureter may be left
posteriorly or carried anteriorly with the peritoneum. The dissection
is carried well to the contralateral side of the aneurysm. The inferior
mesenteric artery is ligated and divided retroperitoneally at its origin.
This approach affords exposure of the bifurcation of both common
iliac arteries and of the aorta as high as the left renal vein.
When the prosthesis has been inserted and hemostasis secured, the

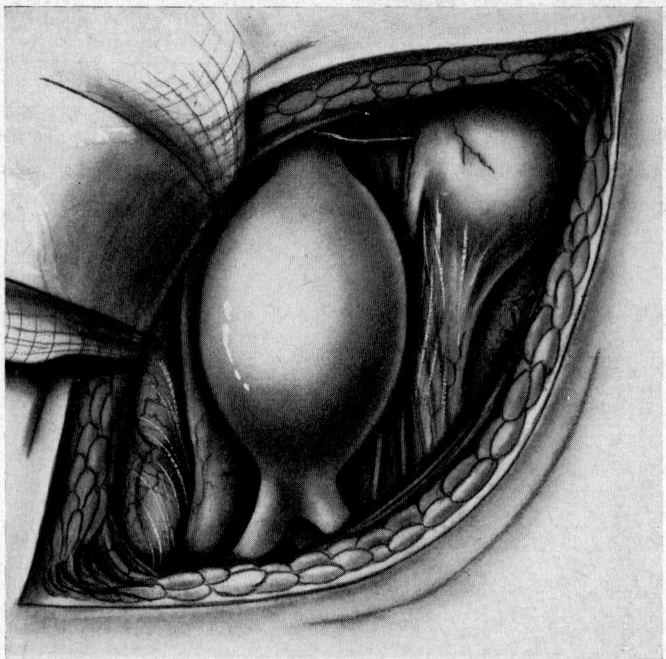

FIG. 4.7. The extra-peritoneal approach can provide access to the bifurcations of both iliac arteries and to the aorta at the level of the left renal vein.

peritoneum is allowed to resume its normal position. The muscle and fascial layers are reconstructed with interrupted 0–0 silk sutures, and the skin is closed with interrupted fine silks.

Aneurysms in Special Sites

Aneurysms of Extremity Arteries

Ideally, aneurysms of the main arteries of the extremities are best treated by excision and construction with autogenous vein. However, in certain areas where the aneurysm may be intimately involved with nerves, venous plexuses, and important muscles, ligation and bypass is better treatment. Popliteal and axillary aneurysms are of this category. In exposing the aneurysm, care is taken to preserve the collateral circulation. The artery proximal and distal to the aneurysm is ligated with heavy suture. A segment of the proximal artery is isolated from the blood stream by cross-clamping at a higher level. A longitudinal incision is made into the lumen of the clamped segment and the proximal anastomosis is constructed, end-to-side, using fine continuous suture technique. The distal anastomosis is carried out in the same manner. The distal clamp is first removed to fill the graft with blood and to expel air, otherwise embolized distally, through the suture lines. Finally, blood flow is restored by removal of the proximal clamp.

Aneurysms of the femoral artery can always be approached through an upper anterior thigh incision. Almost invariably the aneurysmal dilatation begins inferior to the inguinal ligament and a segment of artery of normal diameter is accessible for proximal control by this exposure. It is rarely necessary to divide the inguinal ligament or to extend the incision onto the abdomen.

Upper Abdominal Aneurysms

Exposure of the upper abdominal aorta may be adequate with a long midline incision in thin patients. Far better exposure can be achieved with an oblique thoraco-abdominal incision which extends from the left seventh intercostal space across the costal margin and obliquely

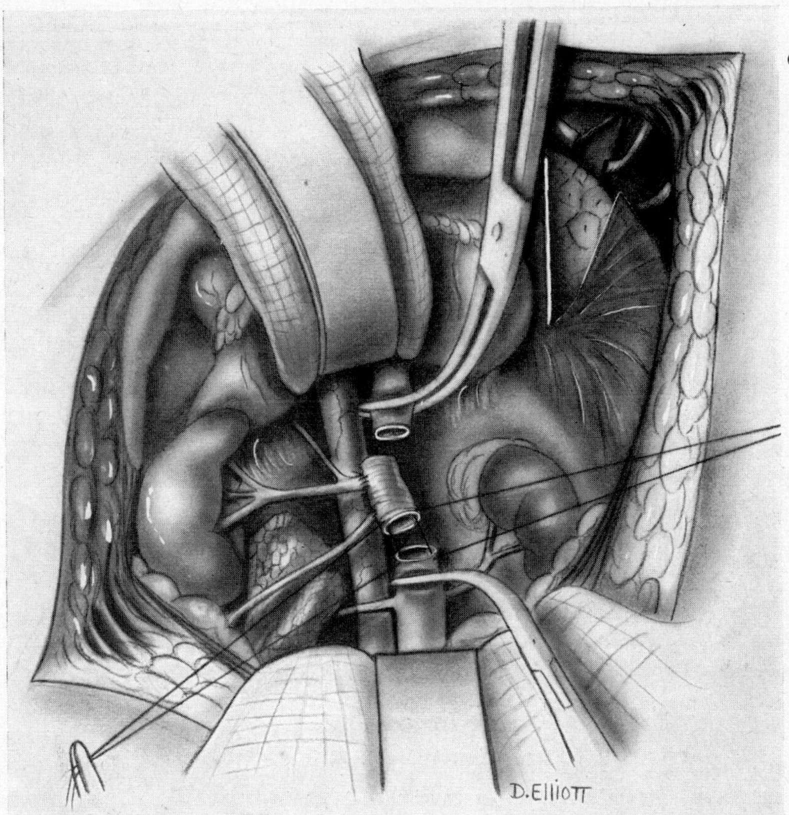

FIG. 4.8. In replacing a segment of the upper abdominal aorta, the visceral arteries should be implanted into the prosthesis before the aortic anastomoses are begun.

across the midline to end at the right costal margin. The aorta is reached by developing the bloodless plane separating the spleen and pancreas from the posterior abdominal wall and reflecting these organs and the abdominal viscera to the right. After excision of the aneurysm, the prosthesis is inserted first by implanting the visceral arteries into it, then by performing the aortic anastomoses (Fig. 4.8).

Aneurysms of the Thoracic Aorta and its Branches

Surgical treatment of aneurysms of the thoracic aorta must include provision for adequate perfusion of the abdominal viscera, the spinal cord, the brain, and the heart during the temporary occlusion of the aorta.

For aneurysms of the descending thoracic aorta a temporary bypass with a fabric prosthesis may be constructed as the initial step in the operation (Figs. 4.9a, b). The aorta proximal and distal to the lesion is side-clamped, and the bypass inserted by end-to-side anastomosis. With the bypass functioning, the aorta may be completely occluded within the limbs of the bypass, the aneurysm excised, and the definitive aortic reconstruction carried out. Finally, the temporary bypass is taken down and normal blood flow restored. Alternatively, partial left heart bypass may be used to assure perfusion distal to the aneurysm. The left atrium and a femoral artery are cannulated, and blood is pumped from the atrium to the femoral artery by extracorporeal means to perfuse the aorta in retrograde fashion. The aortic arch is, of course, perfused by the normal left ventricular outflow.

Saccular aneurysms of the aortic arch can occasionally be treated by side-clamping the aorta and simple excision of the sac. The resultant defect in the aorta is closed with an initial row of 00 horizontal mattress sutures followed by a second row of continuous over-and-over sutures. If bleeding occurs through such a suture line after removal of the clamp, additional sutures may be placed in the everted cuff without reclamping the aorta. Surgical treatment of fusiform aneurysms of the aortic arch requires total cardiopulmonary bypass. Involvement of the ascending aorta is frequently associated with impairment of aortic valve function because of dilatation of the aortic annulus. Thus, valve replacement or annuloplasty may be necessary in addition to treatment of the aneurysm.

Aneurysms of branches of the aortic arch, if the arch is not aneurysmal, are best excised and replaced with a prosthesis. A bypass is first constructed to assure good cerebral circulation while the aneurysmal artery is occluded. The bypass may be left as the definitive reconstruction after excision of the aneurysm and oversewing of its arterial ends. Frequently aneurysms of the branches of the arch are associated with

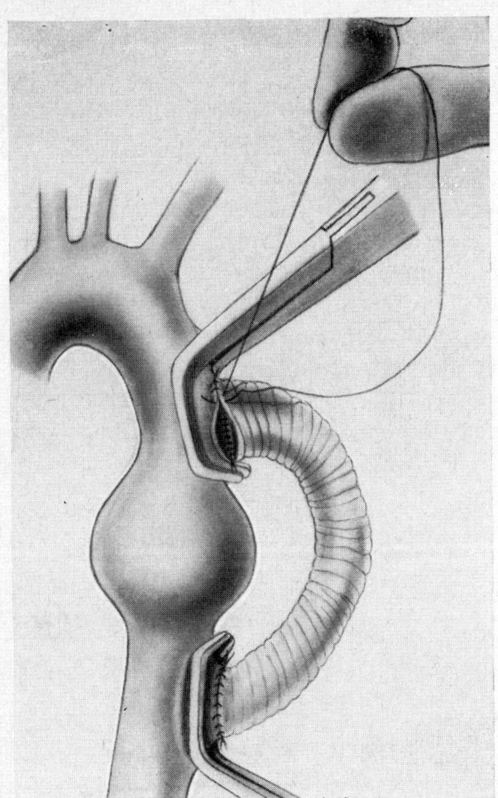

Fig. 4.9a. Provision for distal aortic perfusion in aneurysms of the thoracic aorta may be achieved by construction of a temporary bypass.

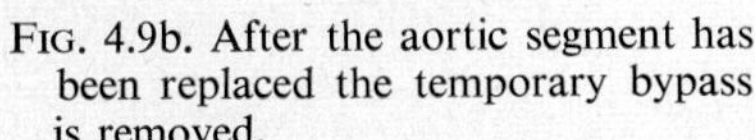
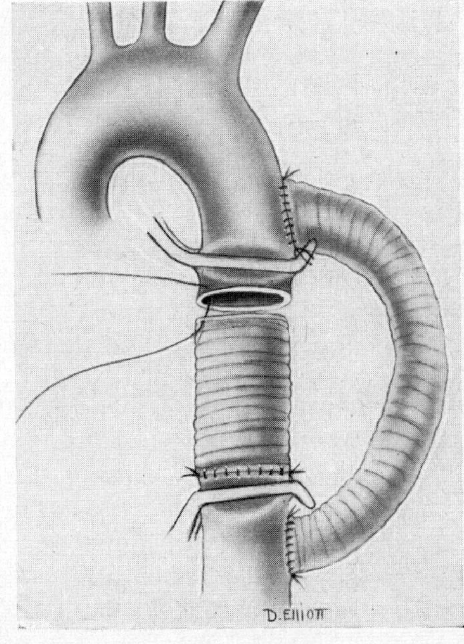

Fig. 4.9b. After the aortic segment has been replaced the temporary bypass is removed.

aneurysmal disease of the arch itself and surgical treatment may require total cardiopulmonary bypass and coronary perfusion.

Dissecting Aneurysm

A dissecting aneurysm results from the formation of a false lumen within the wall of a diseased artery by dissection of blood through an intimal defect. It is not a true aneurysm, and its treatment, therefore, differs in some respects from that of true aneurysm. The intimal defect frequently is a tear associated with an ulcerated atheroma. The process usually originates in the aortic arch above the aortic annulus or immediately distal to the origin of the left subclavian artery. The process may extend proximally to the heart or distally into the arteries of the

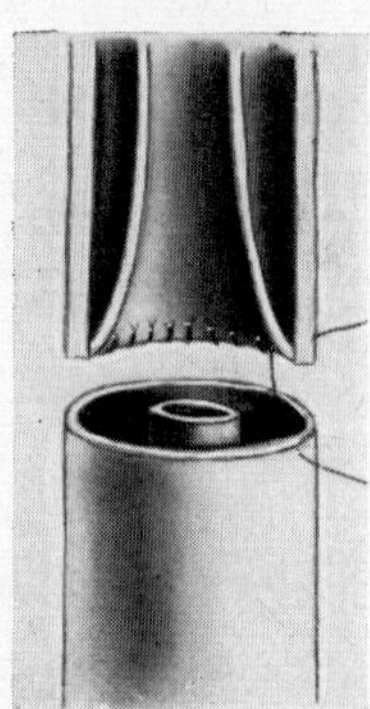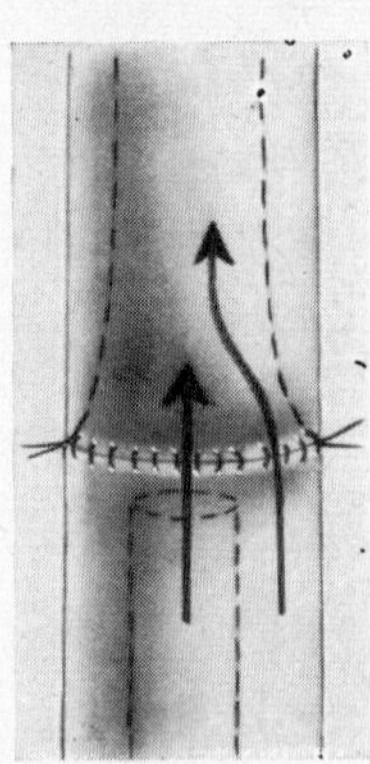

Fig. 4.10. This technique of suturing the true and false lumina of a dissecting aneurysm is designed to prevent progression of the dissection and to decompress the true arterial lumen.

extremities. The true arterial lumen may be severely narrowed or totally occluded by the intramural dissection of blood.

It is sometimes possible to determine rather accurately the origin and extent of the dissection by history and physical signs. Transient vascular bruits and loss of pulses indicate changes in local hemodynamics as the process of dissection proceeds. Occasionally, aortography is necessary to confirm the diagnosis or to demonstrate the extent of the dissection.

Important prognostic signs are the level of consciousness and the state of renal function. Deterioration of either faculty suggests that the dissection has caused occlusion of the cerebral and renal circulations. Death occurs by renal failure, stroke, or, when the dissection ruptures proximally into the pericardial sac, by tamponade.

The lesion may be treated in two ways: First, medically with hypotensive drugs and, second, surgically when one or two procedures have been employed. The false lumen may be "windowed" so that blood is readmitted into the normal lumen and the false lumen is decompressed (Fig. 4.10). In this procedure the lower extent of the dissection is surgically exposed. Vascular clamps are applied to isolate this segment of artery and the vessel is completely transected. The distal artery's inner and outer walls are sewn together with a continuous fine silk suture. This repaired arterial end is sutured end-to-end to the outer wall of the proximal arterial end, so that both its true and false lumina empty into the reconstructed, true, distal lumen. The purpose of this procedure is to decompress the false lumen and thus to prevent further dissection.

The alternative and preferable procedure is to find the intimal defect responsible for the dissection and to transect the vessel through this defect or to excise this segment of artery. Vascular continuity, and a single, normal lumen, is restored by end-to-end anastomosis of the artery or by interposition of a short prosthesis. Because the dissection frequently involves the aortic arch, cardiopulmonary bypass is required for this procedure.

With any mode of treatment this disease carries a high mortality rate.

Post-Operative Care

Most important is the maintenance of an adequate blood volume by transfusion to ensure a good blood pressure and adequate flow through the reconstructed artery. There is otherwise danger of thrombosis in the graft. When persistent hypotension occurs in spite of adequate blood replacement, and continuing blood loss has been ruled out, a pressor drug such as phenylephrine hydrochloride should be used.

Anti-coagulation is never necessary for the post-operative treatment of aortic aneurysms. However, in prosthetic reconstruction for aneurysms of smaller arteries, such as the popliteal, chronic anti-coagulation with Vitamin K antagonists may promote long-term patency of the prosthesis. If heparin is used, anti-coagulation should not be carried out before the 48th post-operative hour. The dangers of haemorrhage or infection of a hematoma are too great.

All oral intake is withheld for one to three days after surgery for abdominal aneurysms. Nasogastric decompression is frequently begun immediately before surgery and continued until evidence of bowel activity is apparent. During this time the patient's water and electrolyte requirements are met intravenously. Early ambulation in moderation hastens return of normal peristalsis. The original dressing need not be changed until the skin sutures are removed on the 7th post-operative day. Retention sutures are left in place for 10 to 14 days.

Special Complications of Aneurysmectomy

The complications that are somewhat uniquely associated with aneurysm surgery stem from interference with blood flow to important organs. Clamping the aorta at any level above the renal arteries requires some provision for protection against distal ischemia. Hypothermia, temporary bypass, internal shunts, or extracorporeal assistance can often provide this protection. But occasionally significant ischemia is not avoided.

Atherosclerotic or intra-operative occlusion of the coeliac axis or proper hepatic artery may diminish the liver's ability to metabolize citrate and make the patient prone to citrate intoxication. Thus, under these circumstances large transfusions of bank blood should be avoided.

Clamping of the upper abdominal aorta may also embarrass adreno-cortical function. It is wise, when this is anticipated, to prepare the patient with cortisone two days before surgery (50 mg. intramuscularly every six hours in multiple sites), to continue the treatment during the operation (100 mg. of hydrocortisone in one litre of intravenous fluid), and to wean the patient from it slowly over a three to five day period post-operatively.

In treatment of aneurysms of the thoracic aorta, ligation of several pairs of patent intercostal arteries may damage the spinal cord by interfering with its blood supply. On the other hand, if these intercostal arteries had already been occluded by mural thrombus in the aneurysm, the collateral circulation will be sufficient to prevent cord damage. Similarly, treatment of coarctation of the aorta may or may not require a temporary shunt or a left heart bypass. If the coarctation is severe, then collateral circulation is usually sufficient to allow aortic clamping without such measures. But if the coarctation is slight, then the lack of collateral circulation may require a shunt to prevent disastrous distal ischemia.

Spinal cord damage has been encountered during temporary occlusion of the thoracic aorta even with the assistance of left heart bypass perfusion. This has been shown to occur when distal aortic pressure did not exceed the cerebrospinal fluid pressure, thus preventing development of a pressure gradient of sufficient magnitude between the arterial circulation and the spinal cord to produce adequate blood flow. This phenomenon can be prevented by lowering the cerebrospinal fluid pressure during temporary aortic occlusion by the intravenous administration of hypertonic urea.

References

CANNON, J. A., VAN DE WATER, J., BARKER, W. F. (1963). Experience with the Surgical Management of 100 Consecutive Cases of Abdominal Aortic Aneurysm. *Am. J. Surg.* **106,** 128–143.

HARDIN, C. A. (1964). Survival and Complications after 121 Surgically Treated Abdominal Aneurysms. *Surg. Gyn. and Obs.,* **118,** 541–544.

MAY, A. G., DeWEESE, J. A., FRANK, I., MAHONEY, E. B., ROB, C. G. Data to be published.

SELVERSTONE, B. (1963). Treatment of Intracranial Aneurysms with Adherent Plastics. *Clin. Neuro.,* **9,** 201–213.

CREECH, O. (1966). Endo-Aneurysmorrhaphy and Treatment of Aortic Aneurysm. *Ann. Surg.,* **164,** 935–946.

ROB, C. G. (1963). The Extraperitoneal Approach to the Abdominal Aorta., *Surg.,* **53,** 87–89.

BLAISDELL, F. W., COOLEY, D. (1962). Mechanism of Paraplegia after Temporary Aortic Occlusion. *Surg.,* **51,** 351–355.

Chapter 5

CARDIAC PACING AND COMPLETE HEART BLOCK

Harold Siddons and Michael Wright

In cardiac muscle as in skeletal muscle, contraction of the muscle fibres is dependent on a wave of depolarization which, once started, will propagate along the muscle cell membrane. The fibres of the atria form a syncytium which is separated from the similar syncytium of the ventricles by a fibrous barrier, bridged only by the bundle of His. Depolarization starting anywhere in the atria will spread over the whole of both atria, but only reach the ventricles when the bundle is intact. In complete heart block, the bundle is interrupted. Ventricular contraction is then dependent on depolarization arising spontaneously in the ventricle.

Normally, this occurs about thirty to fifty times a minute, at a regular rate in any one individual. But the rate is often too slow to provide an adequate cardiac output and, from time to time, no depolarization may occur for an appreciable interval, or there may be bouts of rapid ventricular tachycardia. (See Fig. 5.1.) In either case, the circulation stops, producing the classical Stokes-Adams attack. Periods of arrest long enough to produce some symptoms occur in more than half of all patients in complete block. The longest will be fatal. Shorter periods produce syncope. Very short ones produce transient symptoms which, though usually constant for one individual, vary in pattern from one to another.

Thus, the indications for treatment in complete block lie in the prevention of Stokes-Adams attacks, and in relief of the low cardiac output state. Treatment is directed to increasing the idioventricular rate, either by drugs or by cardiac pacing. The latter, though a considerable undertaking, is much more effective.

It will be seen from the argument above that cardiac pacing can be achieved by inducing depolarization of any small area of the ventricular muscle. This is done by applying a negative-going impulse through an electrode in contact with the ventricle.

Diagnosis of Stokes-Adams Attacks

Since the necessity for treatment in any one patient so often depends on the presence of Stokes-Adams attacks, their accurate diagnosis is important. But from a history they may be difficult to distinguish from vasovagal phenomena or from epilepsy. Sometimes one cannot be certain without E.C.G. monitoring during an attack. The following points may be helpful.

Stokes-Adams attacks may occur at any time and are particularly common on exercise, whereas vasovagal incidents occur in set circumstances, usually when standing. Recovery is sudden and often associated with flushing. Convulsive movements may occur but, unlike epilepsy, only late in the attack. The absence of a pulse during Stokes-Adams attacks establishes the diagnosis; afterwards, the pulse is less informative. A slow pulse suggests a Stokes-Adams attack, but heart block may be intermittent so the pulse may resume a normal rate. Conversely, the presence of heart block does not exclude epilepsy or vasovagal phenomena.

The E.C.G. during a Stokes-Adams attack will usually show p-waves without ventricular complexes. Less often, one finds a rapid ventricular tachycardia, which if prolonged may lead into ventricular fibrillation. Even if sinus rhythm takes over between attacks, the E.C.G. almost always shows some conduction defect, most commonly right bundle branch block.

Aetiology of Complete Heart Block

Complete heart block may develop at any age, but is uncommon under fifty-five. It is estimated that fifty new patients develop complete block per million of population per year. Before the availability of treatment stimulated study, it was thought most often to be a complication of generalized myocardial ischemia. This arose because it certainly occurs in some cases of acute infarction, while in others a Stokes-Adams attack, perhaps associated with chest pains, may have been mistaken for a coronary thrombosis. The E.C.G. may fail to distinguish the two, since the classical features of ischaemia are largely obscured by complete block.

Recently, there has been a more careful analysis of aetiology. Clinically, there is often no clear evidence of infarction. Detailed post-mortem study including coronary angiography shows, in about half the cases, no evidence of coronary narrowing or infarction, or any other gross lesion to explain the block. Such cases have been classified as idiopathic or primary heart block. However, if stained serial sections of the conducting tissue of such hearts are made, an interruption in the bundle of His or its branches is always found, though the interpretation of the disease process causing the microscopic lesions is still open to question. One view regards the lesions as purely degenerative, an extension of a degenerative, often calcific, process affecting the fibrous "skeleton" of the heart. Others consider the lesions to be focal; similar to a myocarditis but affecting the muscle so little as to have no noticeable effect.

Apart from this large group of cases in which the aetiology is uncertain, there are many in which there is a clear explanation for the conduction defect. The underlying causative processes are remarkably diverse.

Congenital complete heart block has been diagnosed in utero and occurs in about 1 in 15,000 live births. Half such patients have other gross congenital cardiac abnormalities; cardiogenic syncope is less common than in acquired block, the idioventricular rate is faster and in particular it speeds more with exercise. Congenital block may not be diagnosed till adult life. Artificial pacing is very rarely required.

Ischaemia causes complete block in 5 per cent of acute myocardial infarcts, but is a rare cause of chronic heart block. Complete block associated with acute infarction carries a high mortality within the first few days, and temporary pacing is indicated. If the patient survives a week, the outlook is relatively good, sinus rhythm returning in most.

Calcification of the aortic or mitral valve ring may extend to involve the conducting tissue.

Iatrogenic complete heart block may follow surgery for septal defects and aortic valve disease. Most recover spontaneously, but if block continues, there is a high incidence of sudden death. Pacing is indicated until stable sinus rhythm returns.

Other aetiological factors are too numerous to list completely but include digitalis intoxication, cardiomyopathies, diphtheria, Chagas' disease, myxoedema, amyloidosis, dermatomyositis and rheumatoid arthritis.

Hypertension is not a cause, but may accompany block. The high stroke volume and long diastole give in any case a high systolic and low diastolic pressure.

Drug Treatment

Isoprenaline raises the ventricular rate in complete block by a few beats a minute and has an inotropic effect; these effects may increase cardiac output enough to obtain significant clinical improvement. That it also prevents syncopal attacks is more difficult to establish, but it is generally believed to do so in some cases. It may however provoke gross arrhythmias, and should first be given as an intravenous drip under E.C.G. observation with apparatus for electrical defibrillation and for pacing immediately available. If no arrhythmias occur it may be given by mouth. Given as a linguet, its action lasts about twenty minutes, but in a sustained release form (Saventrine, Pharmax and Co. Ltd.)

30 mgm. to 60 mgm. four-hourly through the daytime maintains an adequate blood level. It may cause nausea, trembling, sleeplessness and an irregular pulse from ectopic beats. The maintenance dose does not have to be increased with time.

Gluco-corticoids are widely used in the acute infarct and, by a few, in chronic heart block. They also lower the threshold required to pace and are helpful when implanted pacemakers are supplying barely sufficient power.

Digitalis is contra-indicated in intermittent complete block and in partial block but, when complete block is established and when patients are being paced artificially, it need not be withheld; it is often very valuable in failure.

Diuretics can be used when indicated.

Artificial Pacing

Every pacing system must consist of three parts: a power source and pulse generator, a pathway to the heart, and two electrodes; one makes contact with the ventricular muscle, the second completing the circuit can contact any convenient tissue.

The indications and methods used for pacing for short periods differ so markedly from those when pacing is to be prolonged for more than a week or two, that temporary and long-term pacing will be considered separately.

Indications for Temporary Pacing

Prolonged or rapidly recurring Stokes-Adams attacks. The initial emergency treatment of Stokes-Adams attacks is that of any other cardiac arrest; closed chest compression and forced ventilation. The first squeeze of the chest or a sharp blow on it may well re-establish a heart beat. Next an E.C.G. is set up to show whether the heart is in asystole or ventricular fibrillation. Fibrillation must be reversed by electrical defibrillation before pacing can be effective.

Heart block associated with acute myocardial infarction. Sudden death, often in ventricular fibrillation, is common in patients with second degree or complete heart block. If the heart is paced at an adequate rate, ectopic foci may be subdued. As sinus rhythm when it returns may prove intermittent, and the risk of cardiogenic syncope is not immediately over, it is suggested that pacing should be continued for 3 to 4 weeks.

To cover all anaesthetics and operations in patients with established or intermittent complete block. The risk of cardiac arrest when operating on patients with complete block has been estimated as over 25 per cent.

Temporary pacing should be set up before anaesthetizing for any operation including that for implantation of a permanent pacemaker. In a unit well used to emergency pacing techniques, it may be justifiable to stand by with needle electrodes suitable for direct puncture of the heart, ready to institute pacing within seconds of the occurrence of cardiac arrest.

When block occurs during cardiac surgery.

Methods of Temporary Pacing

An external pulse generator is used. One of the following temporary electrode systems is recommended.

Large skin electrodes (such as E.C.G. electrodes) applied at the apex and the base of the heart are used with a pacemaker giving an output voltage of 200 or more. Painful convulsive skeletal muscle contraction will occur with each impulse. The technique is impracticable in the conscious patient except for brief periods in extreme emergency.

A needle inserted through the skin to make contact with the left ventricle will act as an electrode which requires only 5 to 10 volts. An uninsulated lumbar puncture needle is suitable and should be inserted in the 6th space just to the left of the xiphoid and directed towards the second right costochondral junction at 30° to the chest wall. If pacing must be prolonged, a stainless steel wire (preferably insulated except for its last 2 cms.) can be threaded down the needle which is then withdrawn over the wire. Contact has been maintained by this method for periods of days. The circuit is completed either by a similar second electrode in the subcutaneous tissues or by a second electrode contacting the ventricle perhaps through the 4th or 5th space. With two ventricular electrodes, pacing will continue if one of them loses contact with the ventricle provided it retains contact with other tissue. With this method, the risk of damage to coronary vessels and haemopericardium has not been reported to be serious.

The endocardial transvenous electrode, either unipolar or bipolar, is the method of choice for temporary pacing when suitable X-ray facilities are available. If a unipolar electrode is used, the circuit is completed with a wire electrode under the skin near the site of the cutdown for the vein. A bipolar electrode avoids the necessity for a separate indifferent electrode, which saves time in an emergency. Bipolar electrodes are greater in diameter and have two other disadvantages which apply particularly to their long term use:

    (*a*) A positive electrode in the bloodstream attracts platelets, and tends to form clot.

    (*b*) Mechanical breakdown is more frequent with a double wire.

The threshold required to pace should be less than 1 volt at 2 m.secs.

An arm vein is recommended for temporary pacing but some select the external jugular or the saphenous.

If the patient is too ill to move, a transvenous electrode may still be passed without X-ray control. A battery-operated E.C.G. recorder is attached to the electrode and manipulation continues until large ventricular complexes are recorded, indicating that the electrode has reached the right ventricle. When in firm contact with the ventricular wall there is a characteristic "injury pattern" with S.T. elevation.

Indications for Prolonged Pacing

When drugs do not prevent recurrent Stokes-Adams attacks.

In complete heart block causing a heart rate too slow to provide adequate cardiac output. This low cardiac output may result in cardiac failure, renal failure, or inadequate cerebral flow. Symptoms of lethargy, dizziness on exertion and forgetfulness are common. The syndrome is often attributed to senility and, if there is doubt in the diagnosis, a trial of pacing by a temporary method may be worth while. Lethargy may disappear at once and many patients are immediately relieved of symptoms, though those due to cardiac and renal failure, if they are to clear, may take several weeks.

Methods of Prolonged Pacing

The pulse generator may either be implanted with the electrode system or left external to the body. If a power source outside the body is used, impulses can be transmitted to the heart in three ways: through a wire traversing the skin, by induction across the skin from an external coil to a second coil implanted just beneath, or by radio-frequency from an external transmitter to a more complex implanted receiver.

The Electrodes

Electrodes may be applied either to the outside, or the inside of the ventricular muscle, and are referred to as epicardial or endocardial, respectively.

Commonly used systems are illustrated in Figs. 5.1–5.3.

Epicardial electrodes. There are three main types:

(*a*) A loop of platinum wire, about 1·5 cms. long, is laid on the epicardium and secured by non-absorbable sutures.

(*b*) A cat's-whisker of platinum protrudes from a plastic plaque. A puncture in the epicardium is made to accept the cat's whisker; the plaque lies flat on the epicardium and is secured by sutures at its corners.

(*c*) A flexible wire, insulated up to about 5 cms. from the end, bears a small curved atraumatic needle. After passing once or twice through the epicardium, the needle is cut off. The buried loop may be further secured by a catgut or non-absorbable suture. This type is particularly suitable for temporary use after open heart surgery, since it may be withdrawn by pulling gently, after two weeks or so.

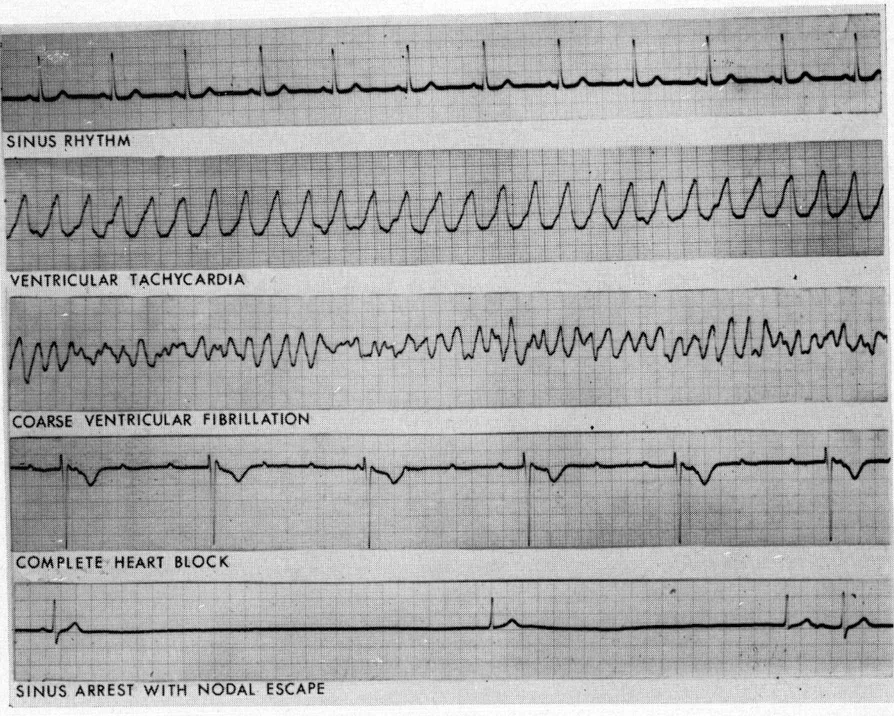

FIG. 5.1.

Ventricular Tachycardia. An irritable ventricle contracts again as soon as its recovery phase is over. There is no time for venous filling; the heart output is negligible, and the peripheral pulse absent. It may revert spontaneously to a slower rhythm, or, due to myocardial anoxia, proceed to ventricular fibrillation.

Coarse Ventricular Fibrillation. Unco-ordinated contractions, with no output: usually irreversible except by a shock which will depolarize the whole muscle mass simultaneously, but occasionally reverts spontaneously.

Complete Heart Block. P-waves representing atrial contractions are unco-ordinated with the slow ventricular complexes and contractions.

Sinus Arrest with Nodal Escape. The first complex is normal. The sino-atrial node then fails to fire. After a long pause the atrio-ventricular node fires spontaneously, producing a normal ventricular complex, but without a P-wave.

Choice of position. Usually three electrodes are placed, two on the heart away from coronary vessels, fat-laden areas, or obvious infarcts, and one indifferent electrode in subcutaneous tissue. If pacing then fails

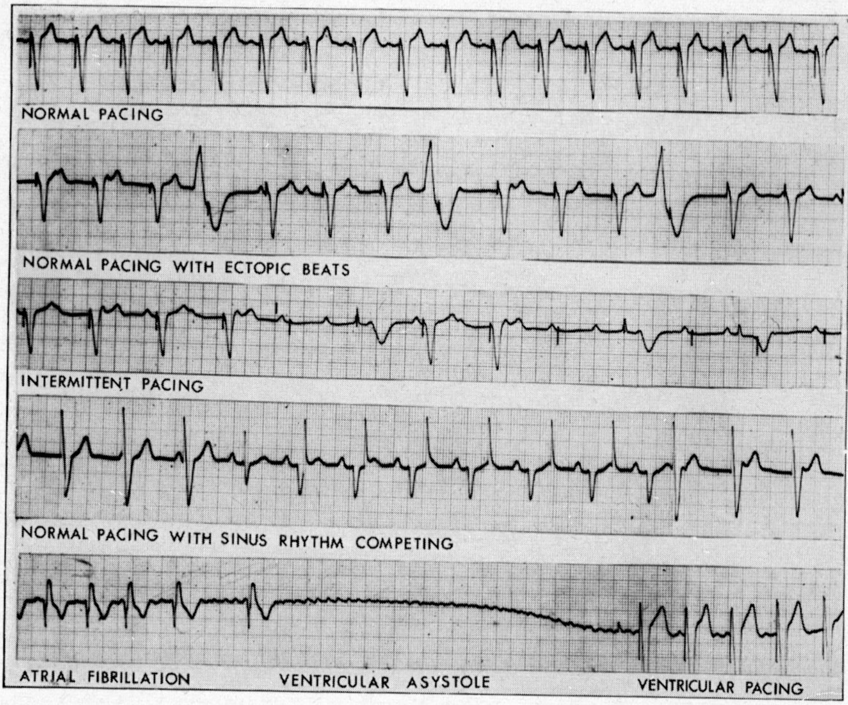

Fig. 5.2

Normal Pacing. The sharp downward deflection is the pacing impulse, followed by a relatively normal ventricular complex. P-waves occur at random through the trace.

Normal Pacing with Ectopic Beats. As above, but with occasional spontaneous ventricular complexes, of abnormal shape, but all the same shape. They are presumed all to arise from the same focus—*unifocal ectopics.* Multifocal ectopics, where the complexes are of different shapes, indicate a greater degree of ventricular irritability, and are more likely to precede ventricular fibrillation.

Intermittent Pacing. Pacing impulses are all of the same size but some are not followed by ventricular complexes. The pacing voltage is close to the threshold required to pace.

Normal Pacing with Sinus Rhythm Competing. The sharp upward deflections are pacing impulses. In the first two complexes the ventricle has been fired. The third pacing impulse falls just after the P-wave, but still fires the ventricle. The fourth and fifth are later, and are superimposed on a normal ventricular complex fired by the P-wave. Not until the eleventh can it again fire the ventricle.

Atrial Fibrillation—Ventricular Asystole—Ventricular Pacing. The pacemaker has been turned on by hand. A Demand pacemaker would cut in after a much shorter period of asystole.

with one electrode, the other may be connected without exposing the heart.

Surgical approach. The heart may be exposed either by a limited antero-lateral thoracotomy or by an abdominal route, incising the central tendon of the diaphragm without opening peritoneum or pleura.

The pacemaker is usually implanted subcutaneously in the axilla

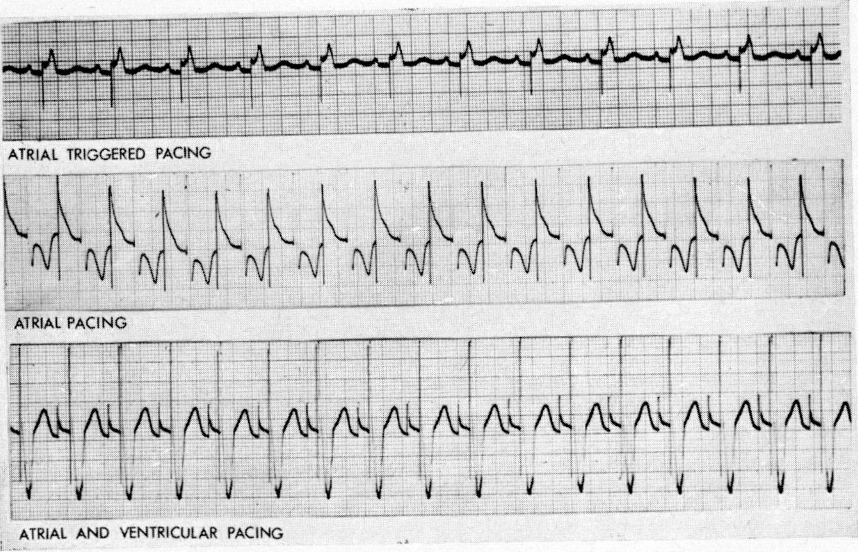

F_{IG}. 5.3

Atrial Triggered Pacing. The P-wave is picked up by a separate atrial electrode, and triggers the pacemaker, which fires the ventricle after a suitable delay (0·16 sec.).

Atrial Pacing. The pacing impulse produces a large and grossly distorted atrial voltage, which is followed by a relatively normal QRS and T.

Atrial and Ventricular Pacing. Both atrium and ventricle are paced separately at regular intervals which are controlled electronically. The atrial complex is similar to that in B above, but smaller.

with the thoracic approach and in the abdominal wall, either subcutaneously or deep to the rectus within its sheath, with the transdiaphragmatic route.

The abdominal approach is a lesser procedure, but wires passing into the abdomen are subject to more movement than thoracic wires and fracture is a common cause of pacing failure. Further, the thoracic approach allows a more complete inspection of the heart and a much wider choice of electrode position.

Endocardial electrodes. Endocardial electrodes have a small bare metal tip on a flexible insulated wire. They are passed like a cardiac catheter through a vein, via the right atrium and tricuspid valve, to make contact with the endocardium among the trabeculae of the right ventricle. Early displacement may require repositioning, but in a few days local tissue overgrowth prevents subsequent movement.

Types of Endocardial Electrode. Failures of endocardial electrodes are due to five main causes:

(1) displacement of the tip
(2) perforation of the myocardium
(3) wire breakage
(4) insulation breakdown
(5) threshold rise without displacement.

Displacement and perforation are reduced by increasing flexibility of the electrode wire, but this increases the difficulty of manoeuvring the electrode into position. A very flexible electrode may be stiffened during positioning by a stilette or an outer tube, but removal of these may be difficult without upsetting the position of the tip. Perforation of the myocardium has not proved to be a dangerous complication. Breakage of wire and insulation are almost eliminated by using a spiral stainless steel wire with polythene or silicone rubber insulation. Threshold rise may be dependent on the material of the tip; while platinum causes least reaction, the joint between platinum and stainless steel is less reliable than stainless steel throughout.

The electrodes commercially available each represent a different compromise between these considerations. In general, each design has its own connection arrangements and pulse generator with pulse width and strength matched to the contact area of the electrode.

Techniques for Placing Endocardial Electrodes

The electrode is inserted into a peripheral vein and then manipulated into position under X-ray control. The threshold required to pace the heart is measured and should be less than 1·0 volt at 2·0 m.secs. The stability of the position is then attested by asking the patient to sniff and cough. It may take many attempts to find a position satisfactory in both respects; the best are usually as far down and out in the apex of the right ventricle as is possible.

If the electrode is to be brought out through the skin for permanent pacing, a tunnel must be made to an exit site at least 4 in. from the cut down site to protect the bloodstream from infection by skin organisms. If a pacemaker is to be implanted, a pocket must be made for it, and a tunnel for the wire from the cut down site. General anaesthesia is best for tunnelling and implanting the unit, unless the patient is unfit.

But as pacing must be established before induction, cut down and manipulation are carried out under local infiltration.

Facilities required. The necessities for this procedure are:

(1) Strict asepsis
(2) Full anaesthetic facilities
(3) X-ray control, with an image intensifier and large screen display.
(4) Good light
(5) Electrical equipment for E.C.G. monitor, internal and external pacing, threshold measurements and defibrillation.

There is no doubt that the proper place to assemble these is an operating theatre, using a portable image intensifier. If an X-ray screening room has to be used, there will be constant compromises with aseptic technique and anaesthetic facilities.

Choice of cut-down site. For long-term pacing, arm veins are not suitable as the arm has to be immobilized to prevent movement affecting the electrode tip, and because of phlebitis.

Usually, the jugular system is most convenient. A 2 in. skin crease incision in the supra-clavicular fossa will expose either the external jugular vein, which may be tied off round the wire, or the internal deep to sternomastoid. In a large vein, the wire is passed through a stab, encircled by a purse string which is tied when the electrode is in satisfactory position.

An incision is now made anterior to the pectoral muscles. Long artery forceps are passed deep to pectoralis major and pushed through the clavipectoral fascia in contact with the under surface of the clavicle, into the neck incision to draw down the electrode. The loop in the neck is immobilized by two non-absorbable sutures to the cervical fascia, and platysma is closed over it.

An electrode, introduced from the arm in an emergency, may be used permanently by exposing the axillary vein and extracting the electrode through a short incision which can be closed round it. That part of the electrode previously exposed at the elbow is sterilized with iodine in spirit and cut off flush with the skin before drawing the rest through. There is an incidence of electrode displacement and axillary vein thrombosis following this procedure, and it is not entirely satisfactory.

The Choice Between Endocardial and Epicardial Pacing

Endocardial pacing has many advantages. The procedures, though they may sometimes be long and tedious, are surgically minor. They can be carried out in an ill patient, even in severe shock. The mortality is negligible and the complications surprisingly slight and infrequent.

Thromboembolism is almost unknown: postmortem examination reveals that the electrode becomes covered by a thin tube of endothelial-like structure, only broken where it passes through the tricuspid valve. Sepsis may sometimes cause the rejection of a buried unit, or force the changing of a subcutaneous course, but minor sepsis may respond to antibiotics, and bacteraemia, septicaemia or endocarditis are extremely uncommon. Nevertheless, valve disease is regarded as a contra-indication to the use of external wires with an endocardial system, because of the increase in the risk of infection.

The chief disadvantage of endocardial pacing is the occasional liability of the electrode to displacement. This is fairly frequent in the first day or two but, if a position appears stable over this time, it seldom shifts later.

In contrast to this, the installation of an epicardial system carries an appreciable early mortality (7–15%). Should sepsis develop, its consequences are more serious than they are in endocardial pacing. Apart from almost certain failure of pacing, sinuses will continue to discharge until the whole foreign system is removed, and the removal of septic wires from the myocardium may be difficult and dangerous. A frank pericarditis may develop and may be fatal.

In spite of this picture, many busy departments, who offer pace-making as an additional service and who may lack the time, equipment and technical assistance necessary for endocardial pacing, have found the installation of epicardial systems a straightforward and predictable procedure, whose results are good enough to justify its continued use on a large scale. This is particularly true in the U.S.A. and on the Continent, whereas in Britain, Scandinavia and in some specializing clinics in the U.S.A. endocardial pacing is more favoured. Epicardial pacing is required in the few patients in whom the endocardial electrode repeatedly displaces.

The Pulse Generator, or Pacemaker, and its Power Source

The smaller the electrode the less electrical current required and the smaller the pacemaker unit to supply it. If pulses stronger than necessary are used, there is an increasing risk of inducing ventricular fibrillation, particularly if a pacemaker impulse should fall during the recovery phase following an intrinsic ventricular contraction. But some margin must be allowed above the threshold measured when an electrode is first implanted. Over the next few days the measured threshold usually rises to double this value. Since the current needed is directly proportional to the area of live muscle membrane it passes through, this effect may be due to death of the tissue in immediate contact with the electrode, through which the current must spread before reaching a larger area of live muscle.

The stimulus required to pace the heart is easily provided by batteries, and to avoid the risk of electrocution, no apparatus connected to a cardiac electrode should be mains-operated, or connected to earth. Strong electrical fields will also induce currents in the electrode wires which may either cause electrocution, or destroy the pacemaker unit. Diathermy should never be used. An implanted unit may survive a defibrillating shock, but cannot be relied on to do so.

External and Implanted Units

Implanted units have the advantage that the user can forget his dependence on an electronic gadget and, once initial healing is complete, the chances of subsequent sepsis are remote. Their designed life is about three years, and is improving. At present, few completely implanted systems run without trouble for the whole three years but, of the failures, less than half are directly due to failure of the pacemaker unit.

Some experimental designs use *biological sources of energy*, e.g. a piezoelectric ceramic crystal, which when distorted by the heart movements develops a voltage, charging a condenser which acts as power source for the pacemaker. If the heart beat fails, the pacemaker can still produce about ten impulses. The U.S.A. Atomic Commission is working on a unit powered by Plutonium 380.

External pacemakers have two main advantages. They are not limited in size or complexity and, if there are signs of trouble, both the unit and the internal electrode system can be tested and the unit replaced immediately, if necessary. They are particularly valuable for patients in variable block whose pacing requirements may alter, when threshold or electrode position are not yet stable, and occasionally when a variation in rate appears desirable. They are of three main kinds:

Boxes for use at the bedside. These are not limited as to size, complexity or versatility and usually carry controls giving a wide range of pulse frequency, strength and duration. They are used for emergency and short-term pacing, for the measurement of threshold and for the testing of the suitability of a given type of pacing in a particular patient.

Units to be carried permanently by the patient. They are small and may be fixed inside the vest or brassiere.

Units providing indirect transfer of energy across the skin barrier. These have the advantages of an external pacemaker, and avoid a wire traversing the skin. In the Lucas system used at Birmingham, the pulse energy is transmitted by induction from a coil glued to the skin to a second coil implanted immediately deep to it. This is connected to the electrodes, either epicardial or endocardial. Glenn, in the U.S.A., uses radio-frequency transmission to an implanted receiver. In spite of their obvious advantages, these methods have not yet gained popularity outside their birthplaces.

Types of Pacemaker Circuit

Fixed rate pacing. If a heart, healthy except for complete block, is paced at a fixed rate, the cardiac output still varies with physiological requirements, since the stroke volume is controlled by the rate of venous return. Normally, a rate of 70 per min. provides an adequate output in the adult for all normal quiet activity. This method is widely used throughout the world, and is satisfactory when block is complete and when there are no ectopic beats arising in the ventricle. But block is often incomplete, or intermittent, and these hearts being abnormal often produce ectopic beats. The resultant cardiac output is irregular, as in atrial fibrillation. There is also a danger of provoking ventricular fibrillation if an impulse arrives in the vulnerable phase of recovery after an endogenous ventricular contraction. Sudden death is more common in paced patients with competing rhythms than when the pacemaker is in complete control, and this is thought to be the mechanism, although many patients with competing rhythms survive years of pacing, when an impulse must fall in the vulnerable period thousands of times a day.

Adjustable implanted pacemakers. Units for implantation have been designed in which rate and power output can be switched from outside between pre-set levels. Some are switched by a fine needle screwdriver inserted through the skin, some by a magnet and some by induction through the skin. An increase in output may revive pacing which is failing due to rise in threshold and different rates may suit different conditions.

One of the many implantable pacemakers now on the market has its circuitry arranged so that an external apparatus, "a threshold analyser", can be placed on the skin over it and alter the power of the impulse. By this means, it is possible to measure the threshold required to pace and the state of the batteries without exposing the unit.

Demand or ventricular-inhibited pacing. In these circuits, an endogenous ventricular complex, whether atrial-induced or ectopic, inhibits the pacemaker. If no complex occurs during a set delay, the pacemaker fires at a fixed rate until further endogenous complexes occur. Such a circuit avoids the danger of stimulation in the vulnerable period and greatly reduces the irregularity of force and rate of the pulse.

Demand pacing is particularly valuable in patients with variable block, as after acute infarcts or open heart surgery, and in patients liable to ventricular standstill though in sinus rhythm between attacks. Most such patients will be on short-term pacing and an external unit is suitable. Experience with implantable demand units is as yet very limited.

Atrial-triggered pacing. If a further electrode is introduced, either attached to the atrium at thoracotomy or placed in contact with it at mediastinoscopy, atrial action-potentials of over 1·0 m.v. can be picked up. This pulse is used to trigger, after a suitable delay corresponding to the P.R. interval, a ventricular pacing impulse applied to the usual epicardial or endocardial electrodes. (See Fig. 5.3.) If no p-wave is sensed as may occur in atrial fibrillation, pacing reverts to a fixed rate. There is also a maximum rate of triggering to avoid trying to make the ventricle follow a rapid atrial tachycardia or flutter.

Atrial-triggered pacing thus avoids the danger of stimulation during the vulnerable period following natural beats of atrial origin, though not following ventricular ectopics. It also restores the use of the atrial transport mechanism and the physiological control of rate. The system is particularly suitable for patients partly in sinus rhythm and for the young and active. It should also benefit those hearts close to failure.

Aftercare

When a satisfactory pacing system is established and the patient is discharged, he is asked to report back immediately on two points:

(1) If a daily pulse count shows speeding or slowing by more than four points in a full minute. Change in rate of the unit may herald electronic breakdown or indicate failure of the heart to follow all stimuli. Rates over 110 per minute may induce ventricular fibrillation and deaths from such runaway pacemakers have occurred. Urgent action is indicated.

(2) Any sign of sepsis in any of his wounds. Minor local sepsis may respond to antibiotics but, if it does not do so, then the whole system may have to be changed. Sometimes, if sepsis is round the unit, the endocardial wire may be preserved and re-routed to a new pacemaker at a new site or exteriorized through a new tunnel for connection to an external pacemaker.

Apart from these instructions, the patient is seen in Outpatients at three month intervals. As well as routine clinical, X-ray and E.C.G. assessment (see Fig. 5.2), the stimulus wave form is measured by means of a calibrated oscilloscope (Tektronix) which may show signs of impending failure from wire deterioration or battery exhaustion.

References

SIDDONS, H. and SOWTON, E. (1967). Cardiac Pacemakers. Pub: C. C. Thomas. Springfield, Ill., U.S.A.

ESCHER, D. J. W. (1967). The Present Status of Clinical Cardiac Pacing. *Amer. Heart J.*, **74,** 126.

CHAPTER 6

EXTRACRANIAL AND MESENTERIC ARTERIAL DISEASE

J. R. KENYON

EXTRACRANIAL ARTERIAL STENOSIS AND OCCLUSION

In 1888 Mehnert quoted by Chiari, observed the high incidence of atherosclerosis of the extracranial carotid and innominate arteries, and in 1914 Hunt drew attention to the association between stenosis and thrombosis of these vessels with neurological syndromes. Moniz *et al.* (1937) established the diagnosis of internal carotid thrombosis of four clinical cases of stroke by arteriography. Eastcott, Pickering and Rob (1954) published the first case report of a patient suffering from intermittent stroke which was successfully treated by surgical correction of an atheromatous stenosis of the internal carotid artery. Rob and Wheeler in 1957 reported on a series of patients treated by vascular reconstruction with satisfactory results, since when many publications have been devoted to the diagnosis and treatment of stenosis and thrombosis of the extracranial arterial system.

Pathophysiology

The brain, being the body's most sensitive indicator of blood flow, or lack of it, and with the extracranial blood supply accessible to arteriography and direct surgery, this system provides an excellent field for research in the process of atherosclerotic stenosis and occlusion. It is surprising that relatively few studies have been directed to it.

The circle of Willis is a collateral arterial system, supplied by four main arteries, the two carotids and the two vertebrals. There are, however, many anatomical variations of the circle, particularly in the calibre of the anterior and posterior communicating arteries, which explains why one group of patients can tolerate common carotid ligation without developing symptoms, whereas another will develop hemiplegia. There are several well documented cases of patients relying solely on one patent carotid or vertebral artery for cerebral blood flow without impairment of neurological function. The efficiency of the collateral flow in the circle can be demonstrated at operation on the carotid bifurcation, when the internal carotid artery is clamped and pressures are measured on either side of the occlusion. In approximately 70 per cent of patients there is a difference of 10 mm. or less in the mean arterial pressure. Mere reduction of arterial pressure is an uncommon cause of attacks of cerebro-vascular insufficiency. A further relevant factor is that a simple stenosis of a vessel must reduce the lumen by 90 per cent before a pressure differential can be measured across the narrowed segment. It is therefore unlikely that pressure differences

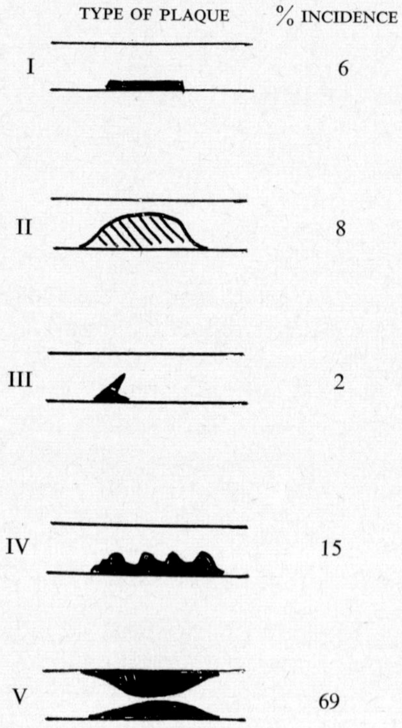

	TYPE OF PLAQUE	% INCIDENCE
I		6
II		8
III		2
IV		15
V		69

FIG. 6.1

produce the attacks, but should the stenosis become extreme, pressures in the internal carotid and the circle of Willis are equalized and stasis and thrombosis result.

Micro emboli have been observed with an ophthalmoscope in the fundi of patients during attacks of intermittent carotid insufficiency and also after corrective surgery. The most likely source is the athero-sclerotic plaque or the arterial suture line. Ross Russell (1964) has demonstrated this experimentally by partially occluding an artery in the rabbit mesentery. The micro emboli, consisting of fibrin and platelet aggregations, form on the stenosed segment and then separate, to be carried by the blood stream to occlude a smaller branch. Gunning *et al.* (1966), in a clinical study of 16 patients have suggested that the emboli form on the smooth atherosclerotic plaque. Moreover, atherosclerotic plaques are not necessarily static entities. Duguid (1954) has shown that they may gradually develop by surface deposition of fibrin and Winternitz (1934) has also demonstrated that haemorrhage into a plaque can produce a local form of dissection, with injury or damage to the vasa vasorum. Kenyon and Thompson (1965) in a study of 49 patients with carotid artery stenosis, classified the plaques into five main types (Fig. 6.1). *Type I* is a flat plaque and seldom produces symptoms. *Type II* is a localized dissection containing altered blood or a paste like autolysed material. *Type III* the web plaque, could possibly arise from rupture of Type II. *Type IV*, the ulcerated plaque and a frequent source of mural thrombi, might arise from degeneration of Type II. The commonest plaque, *Type V*, is built up by platelet deposition and was most frequently associated with the typical history of carotid artery stenosis.

However, the production of micro emboli by atherosclerotic lesions does not entirely explain the consistently focal and repetitive nature of the intermittent stroke; it is difficult to envisage each stream of emboli arriving at the same area of cerebral cortex on each occasion, with subsequent fibrinolysis, or compensation by collateral circulation, with full clinical recovery of the brain. It is probable that cerebral capillary stasis, as suggested by Denny Brown (1961), and demonstrated under physiological and pharmacological stresses in animal brains by Meyer (1959), may be additional factors in producing the characteristic syndrome.

Vessels Affected

(1) The internal carotid is most commonly affected. The atherosclerotic plaque occurs at its origin as shown in Fig. 6.2(i) and may develop to a tight stenosis and ultimate thrombosis as shown in Fig. 6.2(ii). The thrombosis extends along the internal carotid usually to the first collateral, the ophthalmic artery. The plaque also involves the origin of the external carotid but rarely produces appreciable stenosis. These lesions are bilateral in 50 per cent of cases.

(2) The vertebral artery is second in frequency and the plaque invariably occurs at its origin from the subclavian artery. Thrombosis, when it occurs, extends at least to the basilar artery. Occasionally both vertebrals are involved (Fig. 6.2(iii) and (iv)).

(3) The innominate and left subclavian artery are affected as often as the aortic arch but compared with the internal carotid and vertebral arteries they less frequently proceed to thrombosis because of the

relatively greater calibre (Fig. 6.2(v) and (vi)). However, when this occurs, the syndrome of "subclavian steal" results.

(4) The aortic arch is often affected by scattered atheromatous lesions, especially in diabetic patients and cerebral insufficiency is produced when the origins of the innominate and common carotid arteries are narrowed by the sclerosis (Fig. 6.2(vii)). Complete obliteration of the aortic arch, or one or more of its major branches, occasionally occurs in the "pulseless disease" of Takyashu.

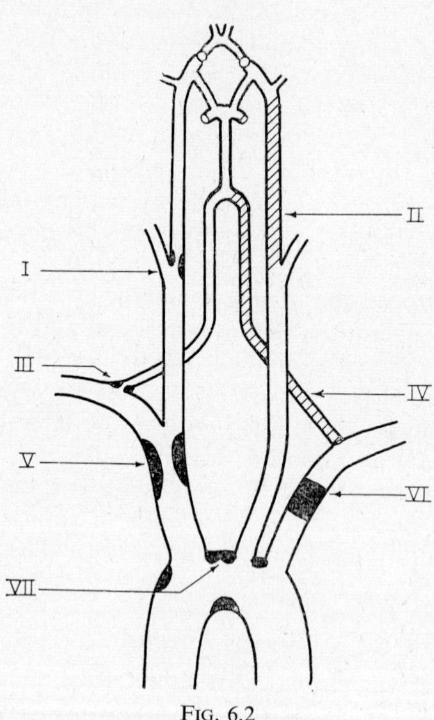

Fig. 6.2

Clinical Features

Atherosclerosis being the common factor, patients usually present in the 6th and 7th decade. In diabetics the age incidence is 10 years earlier. Those with a poor genetic history i.e. one or both parents dying at an early age from coronary thrombosis or stroke, are also affected earlier. Women are affected less often with a resultant sex ratio of five to one.

The clinical presentation can be divided into:

    (i) Impending stroke,
    (ii) Progressing stroke,
    (iii) Completed stroke.

(i) **Impending stroke:** it is helpful to subdivide this group into:

    (*a*) Complete neurological recovery

    (*b*) Partial neurological recovery.

The patient with carotid artery stenosis presents with intermittent attacks of contra-lateral hemiparesis or homolateral loss of vision. The attacks are of short duration, three to five minutes at the most, after which recovery is more or less complete. The frequency is random, varying from monthly to weekly intervals up to several episodes in one day. Occasionally a fall of arterial pressure produced by the vasodilation of a hot bath or an episode of ventricular tachycardia will precipitate an attack.

When the motor functions are affected, the patient experiences inco-ordination, weakness or even complete paralysis of the hand, which may extend to the arm; the leg is usually less affected. Speech defects may occur concurrently or independently when the appropriate side of the brain is affected. These vary from an inability to count or express thought to a complete dysarthria or aphasia. Although loss of vision usually occurs separately it is sometimes associated with motor or speech symptoms in the same individual. Occasionally there is a preliminary loss of colour appreciation, rapidly followed by dimness of vision and then complete blindness of one eye.

Neurological recovery may or may not be complete after the attack. In the latter case there is inco-ordination of fine hand movements which will impair writing or other skilled work, dysarthria, or inability to express thought accurately, although the patient appreciates what he wants to say. When the eye has been affected there may be residual field defects. These sequelae occasionally deteriorate with subsequent episodes.

In patients with complete recovery the neurological examination is entirely negative. Tendon reflexes, sensation and cranial nerve function are normal. Positive signs indicate a small infarcted area in the brain.

When the vertebral-basilar system is primarily involved the patient presents with a history of attacks of similar duration and complains of giddiness, vertigo, inco-ordination of gait or falling to one side. Similarly, recovery may be complete or incomplete; in the latter case, neurological examination will reveal inco-ordination of limb movements, balance or gait.

Tinnitus has been a frequently mentioned symptom in recent publications, but in the writer's experience this has been unusual.

(ii) **Progressing stroke,** this commences with a fully established hemiplegia followed by an increase of the neurological involvement and deepening of the level of consciousness over a period of hours or days, indicating a progressing cerebral arterial thrombosis. The course may continue to death or the progression may stabilize to a completed stroke.

(iii) **Completed stroke,** it may be preceded by impending stroke or progressive stroke or occur *de novo,* in which case the onset is sudden. However, once established there is a steady improvement over a period of weeks to months. Full recovery is unusual, but considerable compensation and adaptation to the sequelae of the hemiparesis, speech defects and visual field involvement, may be expected in the first year after onset. This type of stroke is due to a cerebral embolism or cerebral thrombosis, without extension of the thrombus to the surrounding vessels.

Diagnosis

Only those factors of special importance will be discussed; a full neurological examination, including fundi and optic fields, and a full physical examination are pre-supposed. Similarly the patient should be examined biochemically for diabetes, hypercholesterolaemia, hyperlipaemia and abnormal blood coagulation factors.

Examination of Head and Neck Vessels

An absent carotid or brachial pulse is significant. Mere variations in pulse amplitude are difficult to detect by digital palpation alone, unless there is aneurysmal dilatation of the vessel, therefore blood pressure recordings should be taken simultaneously in each arm and variations of 10 per cent or more may be regarded as significant of local stenosis at the root of the neck.

Arterial auscultation is most helpful in clinical diagnosis and positive findings are present in the majority of patients. Narrowing or irregularity of an artery causes a turbulent blood flow resulting in a rough bruit which can be heard with a stethoscope. A simple bell type is best for this purpose, but care must be taken to avoid compressing the artery thus producing an auditory artefact; also the typical rough bruit must be differentiated from the venous hum frequently heard at the root of the neck in normal individuals. Particular attention should be paid to the conduction of the bruit, alteration of its character, and the intensity in relation to the estimated depth of the artery. The heart is auscultated first and special attention paid to the aortic area to exclude heart murmurs and calcific aortic disease, which bruits may be conducted to the arch or neck vessels. The patient is now placed with the hands clasped behind the head and the chin extended. The manubrium, root of neck, supra clavicular fossae, axillae and carotid arteries to angle of jaw, are auscultated. A few examples of interpretation are illustrated in Fig. 6.3.

A palpable thrill is occasionally present in superficial vessels. A murmur previously auscultated, which subsequently disappears, often indicates thrombosis of the vessel. With experience, a fairly accurate assessment of the distribution of the athero-sclerotic involvement can be diagnosed with the stethoscope.

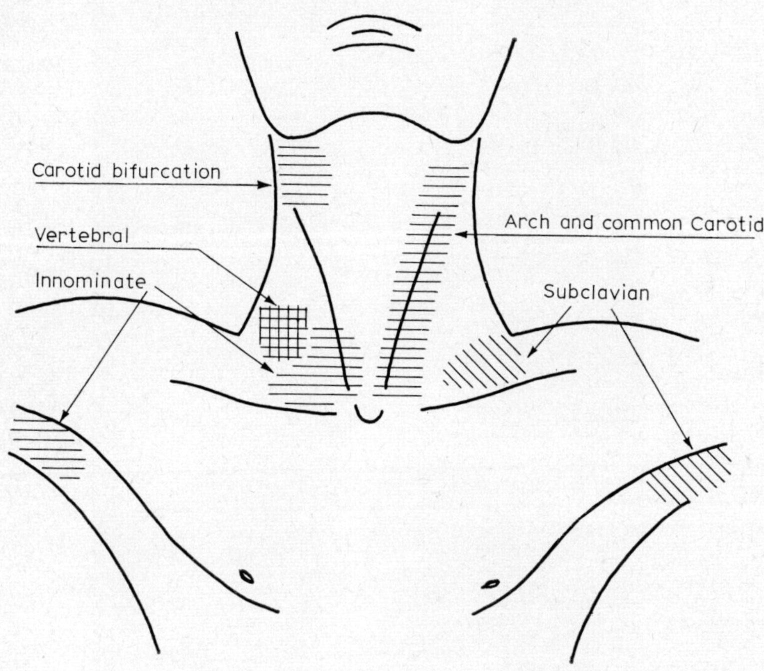

FIG. 6.3

Special Investigations

Angiography. Four vessel angiography is essential for accurate diagnosis of aortic arch syndromes. The arch and its major branches may be opacified by retrograde catheter angiography (Fig. 6.4). Technique and interpretation have been well described and analysed by Sutton and Rhys Davies (1966).

Cerebral angiography (Fig. 6.5) may also be indicated to opacify the intracranial vessels, to exclude cerebral tumour and to visualize the terminal portion of the internal carotid artery. Extension of the disease to the syphon or middle cerebral vessels will carry a less satis-factory prognosis after surgical correction.

E.E.G. The electroencephalogram is valuable for demonstrating and locating focal cerebral lesions such as areas of brain infarction. It is specially helpful in excluding cerebral tumour in patients with suspected vascular disease.

Ophthalmodynamometry. Reduced eye ball tension can frequently be measured in cases of carotid artery stenosis but the significance is

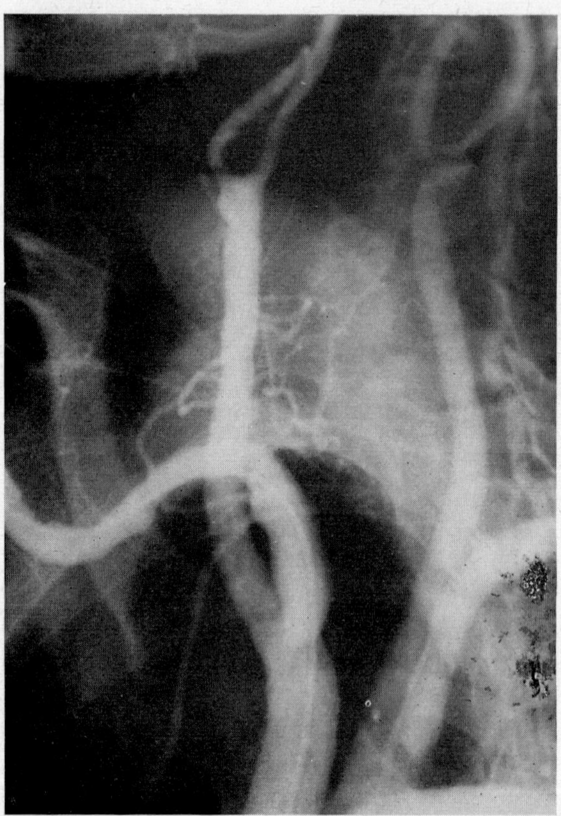

Fig. 6.4. Severe atheroma of both carotids (internal). The right vertebral is occluded and the left tortuous. (Sutton and Rhys Davies, 1966. *Clin. Radiol.* XVIII, 4.)

not always clear. Stenosis is often bilateral to a greater or lesser degree and other methods of investigation, particularly arch angiography, are more valuable.

Cerebral blood flow measurements. Radioactive Krypton and Xenon have been used to measure cerebral blood flow. While offering great promise for the future, these methods are at present insufficiently accurate to demonstrate small focal alterations in blood flow.

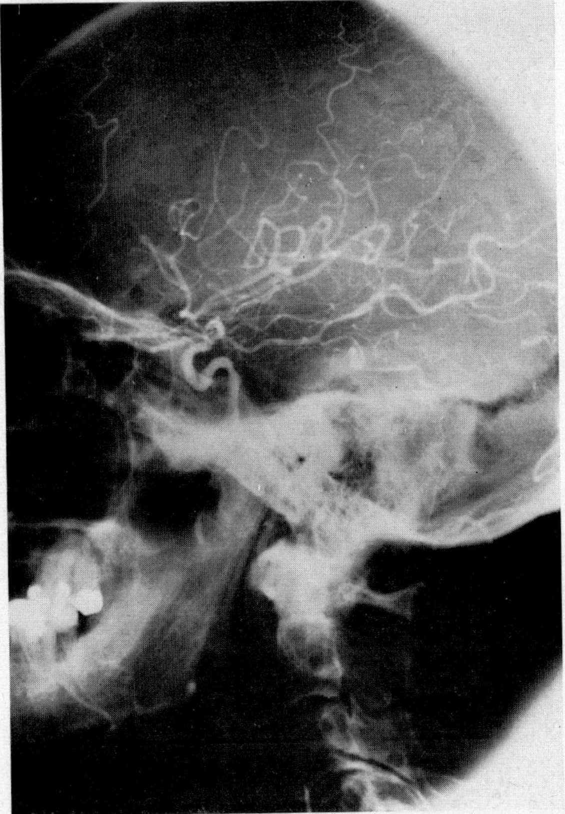

FIG. 6.5. Carotid arteriogram showing atheromatous lesions in syphon.

Treatment

Anti-coagulant Therapy

This has been recommended by some groups notably the Mayo Clinic (Milliken, Seikert and Whisnant, 1958). However, it is well known that patients with an arterial stenosis may develop thrombosis even when on a well controlled anti-coagulant regime. Moreover, for anti-coagulants to be worthwhile, they have to be continued *ad infinitum*. The hypertensive patient, with an area of cerebral softening is particularly at risk from haemorrhage into the infarct and this danger is increased by anti-coagulant therapy. Anti-coagulants therefore, are, reserved for the normotensive patient who is unfit for surgery due to severe cardiac or pulmonary disease.

Reconstructive Surgery

The main indication for surgery is in those patients with a stenosing lesion causing symptoms of impending stroke. Not infrequently the stenosis may proceed to thrombosis without clinical evidence of stroke. In these cases there is no production of micro emboli and consequently the symptoms of intermittent cerebral insufficiency disappear. However, it is not possible to predict in which cases such a "cure" will occur. Operation on the thrombosed side is contraindicated but stenosing lesions elsewhere in the extracranial system should be assessed and treated on their merits to ensure an adequate collateral blood supply.

Carotid artery stenosis. The operation of thromboendarterectomy on the carotid bifurcation, properly performed, offers an excellent prognosis in patients with intermittent stroke without neurological signs; in those with inco-ordination of fine movements of the hands and minor speech and visual field defects, the recovery may not be complete, but improvement may be expected. In both groups, there is a small risk of post-operative hemiparesis, but fortunately this is not severe, and complete recovery usually occurs within three to four weeks.

The carotid bifurcation is exposed through a skin crease incision in the neck; particular care must be taken to avoid injury to the cervical branch of the facial and the hypoglossal nerves. When the vessels are exposed 5,000–7,500 units of Heparin is injected intra-arterially and the common, external, internal and superior thyroid arteries clamped. The plaque is identified and exposed through a vertical arteriotomy. Meticulous care is taken in removing all fragments of atheroma and in closing the arteriotomy with a 5·0 continuous suture. A vein patch is not usually necessary since there is sufficient redundant arterial wall which permits closure without stenosing the internal carotid. After removal of clamps and gentle sponge pressure to ensure haemostasis, the wound is closed in layers with drainage. This procedure takes about 15 min. to complete, and the brain circulation must be protected during this period. Three methods are in common use:

(i) Hypothermia to 30°C by surface cooling.

(ii) Internal shunt by Vinyl or Silastic tube from common to internal carotid during the endarterectomy.

(iii) Operation performed under local anaesthesia, with insertion of shunt if neurological impairment develops.

Since hypothermia is time consuming, and carries a risk of ventricular fibrillation in elderly atherosclerotic patients, it is not recommended. In practise the internal shunt and local anaesthesia have proved equally effective. Several other techniques have been tried but are generally unsatisfactory. Trial compression of the bifurcation should be avoided, since it may detach the thrombus or fragments from a soft arterial plaque. Induced hypertension carries the risk of haemorrhage into an area of cerebral softening after removal of the clamps.

When there is bilateral internal carotid artery stenosis, the operations should be staged. The side causing symptoms is operated upon first and after recovery a prophylactic operation is generally necessary on the opposite side, after an interval of 6–8 weeks. This period appears necessary to permit a potentially diseased cerebral circulation to adjust to the altered haemodynamics following operation.

Internal carotid artery thrombosis causing stroke. Should the patient present soon after onset of a completed stroke, it is often possible to remove both plaque and the thrombus which extends to the syphon, thus restoring carotid blood flow. Several authors have reported good results from this procedure, but in the writer's experience it is seldom the case. Probably the explanation is that nerve cells, deprived of oxygen, die in 4–5 min., and it is impossible to restore the circulation within this time limit. There is also the risk that the increased pressure following the revascularization will produce a fatal haemorrhage into the soft cerebral infarct. The best management would appear to be to treat the stroke conservatively and promote collateral blood supply, by removing any stenosing lesions in the other vessels.

Vertebral artery stenosis. The vertebral artery is approached through a supraclavicular incision extending along the medial two thirds of the clavicle, with division of the clavicular head of the sternomastoid and scalenus anterior muscles. The plaque is accessible through an arteriotomy of the subclavian, immediately distal to the origin of the vertebral. The patient is heparinized, as described previously; a by-pass shunt is not necessary during the reconstruction.

Common carotid, innominate and subclavian arteries. Access to the aortic arch and its major branches is obtained through a median sternotomy. This is done by making a burr hole opposite the 4th costal cartilage. A Gili saw is passed retrosternally and the upper part of the sternum divided and retracted. After mobilization of the thymus and the left innominate vein, good access to the aortic arch and great vessels is obtained. A short stenosis or occlusion of these vessels is best treated with local thromboendarterectomy and a patch graft is necessary to avoid narrowing at the arteriotomy site; a saphenous vein patch is preferable to dacron. For a long stenosis or occlusion, a dacron by-pass graft from the aortic arch to the distal artery involved, is the best procedure. A temporary intra-luminal shunt or external by-pass is necessary to preserve the cerebral circulation during each of these procedures.

Results

The overall mortality rate varies between 2 and 6 per cent; the simpler procedures of carotid and vertebral endarterectomy usually carry less risk than operations on the great vessels.

Surgical correction of internal carotid artery stenosis has a good prognosis with 75–85 per cent of patients either symptom free or improved. A significant number of these have been followed for five years or longer. The result of corrective surgery on the vertebral artery is more difficult to assess, probably because the stenosis is more often associated with other occlusive lesions in the extracranial arteries. Both groups have been critically reviewed by Edwards (1965).

The late results of corrective surgery on the aortic arch, innominate and common carotid arteries are equally difficult to assess. De Bakey, Crawford, Cooley, Morris, Garrett and Fields (1965), and Firt, Kejhel and Michel (1965) have published excellent results in large series of patients.

The main problem is the immediate treatment of the progressing stroke and completed stroke. Crawford, De Bakey and Fields (1961) and De Bakey *et al.* (1965) have had a low operative mortality, with 40–45 per cent of patients becoming symptom free within the follow up period. However, this management is not generally accepted, and several observers believe that surgery in the acute stage may aggravate the stroke. A controlled trial on the treatment of stroke should be interesting and would probably resolve the different views on the best management.

MESENTERIC VASCULAR INSUFFICIENCY

Stenosing or occlusive lesions of the coeliac axis, superior or inferior mesenteric arteries, together or separately, produce a syndrome which has been variously mis-named as "Abdominal Angina, Intermittent mesenteric claudication or mesenteric stroke". In 1868, Cheine reported an autopsy study in which there was complete obliteration of the three main vessels to the viscerae, which, during life, had received a blood supply from extra-peritoneal collaterals. Dunphy (1936) gave an account of the clinical syndrome of mesenteric vascular insufficiency and Mikkelsen (1959) recorded the first case in which stenosis of the superior mesenteric artery was successfully treated by thromboendarterectomy. Morris and De Bakey (1961) have described the clinical presentation in 12 patients, 8 of whom were successfully treated by arterial reconstruction.

Stenosis

Symptoms are caused by an atherosclerotic stenosis affecting one or more of the vessels supplying the viscerae. Morris and De Bakey (1961) have stated that two out of the three main vessels must be involved before symptoms occur. Ageing or elderly male patients are commonly affected and they often have occlusive vascular disease of the limbs or previous episodes of coronary insufficiency. The history is characterized by intermittent attacks of severe abdominal pain usually occurring between meals; the pain may be referred to the xiphisternum and confused with cardiac angina, but is not related to exercise. Later, malabsorption occurs resulting in bulky fatty stools and weight loss. Finally, because of pain, the patient may be afraid to eat and become emaciated, or arterial thrombosis may cause death by mesenteric infarction.

Diagnosis

(1) *An arterial bruit* is usually auscultated over the xiphisternum or epigastrium. This should be differentiated from cardiac murmurs or those produced by a Leriche syndrome.

(2) *Barium meal and follow through* is not often helpful, but may show a delay in the terminal ileum due to inadequate peristalsis. Its main value is in excluding other bowel lesions.

(3) *Stool examination* may show increased faecal fat resulting from malabsorption but this is a late occurrence.

(4) *Lateral aortogram* is the most helpful diagnostic investigation. Since the stenosis is usually situated at the origin of the coeliac axis, or along the first 2 or 3 cms. of the superior mesenteric artery, lateral projections are essential to avoid the aortic shadow concealing the lesion.

Treatment

Laparotomy is indicated in the majority of patients, even though there is reasonable doubt of the diagnosis after clinical investigation.

The superior mesenteric artery is the most commonly affected and while thromboendarterectomy has proved successful, exposure of the origin is difficult and the distal vessel is often friable. An aorto-mesenteric by-pass graft, using autogenous saphenous vein, is the better procedure. Fig. 6.6 is a post-operative arteriogram showing the superior mesenteric artery re-vascularized in this way. This patient, who had suffered many attacks of severe abdominal crises, has been symptom free for four years after this operation. The splenic artery has also been used to re-vascularize the superior mesenteric, but since it may also be involved, or at a risk of being potentially involved, this is not recommended.

The branches of the coeliac axis may be similarly treated with the by-pass principle and autogenous vein is preferred to dacron. The

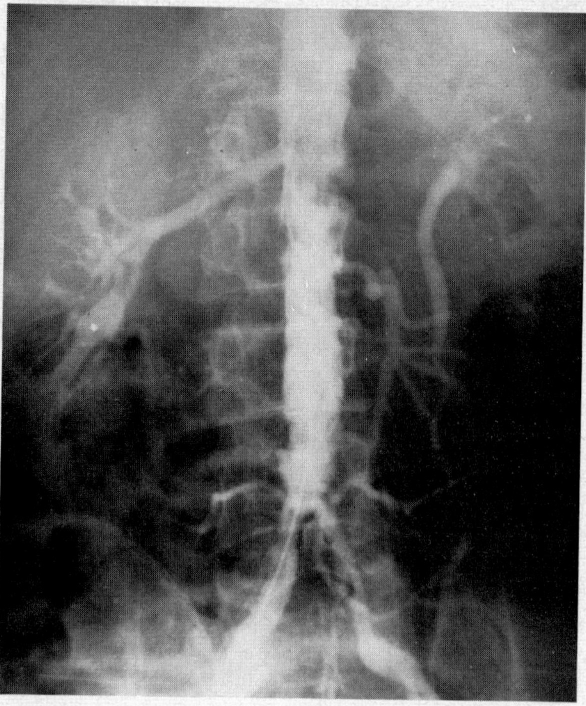

FIG. 6.6. Post-operative arteriogram showing graft from aorta revascularizing superior mesenteric artery.

inferior mesenteric artery is not generally suitable for vascular reconstruction, and ischaemic lesions are best treated by hemicolectomy.

Occlusion

Sudden occlusion of the superior mesenteric artery is caused by embolism or spontaneous thrombosis of a pre-existing atheromatous plaque; occasionally symptoms are secondary to a spontaneous portal vein thrombosis. It presents with agonal abdominal pain, blood in the stools and oligaemic shock. In the early stages the bowel is pale and bloodless, but gangrene rapidly ensues with the typical purple infarcted intestine extending from the duodenal-jejunal flexure to terminal ileum.

For endarterectomy or vascular reconstruction to be successful, early diagnosis and laparotomy are essential. Stewart, Sweetman, Westphal and Wise, (1960), reported two patients recovery after embolectomy but there have been very few subsequent successes. Equally, few patients survive the metabolic debt resulting from the massive resection of infarcted bowel.

References

CHEINE, J. (1868). Address to the British Medical Association.

CHIARI, H. (1905). *Verh. dtsch. path. Ges.*, 326.

CRAWFORD, E. S., DE BAKEY, M. E. and FIELDS, W. S. (1961). "In Cerebral vascular diseases", edited by R. G. Siekert and J. P. Whisnant, p. 178. Grune & Stratton, New York.

DE BAKEY, M. E., CRAWFORD, E. S., COOLEY, D. A., MORRIS, G. C. jr., GARRETT, H. E. and FIELDS, W. S. (1965). *Ann. Surg.*, **161**, 921.

DENNY-BROWN, D. (1951). *Med. Clin. N. Am.*, **35**, 1457.

DUGUID, J. B. and ROBERTSON, W. B. (1957). *Lancet*, **i**, 1205.

DUNPHY, J. E. (1936). *Am. J. Med. Sci.*, **192**, 109.

EASTCOTT, H. H. G., PICKERING, G. W. and ROB, C. G. (1954). *Lancet*, **ii**, 994.

EDWARDS, C. H. (1966). "In Die chirurgische Behandlung der Carotis- und Vertebralisinsuffizienz", edited by C. Kulenkampff and W. Dorndorf., p. 40. Thieme Verlag, Stuttgart.

FIRT, P., HEJHAL, L., HEJNAL, J. and MICHAL, V. (1965). *J. Cardiovasc. Surg.*, **6**, 394.

GUNNING, A. J., PICKERING, G. W., ROBB-SMITH, A. H. T. and ROSS RUSSELL, R. (1964). *Q. J. Med.*, **33**, 155.

HUNT, J. R. (1914). *Am. J. Med. Sci.*, **147**, 704.

KENYON, J. R. and THOMPSON, A. E. (1965). *Br. Med. J.*, **i**, 1460.

MEYER, J. S. (1958). *J. Neurosurg.*, **15**, 653.

MIKKELSEN, W. P. and ZARO, J. A. jr. (1959). *New Engl. J. Med.*, **260**, 912.

MILLIKAN, C. H., SIEKERT, R. G. and WHISNANT, J. P. (1958). *J. Am. Med. Ass.*, **166**, 587.

MONIZ, E., LIMA, A. and DE LACERDA, R. (1937). *Presse Med.*, **45**, 977.

MORRIS, G. C. jr. and DE BAKEY, M. E. (1961). *J. Am. Med. Ass.*, **176**, 89.

ROB, C. and WHEELER, E. B. (1957). *Br. Med. J.*, **ii**, 264.

ROSS RUSSELL, R. W. (1963). *Lancet*, **ii**, 1354.

STEWART, G. D., SWEETMAN, W. R., WESTPHAL, K. and WISE, R. A. (1960). *Ann. Surg.*, **151**, 274.

SUTTON, D. and RHYS DAVIES, E. (1966). *Clin. Radiol.*, **17**, 330.

WINTERNITZ, M. C. (1954). "In Symposium on atherosclerosis", published by the National Academy of Sciences—National Research Council, p. 14. National Academy of Sciences—National Research Council, Washington, Publication 338.

CHAPTER 7

ARTERIOGRAPHY IN THE DIAGNOSIS OF ABDOMINAL DISEASE

LOUIS KREEL

The widespread use of angiography in the diagnosis of abdominal disease is dependent on three separate factors. The first and most important of these is the development of non-toxic contrast media. It has been found that sodium diatrizoate (Hypaque) and sodium iothalamate (Conray) can be used in high concentrations and in large quantities without causing harmful effects. When reactions do occur these are usually immediate, occurring after small amounts as when initial test doses are given. These reactions are probably hypersensitivity phenomena. In their mildest form this is merely nausea and vomiting, but occasionally it may lead to cardiovascular collapse. The mild reactions can usually be controlled with anti-histamines, whereas the more severe reaction requires steroids. These reactions are, however, uncommon.

The second factor that has enabled angiography to become a routine investigation is the development of the percutaneous technique of vascular catheterization first described by Seldinger. All the large peripheral arteries and veins can now be catheterized without resorting to open exposure.

The third major development in vascular roentgenology has been the introduction of the radio-opaque catheter which can be moulded into any shape that may be required. This has produced the situation where almost every branch of the aorta can be selectively catheterized from a distance.

A further development may be mentioned which has proved extremely valuable although not essential. This is the introduction of image intensification and television monitoring. These radiological procedures need no longer be carried out in complete darkness, and a more adequate rapport with the patient can thus be established. In the future, the use of video-tape recordings and a closed circuit television system will enable these examinations to be performed more rapidly and lead to more accurate diagnosis.

4*

Techniques

In any individual case, the ideal method of examination may only become obvious after the diagnosis has already been established or when the procedure has been completed. With the full knowledge of the particular anatomy and pathological state one would be in a position to plan the procedure accordingly. But of course in actual practice, this never happens. This paradoxical state of affairs therefore implies that any given problem must be approached in such a way that the technique can be varied should the indication arise. However, certain general principles may be noted.

Where the pathological lesion has been localized to a definite anatomical organ, a selective arteriographic examination will usually yield the most detailed information. This is particularly true in the examination of the kidneys, liver and spleen, and these organs may have been implicated as the site of disease by a variety of tests—biochemical, radio-isotope studies or radiographic examinations. The major advantage of selective arteriography in these organs is that it shows their vascular pattern in greater detail and unobscured by the arterial patterns of adjacent or overlying organs. Selective examinations are not always possible and a free flush aortogram will then have to be carried out. However, if the pathological lesion is thought to be ischaemic and related to the orifice of the vessel at its origin from the aorta, then a "free flush" aortogram is the essential procedure. Thus in the diagnosis of the aetiology of hypertension or of post-prandial "angina", this is the examination of choice. It is thus essential for the diagnosis of a vascular lesion to show the origin of the vessel. In the case of the renal arteries, a frontal view or a slightly oblique view to superimpose the superior mesenteric artery on the aorta so as not to obscure the origins of the renal arteries, is required. But, to visualize the origins of the coeliac axis, splenic artery or mesenterics, an oblique or lateral view is essential.

The films taken immediately after injection of the contrast medium will demonstrate the arterial pattern, whereas later films show the "blush" phase and markedly delayed films the returning veins. The particular sequence of films to be taken will depend on the lesion suspected, and may vary considerably from case to case. Particular examples will be mentioned, but as a general principle the arterial and arteriolar phase will be shown in the first two seconds, while the origins of the vessels are best delineated in the initial films. The "blush" phase tends to occur at 6–8 sec., and the venous phase is shown about 10–14 sec. after the injection.

Hypersensitivity and toxic effects are uncommon with the newer contrast media such as the diatrizoates and iothalamates. These are usually mild nausea, flushing, and an occasional vomiting. These effects can be rapidly controlled with intravenous anti-histamines such as 10 mg. of Piriton. More severe reactions are very uncommon, but may take the form of circulatory collapse or angio-neurotic oedema. For these patients 50–100 mg. of intravenous hydrocortizone will be required, and the procedure should be immediately discontinued. Furthermore, strict precautions as to the future use of radiographic contrast media must be taken. A further precaution recommended to limit the adverse effects of contrast media is injection of 200–300 ml. of 5 per cent glucose or normal saline at the end of the procedure, and a film of the renal areas and bladder to be sure that the contrast medium is being excreted.

The lesions that can be demonstrated by vascular roentgenology are extremely varied but may be grouped into those pertaining to the arterial system, to the venous system, to space-occupying lesions and to the effect of trauma. The arterial lesions include partial or complete obstruction, aneurysm formation, arteriovenous fistulae and angiomatous malformations. The effects of these lesions will depend not only on the artery affected and the degree of involvement, but also on the rapidity of its onset, and will vary from the completely innocuous as in a slowly progressive stenosis of the splenic artery to a fulminating gangrene in the sudden complete occlusion of the superior mesenteric. The demonstration of the portal and mesenteric veins is an essential pre-requisite in the assessment of cases for shunt operations in portal hypertension.

Space-occupying lesions can be either benign or malignant. Although it is not always possible to distinguish between the benign and malignant lesions radiologically, in most cases this is possible and in many the signs are unequivocal. The typical "malignant circulation" is one in which there is a marked increase in the size and number of vessels, the arteries show increased tortuosity and lose their tendency to taper. Arteriovenous shunting is often present, and small blobs or pools of contrast medium become visible in the tumour area. There is also a more intense "staining" or a diffuse retention of contrast medium in the tumour. As opposed to these signs, there are those of a benign cyst where vascular displacement and a "bare" area or clear region of non-visualization within the organ blush are the only indications of a space-occupying lesion. The typical malignant circulation may occur in any organ but is particularly demonstrable in the hypernephroma and in the solitary hepatoma. The benign cyst most frequently occurs in the kidney, but the hydatid cyst of the liver produces similar appearances. However, in the pancreas the signs of a malignant tumour are much more subtle and require a meticuluos arteriographic technique. Truncated vessels, a faint tumour blush and minimal marginal vascular irregularity may be the only signs visible. These radiological features will be considered more fully in each section.

Traumatic lesions of abdominal organs can be demonstrated arteriographically. This is particularly valuable in the kidney where a very accurate pre-operative assessment of the lesion can be made which will often determine the management of the case. It has also been used in traumatic lesions of the liver and spleen, and recently it has been shown that selective arteriography can be used to demonstrate the source of gastro-intestinal haemorrhage.

Vascular Roentgenology of the Liver

Space-occupying lesions of the liver may affect the hepatic arterial system, the portal venous system or the hepatic venous system. Benign lesions produce vascular displacement which can be shown by examining either the arterial or venous systems, but malignant lesions often produce quite different effects on each of these systems. In malignant liver lesions, particularly with hepatomas, there is often occlusion of the portal venous system. Spleno-portography will then show only a "bare" area which on arteriography may be seen as a highly vascular lesion having the pattern of a malignant circulation. (Fig. 7.1(*a*) and (*b*).) Such malignant lesions can also on occasion be shown by hepatic venography. The choice of the initial vascular examination frequently depends on whether or not there is associated splenomegaly. Where the spleen is enlarged and the prothrombin time is normal, spleno-portography is a safe procedure. In the presence of a small spleen, coeliac axis arteriography is not only safer but will usually show both the arterial pattern of the liver and the portal venous system. (Fig. 7.2(*a*) and (*b*).)

Bare areas with distortion of the vascular pattern due only to vascular displacement occurs in hydatid cysts, amoebic abscess and with secondary deposits in the liver. Frequently the correct diagnosis has already been established and the object of the arteriographic examination is to indicate the size and number of lesions and their relationship to the hepatic vasculature, prior to operation. In this respect, coeliac axis arteriography is particularly valuable in hydatid disease. (Fig. 7.2.) On occasion, however, the problem is one of diagnosis in a case with fever and liver enlargement. A definite malignant circulation within a mass (Fig. 7.1(*b*)) will then distinguish between an amoebic abscess and a malignant lesion.

Various radiographic patterns may occur in malignant hepatic lesions. The hepatomas tend to be more vascular and frequently give

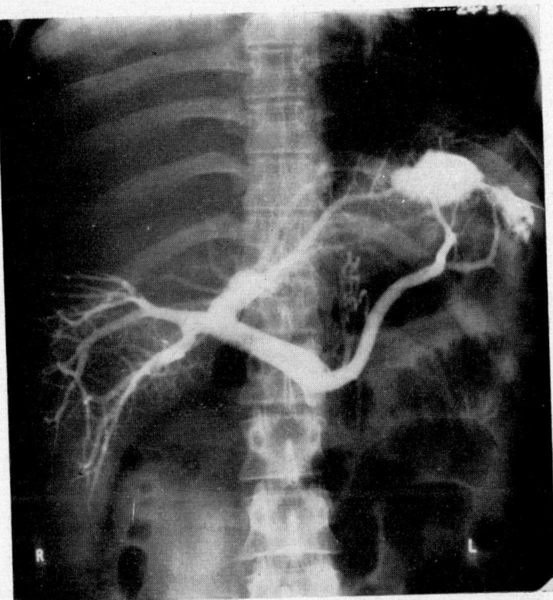

FIG. 7.1(*a*). Spleno-portography demonstrates a large "bare" area of the liver in the upper part of the right lobe with some displacement of the remaining portal veins.

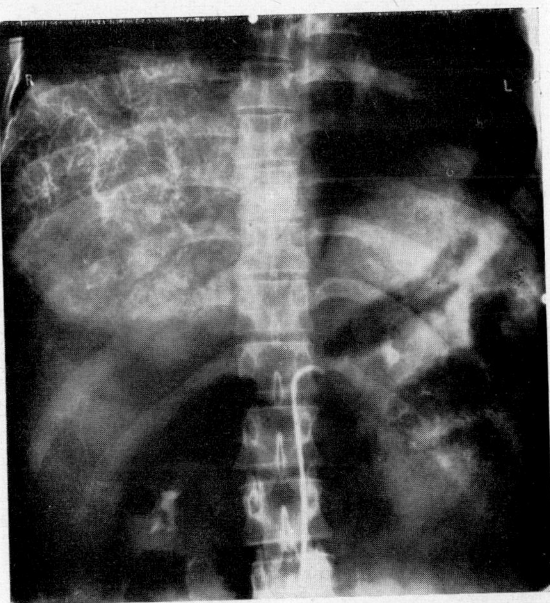

FIG. 7.1(*b*). Late arterial phase of a selective coeliac axis arteriogram in the same patient. The upper part of the right lobe of the liver is shown to have a malignant circulation with "tissue staining" indicating that the lesion is a hepatoma. It also shows the extent of the lesion.

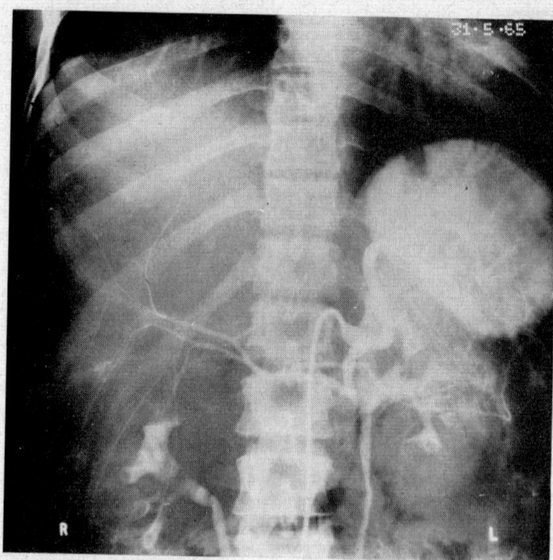

FIG. 7.2(*a*). Arterial phase of a coeliac axis arteriogram. The hepatic arteries are stretched, narrowed and displaced by two large hydatid cysts, one above and the other below the main hepatic artery.

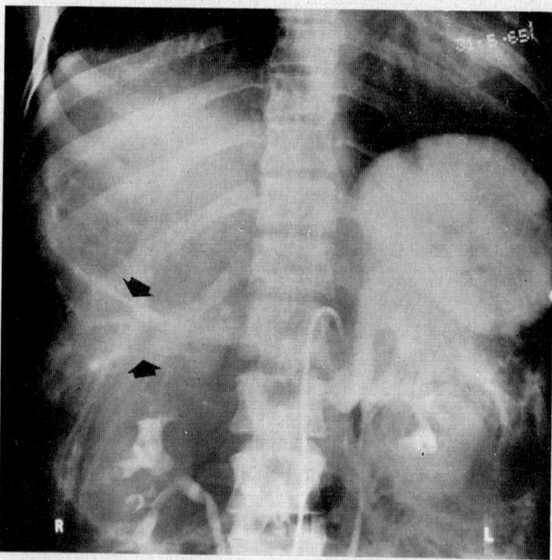

FIG. 7.2(*b*). The venous phase showing the splenic and portal veins. The portal veins show displacement similar to that of the arteries indicating the site of the cysts. There is also a slight marginal blush of contrast medium as indicated by the arrows.

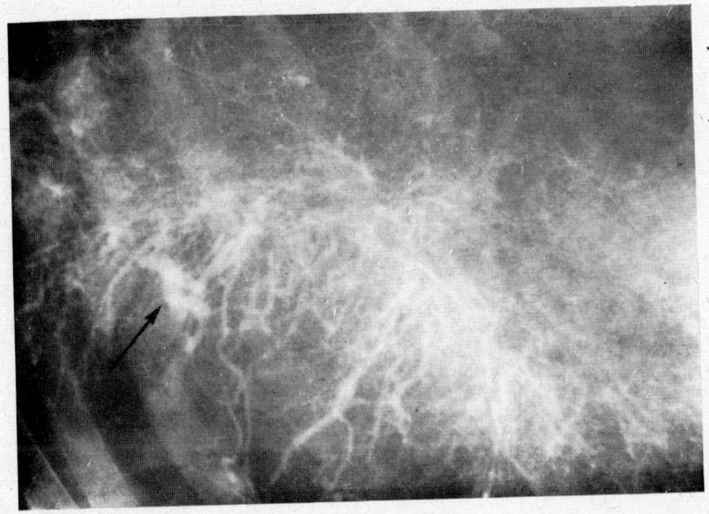

Fig. 7.3(*b*). Late arterial phase showing a large pool of contrast at an arteriovenous shunt (shown by arrow).

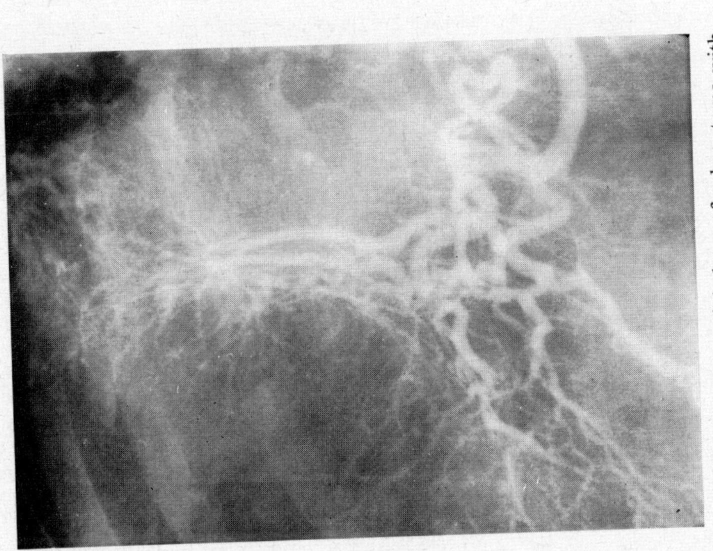

Fig. 7.3(*a*). Early arterial phase of a hepatoma with vascular displacement and marked increase in the number of vessels, many of which are irregular and tortuous.

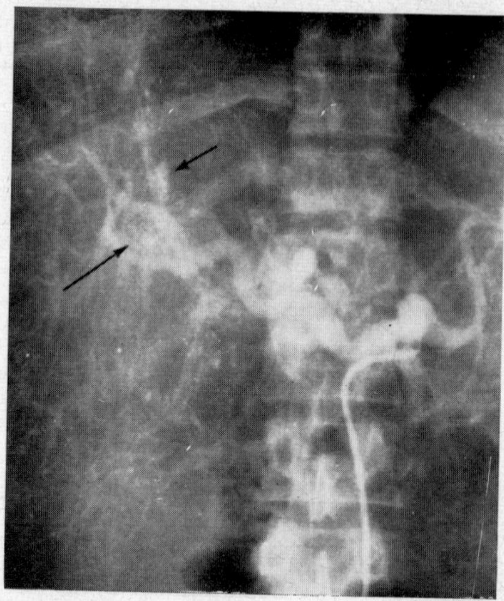

FIG. 7.4(*a*). Arterial phase of a selective coeliac axis arteriogram. The arrows point to localized areas of tumour circulation in the region of the hilum of the liver.

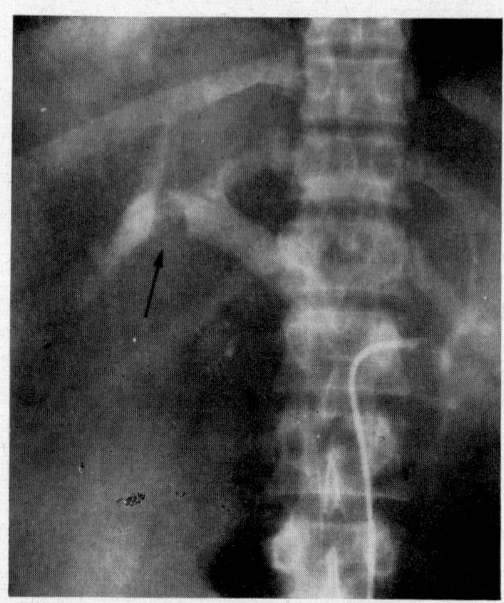

FIG. 7.4(*b*). Slightly later film which demonstrated filling of the portal vein from the liver indicating an arteriovenous shunt. There is a filling defect in the portal vein as indicated by the arrow, caused by tumour tissue.

appearances which make a definite diagnosis possible. At the one extreme there is the single, highly vascular mass with numerous tortuous and irregular arteries, contrast blobs, arteriovenous shunts and a late irregular tissue blush (Fig. 7.3). The exact delineation of this type of tumour is usually required as a pre-operative investigation with a view to partial hepatectomy. On the oblique views the relationship to the spine and posterior abdominal wall can be established and the vascular anatomy can be shown in relationship to the tumour. This is particularly important if the major arterial supply to the liver arises from the superior mesenteric, or if there are two separate hepatic arteries.

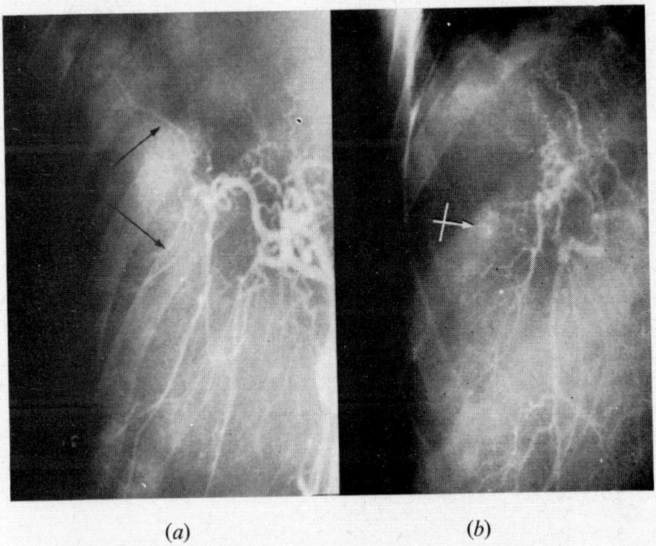

(a)   (b)

FIG. 7.5(a). Vascular displacement (shown by arrows) indicating the site of a space-occupying lesion.

FIG. 7.5(b). Central area of this lesion shows small irregular tortuous arterial pattern as occurs in a hepatoma.

When chemotherapy is being considered this information is of the utmost importance. Cytotoxic agents are most effective if their effects are limited to the tumour. To achieve this the arterial supply to the mitotic lesion must be delineated and any anatomical variations particularly noted. Selective catheters may be left in position for up to two weeks and the chemotherapeutic agents given in this way. Another definite sign of a primary hepatoma is an arteriovenous shunt to the portal vein with a filling defect within the portal vein. (Fig. 7.4 (a) and (b).)

Primary malignant lesions of the liver, on the other hand, may also be relatively avascular or they may be multiple. The multiple primary lesions are usually associated with cirrhosis. Multiple or single filling defects in cirrhosis may, showever, also be due to regenerating nodules, but the presence of an abnormal arterial pattern in the central part of the lesion favours the diagnosis of a hepatoma (Fig. 7.5) as does a residual contrast blush in the area of abnormal vascularity (Fig. 7.6). Primary cholangiomas are avascular tumours and on arteriography are shown only as a space-occupying lesion with vascular displacement.

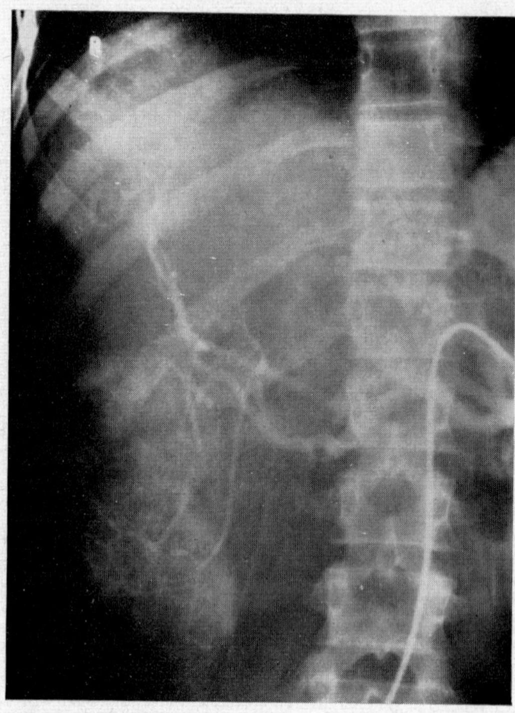

Fig. 7.6. Multiple areas of "tissue staining" due to contrast medium producing a "blush" effect. This indicates the presence of a malignant lesion which in this case was a hepatoblastoma.

In one case this was associated with infiltration of the arterial walls causing localised areas of narrowing—'stenotic' lesions. In liver cirrhosis a pattern of arterial 'reduplication' of the smaller vessels may occur. This can be associated with malignancy, but probably only indicates an associated block of the portal veins, which is common in hepatomas. Tumour infiltration of the major portal venous channels, producing actual filling defects, has been demonstrated by spleno-portography, and will also be demonstrated by hepatic arteriography in the presence of an arterio-venous shunt to the portal vein (Fig. 7.4(b)). Another sign which has been noted in cirrhosis which could lead to an incorrect diagnosis is the presence of an isolated arterio-venous shunt. An isolated arterio-venous shunt can occur in a cirrhotic liver without malignant transformation.

Metastatic deposits in the liver can be shown as areas of vascular displacement (Fig. 7.7), which may be associated with an increased

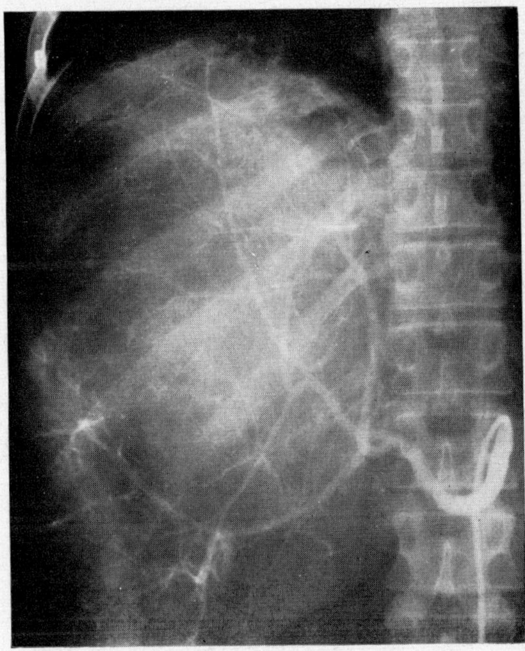

FIG. 7.7. Selective hepatic arteriogram. Marked displacement of the intrahepatic branches of the hepatic artery by a large metastatic deposit from a carcinoma of the colon.

number of irregular and distorted arteries (Fig. 7.8) or as large irregular patterns of low and high density contrast staining on the late films. Only the margin may be of increased density producing a thick rim of increased density (Fig. 7.9). The central part of a secondary deposit or a hepatoma may be so avascular as to produce necrosis, rupture and haemorrhage. This will then be seen as an area of diminished density at the centre with peripheral arterial displacement (Fig. 7.10).

Coeliac axis arteriography can also be used in the pre-operative assessment for portal hypertension. Where splenic puncture is contra-indicated, as in the presence of a prolonged prothrombin time, where previous splenectomy has been performed and where there is an extra hepatic portal vein block, arterio-portography is at present the method of choice in the demonstration of the portal venous systems. The opacification of the splenic and portal veins is not as marked as that obtained with spleno-portography, but is usually adequate for diagnostic purposes.

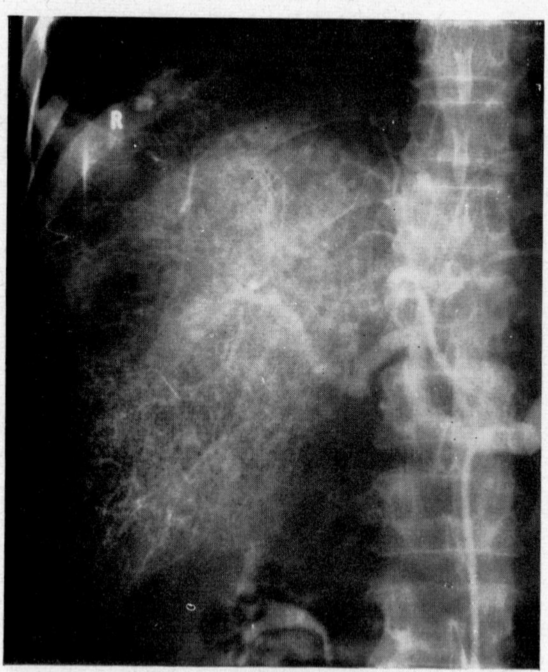

Fig. 7.8. Coeliac axis arteriography. Marked increase in the number of small hepatic arteries, many of which are irregular in direction and calibre. There are also many bare areas with peripheral vascular bowing. The appearances are due to multiple metastatic deposits in the liver.

Where the spleen is enlarged, at least 50 ml. of "Conray" 420 or equivalent iodine containing contrast medium must be used. Where a portal vein block is present or after splenectomy, the superior mesenteric artery must be injected to obtain the required arterio-portography.

The presence of a normal and patent portal vein can be shown, (Fig. 7.11) or it may be patent but narrowed (Fig. 7.12). On the other hand, the size and position of the superior mesenteric veins can be shown and whether or not these would be adequate for the establishment of a successful shunt (Fig. 7.13).

Hepatic venography is not often used in the diagnosis of liver disease, but lesions such as tumours, cysts and post-necrotic regeneration

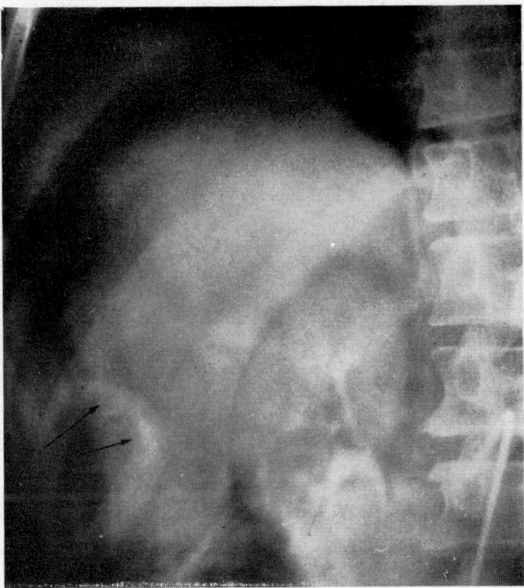

Fig. 7.9. Late phase of a hepatic arteriogram. A thick rim of increased density indicates the site of a secondary deposit, the centre of which is completely avascular.

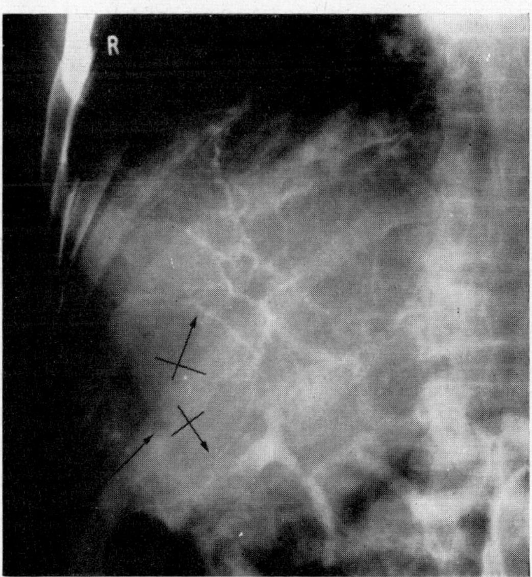

Fig. 7.10. A hepatoma secondary to liver cirrhosis causing displacement of arteries (shown by crossed arrows) outlining the margin of the lesion. The centre of the lesion is translucent (arrowed) due to necrosis and haemorrhage of the tumour. This case presented with a sudden intra-peritoneal haemorrhage.

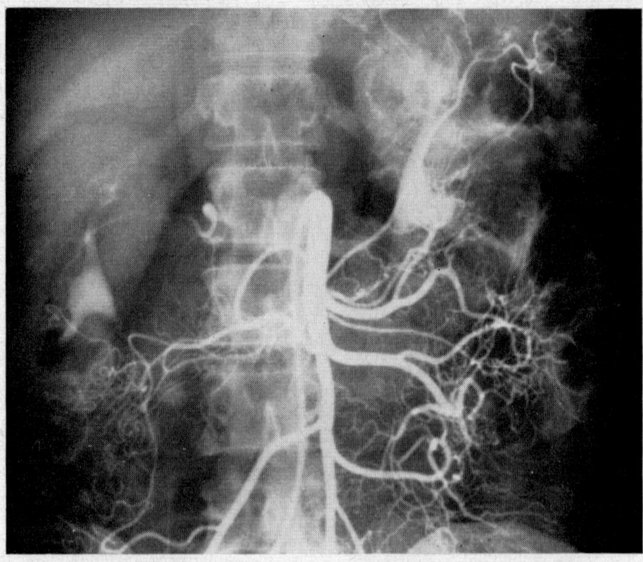

FIG. 7.11(*a*). Arterial phase of superior mesenteric arterio-portography in a patient who had had a splenectomy.

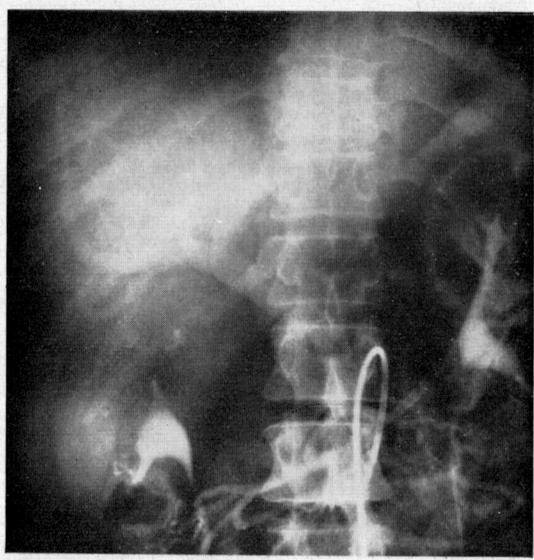

FIG. 7.11(*b*). Venous phase 10 seconds later showing a patent portal vein of normal calibre. The portal system is never as densely shown by this method as on spleno-portography, but obviously after splenectomy the latter examination cannot be performed.

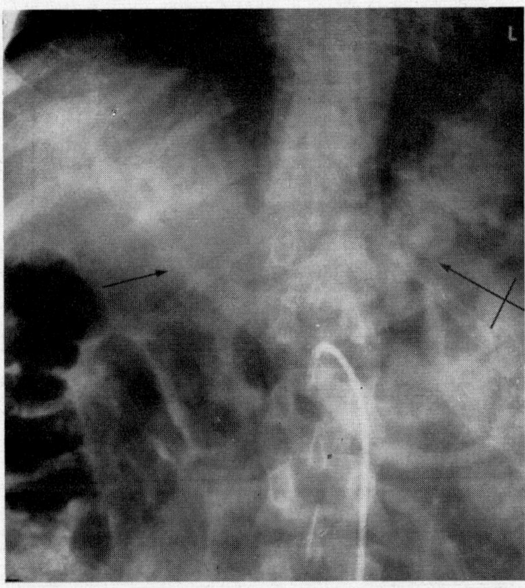

Fig. 7.12. Venous phase of arterio-portography. The portal vein is patent but of diminished calibre (arrowed) as usually occurs in periphlebitis. This usually precludes the use of such a vein for a portacaval anastomosis. Large paravertebral collateral vessels are seen on the left side.

nodules have been demonstrated by this means. Recently specific radiographic signs have been described in hepatic vein occlusion (Budd-Chiari syndrome). An actual stricture of the hepatic vein may be visualized and collateral venous channels can be seen producing a spider network pattern (Fig. 7.14).

The Splenic Artery and Spleen

The splenic artery is frequently involved in "degenerative" disease—calcification, atheromatous plaques, strictures and aneurysm formation (Fig. 7.15). These lesions rarely cause symptoms. This is particularly true of splenic artery aneurysms which can be found in approximately 10 per cent of elderly females. These splenic artery aneurysms will only be found at post mortem if the artery is carefully dissected. They often have extremely thin walls but are protected from rupture by the peri-pancreatic and splenic hilar fibrous tissue. These aneurysms frequently calcify but seldom rupture, thus behaving quite differently from the cerebral aneurysms. However, the uncommonly occurring rupture of a splenic artery aneurysm is particularly associated with the third trimester of pregnancy.

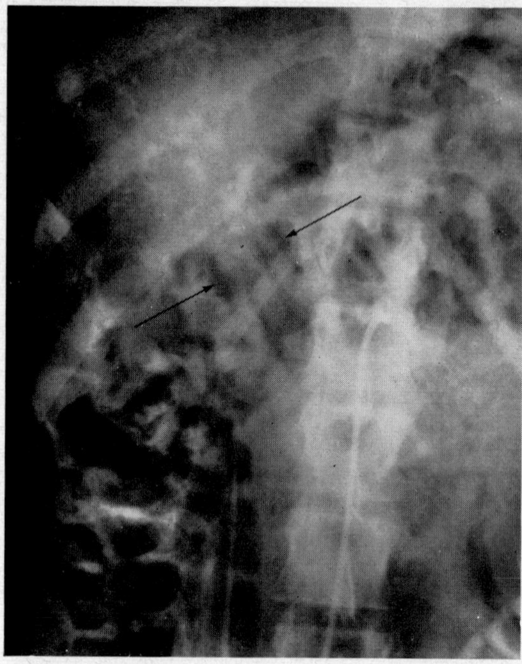

FIG. 7.13. Venous phase of mesenteric arterio-portography showing "cavernous transformation" of a portal vein following portal vein occlusion in childhood. Three mesenteric veins lie alongside each other to the right of the spine (arrowed). The largest of these measured 0·9 cm. and was used to perform a mesenterio-caval shunt to relieve the portal hypertension.

Radiographically these aneurysms can be diagnosed by virtue of their propensity to calcification. They may be seen as ring shadows or as multiple overlapping ovoid and ring shadows—'egg-shell calcifications' in the left upper quadrant. They can also be demonstrated by splenic arteriography, and there is a report of such a case being diagnosed in the stage of partial rupture. However, unless the aneurysms are causing symptoms, there would appear to be no need to undertake special investigations or to resort to surgical intervention.

Another interesting feature concerning splenic artery aneurysms is their very common occurrence in portal hypertension where there is marked splenomegaly. In this context they are most commonly found inside the spleen as bifurcation aneurysms. These intrasplenic bifurcation aneurysms associated with marked splenomegaly in portal hypertension can only be shown by selective arteriography or in specimens by an injection technique.

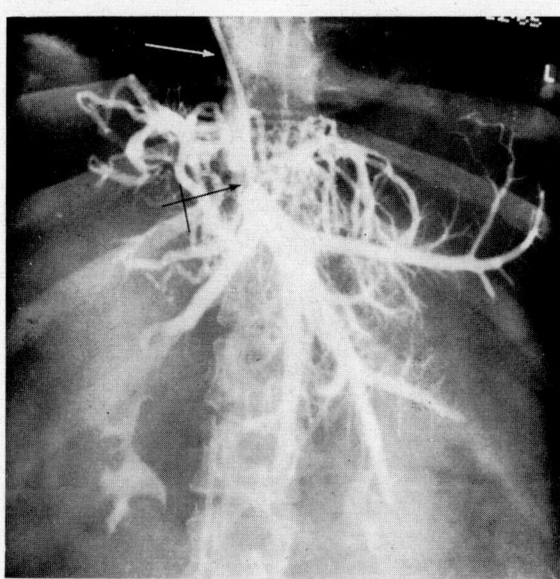

FIG. 7.14. Budd-Chiari Syndrome. The hepatic vein has been catheterized from
the right arm via the superior vena cava. The catheter (arrowed) has traversed
a stenosis of the left hepatic vein (shown by crossed arrow) and filled the
hepatic veins beyond. A coarse network of collateral veins can be seen on
either side of the hepatic vein block.

The arteriovenous aneurysm is a rare but surgically curable cause of
portal hypertension. This lesion should be suspected if there is a
prominent left upper quadrant bruit in the presence of marked splenomegaly. Arteriovenous aneurysms are well demonstrated by selective
arteriography, as are other rare causes of 'surgical' splenomegaly
including splenic cyst, haematoma and rare tumours such as lympho-
sarcoma of the spleen. Although the indications for arteriography in
diseases of the spleen do not often arise, there is no doubt that this is
an effective method in the delineation of the conditions just mentioned.
It is also of particular value in delineating post-traumatic lesions such as
partial rupture of the spleen and peri-capsular haematomas (Fig. 7.16).

Mesenteric Arteriography

Vascular lesions of the bowel may manifest themselves as an 'acute
abdomen' or as a chronic condition. In the former category one may
include those cases presenting as perforation, obstruction, ileus or
haemorrhagic 'colitis', while the chronic states include cases of malabsorption, post-prandial pain—'abdominal angina'—ascites and
chronic obstructive lesions. Vascular pathology will therefore frequently

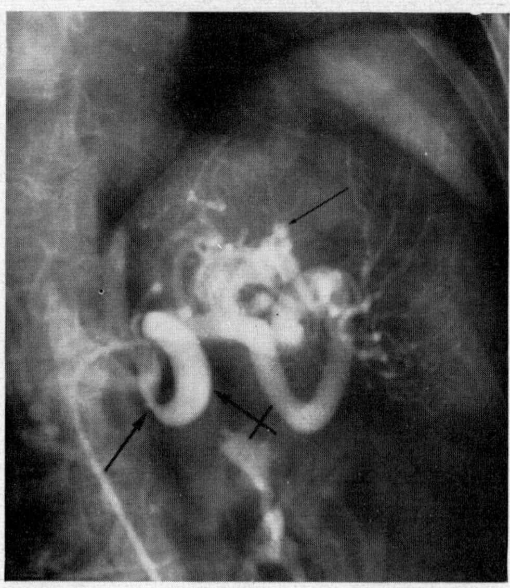

FIG. 7.15. Oblique view of the splenic artery in a patient who was being investigated for ? pancreatic tumour. The proximal part of the artery is markedly narrowed (shown by thick arrow) and beyond this there is a fusiform "aneurysm" (crossed arrow)—a post-stenotic dilatation. At the hilum of the spleen there is a small berry aneurysm (thin arrow). These arterial lesions are not uncommon in the splenic artery and are usually asymptomatic.

be considered in the differential diagnosis of abdominal disease, however low on the list it may come. The lesion most frequently diagnosed by arteriography of the mesenteric vessels is partial or complete occlusion at the orifice.

However, it is important to bear in mind the large range of pathological states covered by the designation of vascular lesions. Ischaemic or vascular insufficiency may be caused by general circulatory collapse, thrombosis, embolism, arteritis, mechanical factors and trauma. The iatrogenic causes require a special mention as these are liable to occur more frequently in the immediate future. Surgeons may find these cases after cardiac and aortic operations. These occlusive lesions give the characteristic pathological appearance of cholesterol emboli. Physicians prescribing enteric coated potassium chloride tablets will sooner or later find cases with bowel strictures. The mechanism is said to be that of venous spasm causing tissue ischaemia and later fibrosis. Radiotherapists should also be aware of this type of lesion, as in their cases bowel obstruction may be due to benign post-radiation strictures and not a recurrence of malignancy. Again these lesions have an ischae-

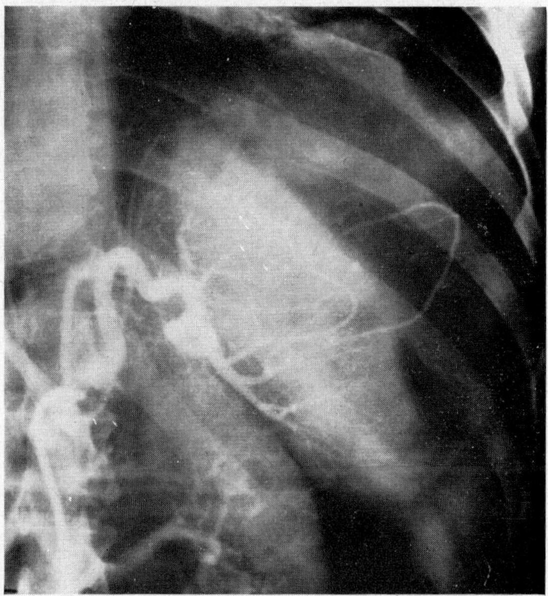

FIG. 7.16. Arterial phase of coeliac axis arteriogram. There is a large gap between the splenic vessels and the dome of the diaphragm. The splenic "blush", indicating the position of the spleen, shows that it is displaced downwards and medially by a large pericapsular splenic haemorrhage.

mic basis. Diagnostic radiologists are also far from blameless in this respect as their procedures, especially translumbar aortography, may also lead to small bowel vascular lesions.

There are three main groups of conditions for which mesenteric arteriography could be used, namely portal hypertension, tumours and vascular lesions. The role of arterio-portography in portal hypertension has been mentioned previously. As far as tumours of the small bowel are concerned, just occasionally these may be demonstrated as a localized tumour blush. These lesions are extremely rare, whereas colonic tumours are common. In the descending and sigmoid colon the barium enema will, for the immediate future, remain the diagnostic method of choice. However, tumours of the caecum are often difficult to diagnose either by barium enema or by follow through examination. Selective superior mesenteric arteriography, by demonstrating the ileo-colic artery, can demonstrate these lesions, and where doubt exists after conventional radiographic examinations arteriography may well give the answer. It is, however, in vascular lesions of the small bowel that superior mesenteric arteriography has its major role. It is said that

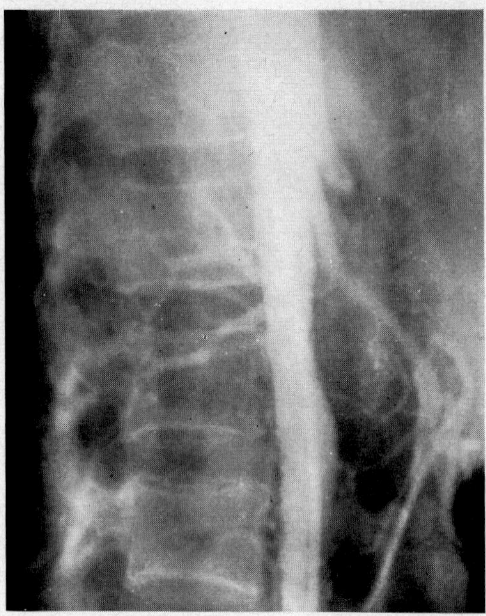

FIG. 7.17(*a*). Occlusion of the splenic artery shown on a lateral view of a "free flush" aortogram. The inferior mesenteric artery also cannot be seen.

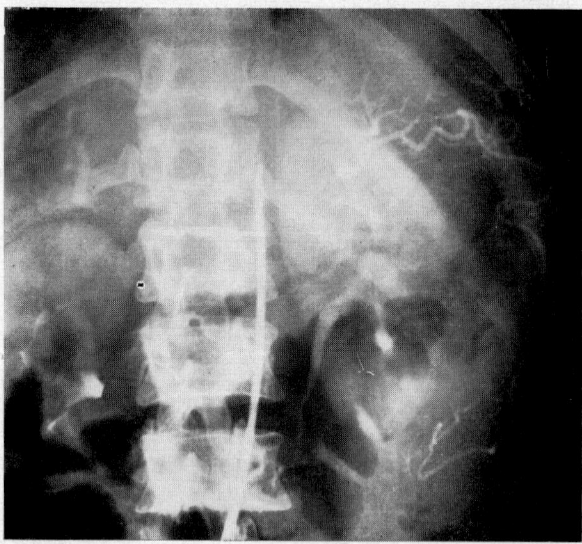

FIG. 7.17(*b*). Late arterial phase on the frontal view showing the collateral arterial supply producing retrograde filling of the splenic artery distal to the occlusion.

at least two of the main alimentary tract arteries must be compromised before symptoms occur. Indeed most of these lesions are detected in patients being examined for other conditions. Pathologists have reported similar findings, namely the frequent cocurrence of symptomless vascular occlusion of the alimentary system. The onset of symptoms depends not only on the degree of the obstructive lesions but on the rapidity of its onset, and thus on the ability of the collateral blood supply to take over.

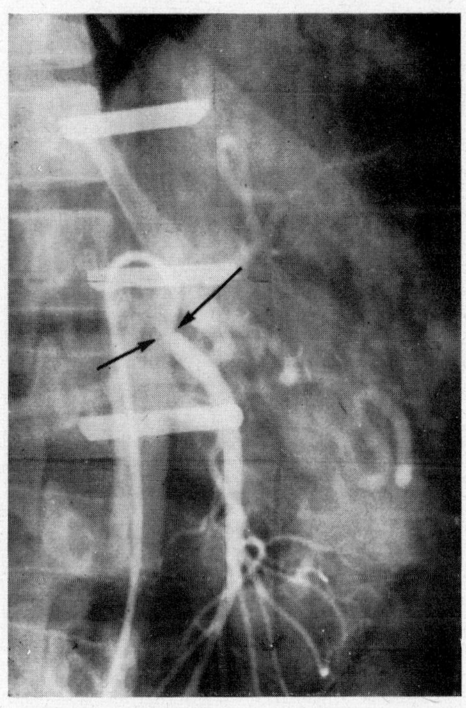

FIG. 7.18. Test injection into the aorta taken in the oblique position (supine with the right shoulder raised to 45°). Stenosis of the superior mesenteric artery in an elderly female who suffered from attacks of post-prandial angina.

As mentioned earlier, to adequately demonstrate lesions of the orifices of the superior mesenteric, coeliac axis and inferior mesenteric arteries, lateral or oblique views with a free flush aortogram are necessary. A selective examination may in fact hide such a lesion, as the end of the catheter may go through the narrowed orifice and not show the proximal part of the artery. The late films in the series will show the adequacy of the collateral supply and the route that it takes. (Figs. 7.17, 7.18 and 7.19.)

These vascular lesions may affect not only the origins of the vessels, but also the larger branches, and may be multiple. Furthermore, atheromatous or degenerative arterial disease may occur in combination—stenosis with post-stenotic dilatation or stenosis with actual aneurysm formation (Fig. 7.15).

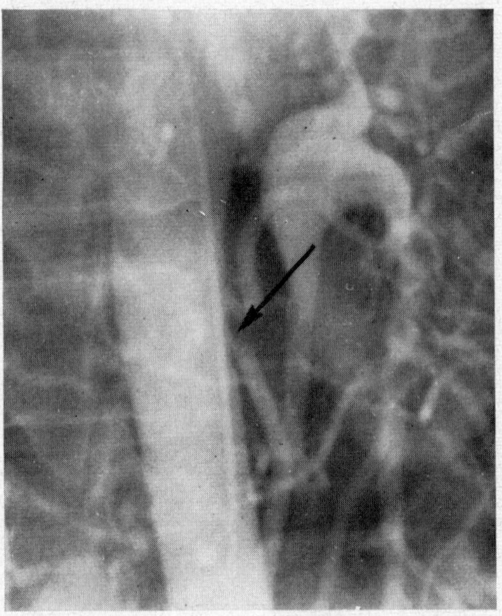

FIG. 7.19. Asymptomatic stenotic lesion at the orifice of the inferior mesenteric artery as shown on a "free-flush" aortogram, taken in the oblique position.

Arteriography in the Diagnosis of the Site of Gastro-Intestinal Haemorrhage

In the vast majority of cases of haematemasis or melaena the cause is peptic ulceration or gastric erosions, and most of these cases can be managed conservatively. The site and nature of the lesions producing the haemorrhage can usually be diagnosed by conventional investigations including the barium swallow and meal, oesophagoscopy, gastroscopy and modifications of the string test. However, where haemorrhage continues, in the absence of a definite diagnosis this can now be obtained by selective arteriography. It has been shown that in active gastro-intestinal haemorrhage, where the appropriate vessel is catheterized—the coeliac axis for the stomach and duodenum, the superior mesenteric for the small bowel and caecum—contrast medium will seep into the cavity of the organ and will be visible on the late films in the series provided the bleeding is not less than 0·5 ml. per minute. The seepage of contrast medium produces an irregular opacity which localizes the site of the haemorrhage. In some cases the nature of the lesions will also become manifest, a round disc-like opacity indicating an ulcer crater, a localized collection of large vessels indicating an angiomatous malformation, or a "malignant" circulation in the case of a vascular carcinoma.

Selective arteriography can thus be recommended for the diagnosis of difficult cases of gastro-intestinal haemorrhage as it is likely to prove of considerable help in locating the site of haemorrhage. It is particularly valuable in the patient in whom a prolonged exploratory laparotomy is considered undesirable. By the means of pre-operative localization of the source of the gastro-intestinal haemorrhage, the operative time can be greatly reduced.

The Pancreas

The arterial supply to the pancreas is derived from the coeliac axis and its branches and from the superior mesenteric artery. The gastro-

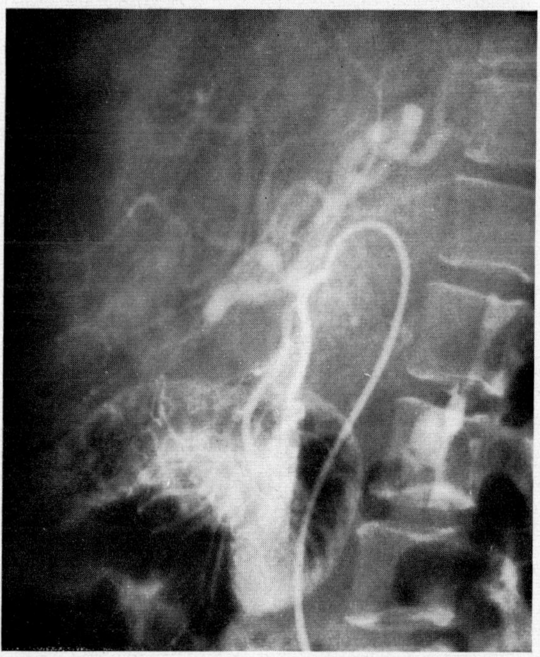

Fig. 7.20. The tip of the selective coeliac axis catheter lies in the gastro-duodenal artery and there has been overfilling of this vessel. This has produced an intense blush of the duodenum which obscures the adjacent pancreas and the small vessels in this area.

duodenal artery, which is a major branch of the hepatic artery, gives off the anterior and posterior duodenal arcades which often rejoin to form the inferior pancreatico-duodenal artery. This inferior pancreatico-duodenal artery arises from the superior mesenteric. The anterior and posterior duodenal arcades give off branches to the head of the pancreas while the body and tail tend to be supplied from the splenic artery. It is also to be noted that the splenic and portal veins lie in close juxta-position to the pancreas.

To achieve adequate visualization of the pancreas, both the coeliac axis and superior mesenteric arteries may have to be catheterized. This has been achieved by the Swedish workers by simultaneous coeliac axis and superior mesenteric injection of contrast. However, it has also been shown that if 'superselective' catheterization is performed, namely selective catheterization of the gastro-duodenal or inferior pancreatic artery, small amounts of contrast medium (10 ml. of

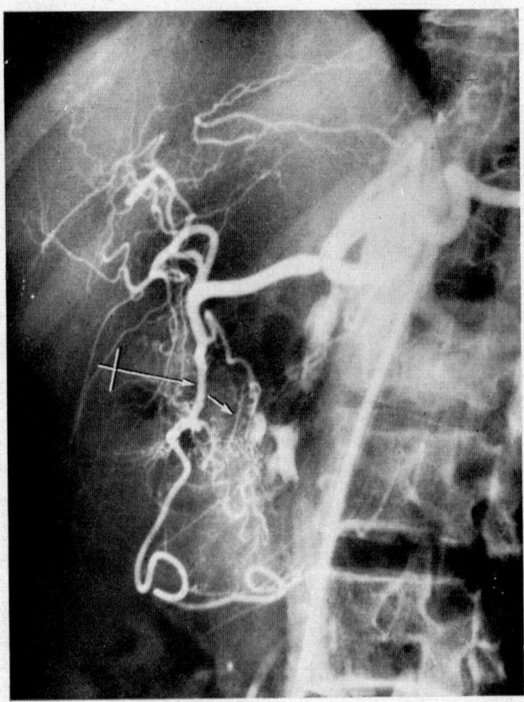

FIG. 7.21. Coeliac axis arteriography in a case subsequently proved to have carcinoma of the pancreas. There is a straightened vessel with marked irregularity of its walls (shown by arrow) and near this there is another vessel with a sharp cut-off. There is also early irregularity of the margins of the gastro-duodenal artery (crossed arrow). There are numerous small irregular vessels in the head of the pancreas.

Hypaque) will demonstrate the whole arterial supply of the pancreas. Frequently, however, there is over-filling of the gastro-duodenal arteries with an intense blush of the wall of the stomach and duodenum. This may obscure a pancreatic lesion (Fig. 7.20).

Malignant tumours of the pancreas only rarely give the typical arteriographic signs of increase in the number and size of vessels, contrast pooling and arteriovenous shunting. These are usually vascular adenocarcinomas of the pancreas. However, in most malignant tumours of the pancreas the signs are much more subtle, although equally valid. Arterial deformity with narrowing of the vessels, irregular margins and sharp truncation of arteries occurs (Fig. 7.21). There may also be vascular displacement and a late contrast blush.

Hypoglycaemia can be due to many causes and to a variety of tumours in various organs. However, the insulinoma is important in connection with arteriography of the pancreas. This may be demonstrated as either a localized area of hypervascularity or as a late nodular blush in the region of the pancreas.

Arteriography in Renal Disease

Initially abdominal arteriography was used particularly for the elucidation of the causes of hypertension and in renal disease. The appreciation that there were cases of malignant hypertension that could be cured by direct surgical correction of renal vascular lesions led to the widespread use of this examination. It was also found to be of particular value in space-occupying lesions of the kidney.

To adequately visualize the renal arteries it is important to demonstrate their orifices, in profile and free of overlying vessels. This can only be achieved on a free flush aortogram with a catheter technique, and the use of a pressure injector is preferred (P.E. 240 catheter, 30 ml. "Conray" 420, in a 50 ml. syringe at 30 lbs./sq. in.). The orifices of the major vessels are best shown on the early films. The superior mesenteric artery may overlie a renal artery, but this effect can easily be overcome by 5–10° rotation of the patient to superimpose the superior mesenteric artery on the aorta. Vascular lesions of the renal arteries may be caused by atheromatous plaques, fibromuscular hyperplasia, sharp kinks with associated extrinsic bands and even by a pheochromocytoma compressing a renal artery. However, the presence of arterial narrowing is not necessarily the cause of the hypertension, nor will the hypertension necessarily be cured by its correction. The pre-operative assessment of the pressure gradient across the stenotic lesion has been recommended; this would require selective catheterization of the renal artery.

Fibromuscular hyperplasia occurs particularly at the renal arteries and produces an appearance of irregular narrowing like a string of sausages with undulating margins (Fig. 7.22). The sharply angulated renal artery may be associated with an extrinsic band which on release can restore the blood flow to normal. Ischaemic renal lesions are usually, however, caused by occlusive disease of the main renal arteries or their branches, or by occlusion of intra-renal vessels. Occlusion of intra-renal vessels tends to produce localized defects in the renal outline at the site of renal infarction. This is best seen on the late films during

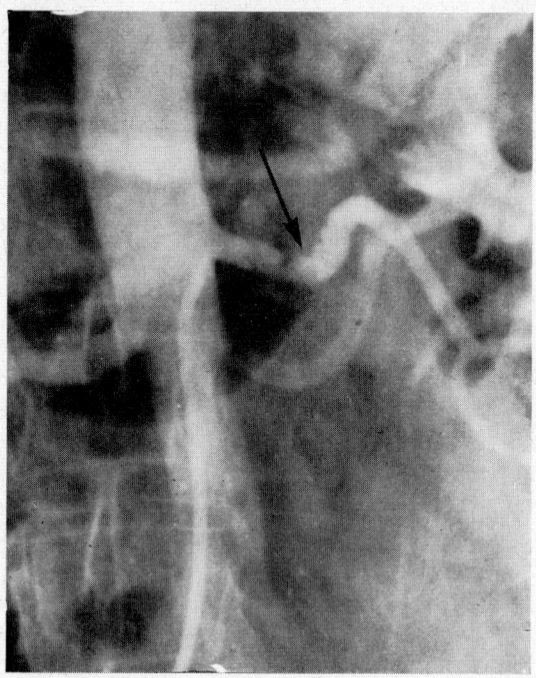

Fig. 7.22. There are two separate renal arteries on the left side. The upper artery shows irregular sausage-like narrowings indicative of fibro-muscular hyperplasia.

the nephrographic or blush phase of the arteriograph. However, larger areas of renal shrinkage are caused by occlusion of the large renal artery branches. Complete occlusion of the renal artery produces a "non-functioning" kidney on the intravenous pyelogram, with a normal pelvi-calycine system as shown on the retrograde pyelogram. This kidney is smaller than normal. Besides the demonstration of the actual arterial occlusion by arteriography, the late films frequently show the collateral circulation along the ureter which forms in these circumstances. The renal artery distal to the occlusion may be

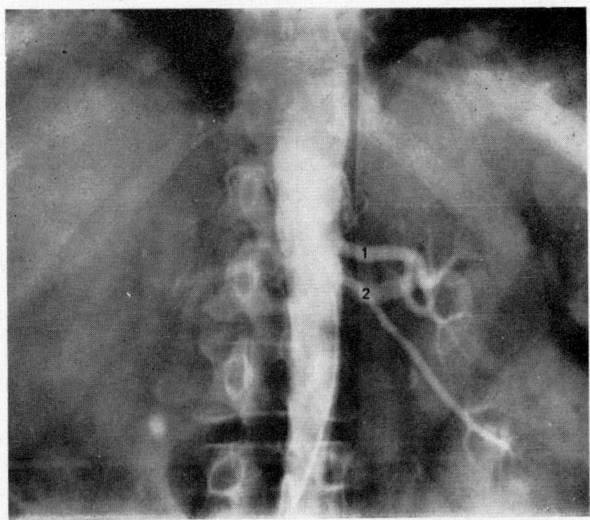

FIG. 7.23(*a*). Very early arterial phase of free-flush aortogram in a patient with marked hypertension. There are two left renal arteries, labelled 1 and 2, the lower artery (2) is superimposed on the tortuous splenic artery. No right renal artery is visible, indicating a complete occlusion.

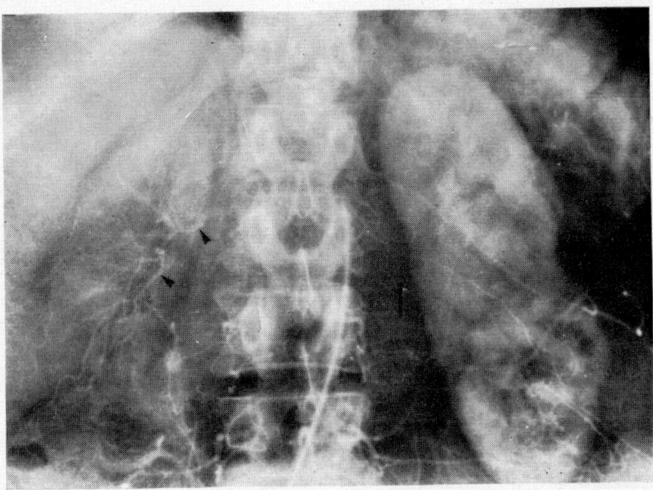

FIG. 7.23(*b*). Late film demonstrating the nephrogram phase on the left side with a defect due to an infarct. The right kidney is markedly diminished in size and there is late filling via collaterals to the renal artery on this side.

demonstrated as well as the intra-renal vascular pattern (Fig. 7.23). The hypertrophied ureteric artery which acts as the collateral channel may produce an undulating pattern on the contour of the renal pelvis.

"Space-occupying" lesions of the kidney are a frequently recurring problem. The distinction between a benign cyst and a hypernephroma is frequently not possible on clinical or pyelographic grounds. Arterio-

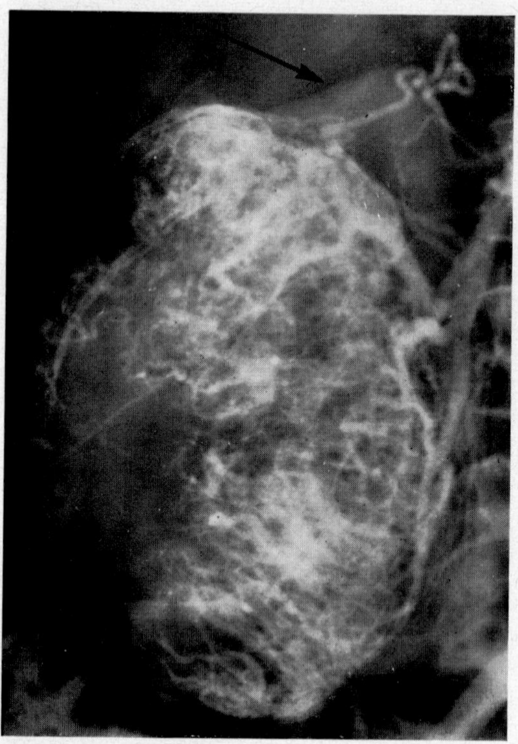

FIG. 7.24. Gross malignant circulation in a hypernephroma. The vessels are irregular, tortuous, and produce large irregular areas of tissue staining. A small area of normal kidney tissue can be seen representing the remains of the upper pole of the kidney (arrowed).

graphy often produces definite evidence of a malignant circulation where the lesion is a hypernephroma (Fig. 7.24). But if an avascular lesion (Fig. 7.25) is shown, the lesion cannot be assumed to be a benign cyst. Occasionally a small tumour can arise on a cyst wall or the "space-occupying" lesion is found to be a necrotic avascular neoplasm. It is thus recommended that immediately after a "cyst-like" lesion has been demonstrated, a percutaneous puncture of the lesion should be undertaken, the "cyst" aspirated, the fluid subsequently examined and

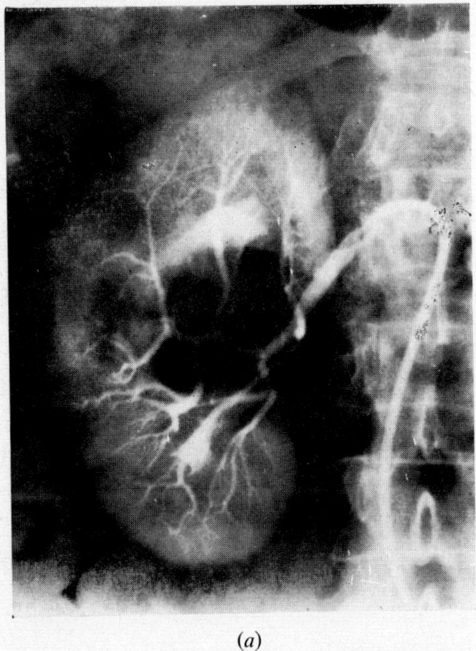

(a)

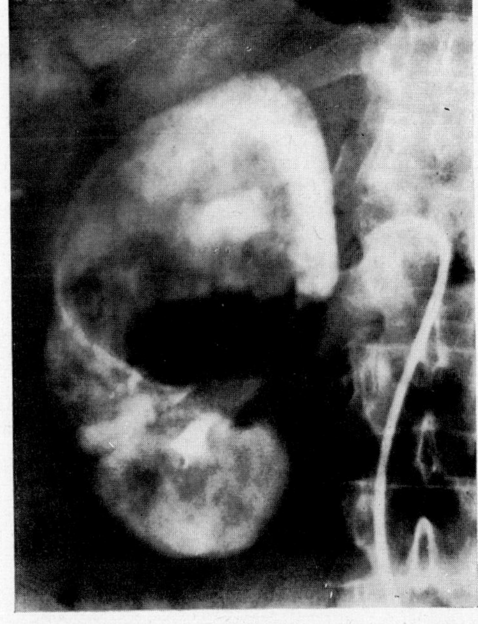

(b)

Figs. 7.25(a) and (b). Space-occupying lesion of the kidney producing vascular displacement in the arterial phase (a) and a bare area in the blush or nephrographic phase (b). Such lesions are usually benign cysts but can be avascular masses or an abscess.

also contrast medium injected into the cyst. Films of the contrast filled "cyst" are then taken and the outlines of the lesion particularly scrutinized. Irregular margins of the "cyst" wall will indicate the presence of a tumour.

Supra-Renal Glands

The supra-renal glands may undergo hyperplasia or be the site of adenomas or carcinoma. These lesions usually manifest themselves as a result of the effects of excessive secretion of various hormones as in Cushing's disease, Conn's syndrome or pheochromocytomas. The presence of these lesions is usually diagnosed by clinical and biochemical means. Following the definitive bio-chemical diagnosis, localization of the lesion as a pre-operative procedure is required. In some cases, such as the adenomas of Conn's syndrome or in Cushing's disease, this is most clearly shown by peri-renal air insufflation, but in others, especially in pheochromocytomas, these tumours are best shown on arteriography. Recently, selective retrograde venous catheterization has been shown to be a useful method of locating supra-renal lesions.

Where arteriography is being undertaken to exclude a pheochromocytoma, certain definite precautions against an overwhelming attack of hypertension must be taken. The pre-arteriographic blood pressure must be established and frequent readings after the contrast injection must be taken. An intravenous 5 per cent glucose drip must be established and an adrenolytic agent such as Rogitine must be available for urgent injection into the glucose drip should a hypertensive attack occur.

The presence of a pheochromocytoma is shown by increased vascularity of the supra-renal, localized enlargement of the organ and a late tumour blush. Rarely pheochromocytomas lie outside the suprarenal and may even be the cause of renal artery narrowing by pressure when it is situated in the hilum of the kidney.

Retroperitoneal Lesions

Abdominal masses requiring elucidation as to their site and nature can on occasion be diagnosed by angiography. Where such a tumour arises within the liver, spleen or kidney, it can usually be accurately located and its nature surmized as previously mentioned. In retroperitoneal lesions this is often more difficult. Selective catheterization cannot be performed and thus the tumour region is often obscured by the overlying mesenteric vessels. This is particularly so in avascular lesions, but just occasionally the extent of a retroperitoneal tumour can be shown as in a retroperitoneal sarcoma. Occasionally, too, an unsuspected vascular metastatic deposit may be demonstrated particularly in the iliac bone. However, retroperitoneal tumours are most frequently located either by simple clinical examination or by intravenous pyelography or lymphangiography.

Arteriography in Chorion Epithelioma

This is a highly vascular tumour and the extent of the lesion is well shown on a free-flush arteriogram of the pelvis with the catheter tip just above the bifurcation of the aorta.

Positive Scintillography

By combining selective arteriography with the injection of ^{131}I-macro-aggregated albumen, it is possible in many cases of malignant disease to show the site and extent of the tumour. Injection of this isotope into the supplying artery demonstrates the neoplastic lesion, one to six days later, as a positive or "hot" area on scintillation scanning. This will almost certainly become a widely accepted technique in the near future.

Summary and Conclusions

Abdominal arteriography is now a well-established, safe procedure which is available to most clinicians. Many pathological lesions can be demonstrated, but it is particularly of value in space-occupying lesions both to establish the diagnosis and for defining their size, number and position. Vascular lesions as such can be shown with great clarity and where operative intervention is contemplated for their correction, this examination is an essential pre-requisite. Traumatic lesions such as lacerations of internal organs or pericapsular haemorrhage can be demonstrated and the resultant findings will determine the management. Although the exact pathological diagnosis can often not be made, it can aid both in locating the lesion to a specific organ, and in defining its blood supply. However, in many abdominal organs it is the only pre-operative method available for the demonstration of disease and does on occasion pin-point pathology which would otherwise escape one's attention at even the most careful exploratory laparotomy.

References

BAUM, S., ROY, R., FINKELSTEIN, A. K. and BLAKEMORE, W. S. (1965). Clinical applications of selective coeliac and superior mesenteric arteriography. *Radiology*, **84**, 279.

BIERMAN, H. R., MILLER, E. R., BYRON, R. L. JR., DOD, K. S., KELLY, K. H. and BLACK, D. H. (1951). Intra-arterial catheterization of viscera in man. *Am. J. Roentgenol. & Rad. Therapy*, **66**, 555.

BOIJSEN, E., JUDKINS, M. P. and SIMAY, A. (1966). Angiographic diagnosis of hepatic rupture. *Radiology*, **86**, 66.

EVANS, J. A. (1965). Techniques in the detection and diagnosis of malignant lesions of the liver, spleen and pancreas. *Radiol. Clin. N. America*, **3**, 567.

KANEKO, M., SASAKI, T. and KIDO, C. (1968). Positive scintigraphy of tumour by means of intra-arterial injection of radio-iodinated macroaggregated albumin (M.A.A.). *Am. J. Roentgenol.*, **102**, 81.

KISADA, K., KIBAKI, T. and OHBA, S. (1966). Positive delineation of human tumours with ^{131}I human serum albumin. *J. Nuclear Med.*, **7**, 41.

KREEL, L., JONES, E. A. and TAVILL, A. (1968). A comparative study of arteriography and scintillation scanning in space-occupying lesions of the liver. *B.J.R.*, **41**, 401.

KREEL, L. and WILLIAMS, R. (1964). Arteriovenography of the portal system. *B.M.J.*, **2**, 1500.

LUNDERQUIST, A. (1965). Angiography in carcinoma of the pancreas. *Suppl. Acta Radiol.*, 235 (Stockholm).

MICHELS, N. A. (1955). "Blood Supply and Anatomy of the Upper Abdominal Organs." J. B. Lippincott Co. Philadelphia 1955.

ÖDMAN, P. (1958). Percutaneous selective angiography of coeliac artery. *Acta Radiol. Suppl.*, 159.

RÖSCH, J. (1966). Tumours of the spleen: the value of selective arteriography. *Clin. radiol.*, **17**, 183.

RÖSCH, J. (1967). "Roentgenology of the Spleen and Pancreas." Charles C. Thomas, Illinois, U.S.A.

SAMMONS, B. P., NEAL, M. P., ARMSTRONG, R. H. JR. and HAGER, H. G. (1967). Ten years experience with celiac and upper abdominal superior mesenteric arteriography. *Am. J. Roentgenol.*, **101**, 345.

SELDINGER, S. I. (1953). Catheter replacement of needle in percutaneous arteriography: new technique. *Acta radiol.*, **39**, 368.

WILLIAMS, R., KREEL, L. and BLENDIS, L. M. (1967). Coeliac axiscatheterization: uses and value in portal hypertension. Colson papers: Liver diseases. Ed. A. E. Read. Blackwell, Oxford.

Chapter 8

PORTAL HYPERTENSION

A. H. Hunt

Sustained increase of pressure within the portal venous system is the result of an obstruction to the free flow of blood through the portal vein or in its passage through the liver. These conditions are referred to as the extra-hepatic (or pre-hepatic) and the intra-hepatic types of portal obstruction respectively. Whipple, Blakemore and Lord (1945) drew attention to the possibilities of clinical cure by surgical means of patients suffering from both types, though removal of the cause or pathological cure is rarely possible. They demonstrated the successful clinical application of the Eck fistula, by constructing anastomoses between portal and systemic venous systems. Interference with the return of blood from the liver to the heart (as in idiopathic thrombosis of the hepatic veins or Chiari's disease, constrictive pericarditis, etc.) causes the pressure to build up within the liver and this is reflected in the portal venous pressure. This condition is referred to as post-hepatic obstruction. It is but rarely the concern of the surgeon.

The majority of patients have certain definite symptoms conforming to the syndrome which carries the name of Banti—haemorrhage from gastro-oesophageal varicosities associated with an enlarged and over-active spleen, as shown by persistent anaemia (apart from haemorrhages), leukopenia and thrombocytopenia. To this may be added the symptoms of advanced liver disease, which may develop to the exclusion of part or all of the typical syndrome, depending on the severity of the cirrhosis. For example, a patient with a rapidly advancing cirrhosis may have a raised portal venous pressure but may not develop oesophageal varices or an enlarged spleen. By contrast, the purest examples of Banti's syndrome occur in patients who have livers which are normal in fact or function; that is, those with extra-hepatic or mild static intra-hepatic obstruction. It is on this account that certain writers exclude from their definition of the symptom-complex patients with ascites or icterus or other evidence of gross hepatic derangement. From time to time cases occur in which not only is the liver cirrhotic, but also the portal vein itself becomes obliterated by clot. Yet again, only a tributary of the portal vein may be permanently obliterated, whether or not the liver is cirrhotic.

5*

In considering portal hypertension, therefore, it is necessary to group the patients according to the causes and effects of the portal obstruction and to assess the results of treatment in relation to each group; bearing in mind that each patient is an individual problem within his particular group.

The normal portal venous pressure varies between 50 and 150 mm. of 3·8 per cent sodium citrate solution when taken from an accessible radicle of the portal vein. It is dependent to some extent on the systemic arterial pressure and the pressure within the inferior vena cava. It can

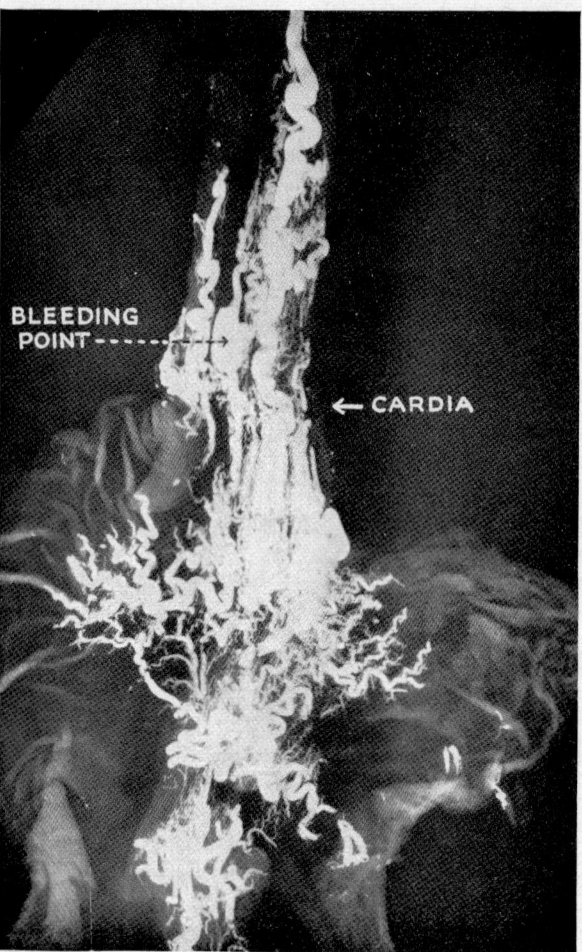

Fig. 8.1. Stomach and oesophagus showing veins injected with bismuth suspension (postmortem) showing continuous nature of oesophageal varices (*Royal Coll. Surg. Museum.*)

be estimated by means of a manometer to give a direct reading, or by rapid electrical recording of the pressure itself (Gray, 1951), by needling of the spleen (Leger, 1966) or by opening up the umbilical vein and catheterization of the portal vein itself (Bayly, 1964; Lavoie *et al.*, 1966). The pressure of the outflow of hepatic venous blood, the "wedged hepatic venous pressure", is a reflection of the portal venous pressure. In portal hypertension, the pressure varies from just above normal to 600 mm. of citrate (Hunt, 1952a).

The most significant and vulnerable of the *anastomotic channels*, which connect the portal with the systemic venous systems (Figs. 8.1 8.2 and 8.3.) develop at the lower end of the oesophagus and the cardiac end of the stomach (Butler, 1951). Their extent may bear little relation to the height of the portal pressure. Large varices which have bled profusely have been encountered with a pressure of no more than 180 mm., whereas in other cases, with portal pressures extending up to 400 mm., no oesophageal varices have been found.

It is often possible at operation to demonstrate a rapid fall in pressure along collateral anastomotic channels, however large these may be or wherever they are situated. Such a circumstance may be encountered in the region of the umbilicus. The size of a caput medusae, which is even more inconstant in development than oesophageal varices, may be no indication of the size of the other communicating channels. Thus large veins at one site often develop to the exclusion of others. However, all surgical approaches to deal with portal hypertension should be placed so as to conserve as many collaterals as possible with the exception of those around the cardiac end of the stomach, so that the natural compensatory channels, such as they are, are preserved.

Causes of Portal Hypertension

Extra-hepatic obstruction (pre-hepatic) occurs in 12·5 per cent of cases of portal hypertension. They may be classified as follows:

(*a*) Congenital obliteration (Thompson, 1940) (Fig. 8.2).

(*b*) Thrombosis following neonatal umbilical sepsis (Shaldon *et al.*, 1962).

(*c*) Thrombosis following intraperitoneal infective conditions, e.g. portal pylephlebitis following appendix abscess, suppurative cholangitis etc. with or without intra-hepatic abscess formation.

(*d*) Thrombosis associated with blood dyscrasias, e.g. polycythaemia rubra vera, myeloid leukaemia, thalassaemia minor.

(*e*) Thrombosis consequent on trauma.

(*f*) Compression or invasion of the portal or splenic vein, with or

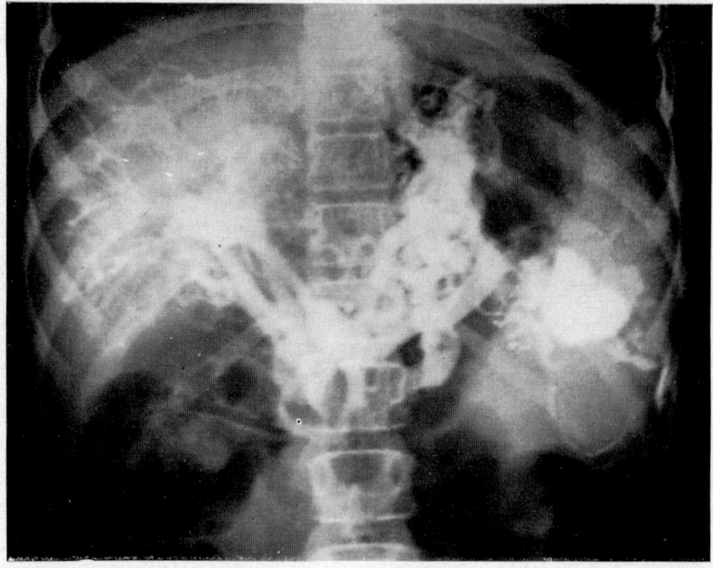

Fig. 8.2. A portal "cavernoma" demonstrated by splenic venography.

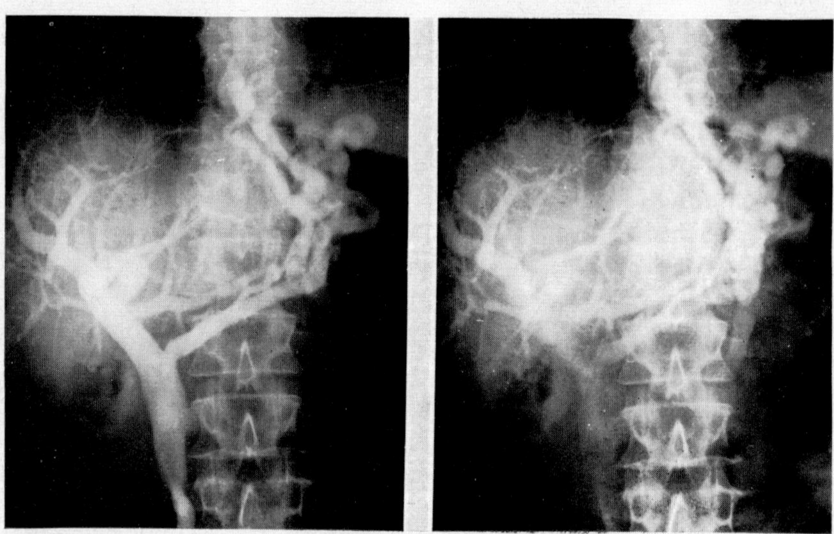

Fig. 8.3. A double portal venogram in cirrhosis hepatis, to show a relatively normal portal vein, the left gastric leading to the gastro-oesophageal varicosities.　　　　　　　　　　　　(The splenic vein shows in neither picture.)

without thrombosis, by malignant tumours (cancer of the stomach, pancreas, hypernephroma, retroperitoneal growths), cysts of the pancreas, aneurysm of splenic artery etc.

Traumatic thrombosis and compression or invasion may lead to segmental portal hypertension affecting only the splenic bed and contiguous drainage areas. Portal hypertension without obstruction may rarely be encountered in association with a splenic arteriovenous aneurysm.

Intra-hepatic obstruction (Fig. 8.3). Cirrhosis of the liver, in its broadest sense, accounts for 87 per cent of cases of portal hypertension. In Britain cryptogenic cirrhosis, in which there is no pre-existing condition to account for the cirrhosis, is the commonest type (42 per cent). In other parts of the world alcoholism or malnutrition may be the commonest. Infective hepatitis precedes the cirrhosis in 17·3 per cent of cases. Toxipathic cirrhosis, primary and secondary biliary cirrhosis, Wilson's disease, haemochromatosis, cardiac cirrhosis, syphilis, amyloidosis, chronic lupoid hepatitis, even schistosomiasis in immigrants, are all encountered from time to time. In some, as with alcoholism, it may be possible to remove the cause, but in most the damage to the liver is already done by the time the patient is referred to the surgeon. Often the aetiological factor of significance is a matter of guess-work, as with the patient who had congenital syphilis, had been overtreated with mercury and arsenic, contracted viral hepatitis, became an alcoholic, contracted schistosomiasis and was then found to be suffering from haemochromatosis. He died of haemorrhage from varices of the oesophagus, with ascites and jaundice. There was a large primary hepatic carcinoma within his cirrhotic liver.

All in all, the cirrhotic patient must be accepted as he comes and the physician and the surgeon concerned with his case must make the best of the situation as they find it.

Thrombosis of the portal vein has been encountered in about 10 per cent of the cases of cirrhosis, particularly following splenectomy when the platelet count is high (Hunt, 1958). The comparatively common complication of mesenteric thrombosis is another aspect of this problem which must always be borne in mind when intestinal obstruction (usually sub-acute or insidious in its onset) develops in the presence of portal hypertension. Abdominal distension following operations for portal hypertension is also commonly encountered and it cannot yet be said to what extent this is due to interference with intestinal conductivity brought about by partial venous occlusion. The problem is complex and emphasizes the need for most careful and complete investigation and supervision at all stages of treatment of these patients.

The extent of portal hypertension appears to bear little relationship to the extent of the liver disease or of the ascites (Hunt, 1952a). The prognosis following major operative procedures to relieve portal hypertension depends on the extent of the liver damage irrespective of the cause of the cirrhosis. However, in comparable patients, the outlook appears to be better for those in whom the cause of the cirrhosis is removable (as in toxic conditions) than for those who must be presumed to have a post-necrotic cirrhosis.

In some cases, the hepatic fibrosis is mild and appears to have reached a static phase (cf. Walker, 1952). Compensatory changes occur which enable the liver to function apparently normally. Clinically and as a result of bio-chemical investigation these patients are difficult to distinguish from those with extra-hepatic portal obstruction except that they are usually adult. From the point of view of surgical treatment, however, they are a more favourable group in that both the portal and the splenic veins are available. Only those with an associated portal thrombosis give rise to the mechanical difficulties which are encountered in patients with the congenital type of obliteration.

It is necessary that all patients with hepatitis shall receive sufficient medical treatment to enable the liver to recover as much as possible before elective major surgery is undertaken. Reversible parenchymatous changes should be given time to resolve under treatment with a diet containing a high proportion of animal protein. Anaemia should be treated with iron and transfusions of fresh blood. Deficiencies of blood prothrombin should, if possible, be made good. All vitamins, especially B and C, should be taken liberally. Gross ascites should be relieved by salt restriction and diuretics, with paracentesis abdominis reserved for the intractable case.

Secondary biliary cirrhosis is a somewhat different problem in that it may be possible to remove the cause of the biliary obstruction and allow the liver to recover. In this type of cirrhosis relief of congestion within the biliary passages also appears to have a beneficial effect on the increased pressure within the portal vein and it may not be necessary to resort to surgery to relieve the associated portal hypertension. It is through the portal tracts that blood is conducted to the liver lobules from the branches of the hepatic artery and the portal vein, in close association with the lymphatics and the bile passages. When these tracts become fibrotic, inelastic and distorted, as they do in cirrhosis (Kelty *et al.*, 1950), it is probably correct to deduce that relief of congestion in one of these channels will enable the blood or bile or lymph to flow more readily in the others. The converse of relief of portal hypertension following restoration of biliary flow can be observed in the amelioration of icterus that occurs following the successful construction of a portal-to-systemic venous anastomosis or common hepatic arterial ligature.

Congenital biliary atresia, in which no serviceable biliary passage can be discovered at operation, is a circumstance which has so far defied all efforts at successful treatment, short of transplant.

Patients with mild or moderate cirrhosis will tolerate a diversion of the portal blood from the liver very well indeed. After such a shunt operation, the liver may pass through a phase in which its function is temporarily impaired, but later to improve. Prolonged follow-up of such patients over the years has shown that such improvement is maintained (Hunt, 1965; Milnes Walker, 1967).

Patients with more advanced cirrhosis, particularly those suffering from gross ascites, will not usually tolerate diversion of the portal blood stream. The liver fails within the first few days of operation. It is this group which requires the most careful medical treatment, for at least three months, before operative intervention is seriously contemplated. The type of operation to be done must be designed with the failing liver constantly in mind. The problem is in the nature of a dilemma, because the most effective way of preventing further oesophageal haemorrhages—reduction of portal hypertension—is also, unfortunately, the very procedure most liable to precipitate acute hepatic failure.

Classification of these patients according to the intimate pathology of the cirrhotic process and according to the degree of liver damage will undoubtedly enable those with good prospects to be separated from those for whom the operative risks are prohibitive. It is justifiable to take risks, however, because many cirrhotic patients live useless, miserable, invalid lives, with such time as remains to them usually limited to a matter of months.

Further, the dangers associated with the treatment of the advanced case must not be allowed to prejudice clinicians against the radical surgical treatment of Banti's syndrome in the mild or moderate cirrhotic, in whom the prognosis is excellent, provided that the portal pressure is reduced. Age in itself is no contraindication to operation.

Post-hepatic obstruction occurs in less than 1 per cent. Chiari's disease presents as acute ascites in a younger person, associated usually with a painful, tender and enlarged liver. The Budd-Chiari syndrome, in which inferior vena cava and the hepatic veins are obstructed, is either a more chronic and extensive type of Chiari's disease or is due to malignant invasion of the hepatic veins and inferior vena cava at the level of the diaphragm. In constrictive pericarditis with ascites, oedema extends higher than in other conditions, and is associated with a high jugular venous pressure. Calcification or rigidity of the pericardium are characteristic.

Investigation of Patients suffering from Portal Hypertension

The investigation of patients who suffer from portal hypertension must of necessity be elaborate in order to decide whether or not the liver is diseased and how extensive this disease is; whether or not the effects on the spleen are sufficient to produce a material degree of secondary hypersplenism; what the intimate nature of the underlying disease process may be; whether or not the portal hypertension *per se* is of material significance; and perhaps to demonstrate an anatomical anomaly. Extensive and valuable co-operation with the ancillary departments, radiological, bio-chemical and haematological, must not lead to neglect of full and careful clinical assessment. For instance, where the liver apparently functions normally, a decision as to whether mild cirrhosis is present or not often rests on an accurate physical examination of the liver. An enlarged, adherent spleen may not extend below the costal margin, but may be detected by deep percussion of the left chest. That the liver is at fault must not blind the clinician to the fact that other vital organs may also be seriously deranged.

Investigation:

Haematological. It is necessary to have the full blood count with platelets, prothrombin, group and serum for cross-matching.

Serological tests for syphilis should be done as a routine.

Biochemical. Liver function tests are essential to help in distinguishing the cirrhotic from the normal liver and to define the functional state of the liver. If the serum albumin is below 3·2 gm./100 ml. (Biuret method), the condition of the liver is not good enough to suggest that the outcome of a portal decompression operation will be successful. A bromsulphthalein retention of 25 per cent at 45 mins. is of similar prognostic value. The serum bilirubin and alkaline phosphatase should also be estimated, and the transaminases may give good evidence of the degree of active parenchymatous disease. Other liver function tests may be helpful in some circumstances but are not essential.

Clinical assessment and pathological investigation are not only of value diagnostically, but also provide valuable information as to when the operation should be done. In this respect good risk patients do not present a problem. They should be operated upon as soon as their physical state has reached a point at which they may be judged capable of withstanding any major surgical procedure. It is the bad risk patients that require the most careful treatment and considered judgment. The general well-being of the patient, reduction of anaemia and improvement in secondary hypersplenism are satisfactory findings. An assessment of the rapidity of the formation of ascitic fluid related to repeated estimations of its protein content will provide valuable information as to the patient's progress or deterioration.

Radiological. Barium studies of oesophagus, stomach and duodenum are essential. X-ray of the chest and intravenous pyelography also provide necessary information.

There are, besides, many complicated investigations that may be required in certain circumstances—liver scan, liver biopsy, peritineoscopy and wedged hepatic venous pressure, to mention but four. Many radiologists do percutaneous splenic venography under local anaesthetic, but it is the author's opinion that this carries an appreciable risk. Material haemorrhage occurs in 2 per cent and emergency splenectomy is necessary in 1 per cent (Leger, 1966). Further, a splenic venogram, however elaborate (and expensive) the radiological apparatus, does not necessarily outline the portal vein, nor is it so informative as combined splenic and portal venography obtained safely at operation. Investigations required only to assist in deciding what operation to do and how to set about it are, therefore, best left until the actual operation.

Indications for Operation

Haemorrhage. Gastro-oesophageal varices bleed, sometimes with lethal effect (Fig. 8.1). The interval between haemorrhages varies, but tends to become shorter and the haemorrhages more profuse. The immediate risk to life is considerable, at least 30 per cent in the cirrhotic patients. For those who survive, work and activities are seriously interfered with. The patient and his relatives live in a state of constant anxiety and rightly feel that they must always remain within easy access of skilled haematological treatment. When the liver is cirrhotic, each haemorrhage produces a further deterioration of liver function. Ascites or irreversible liver failure is often precipitated by a haemorrhage. For all these reasons, it is imperative to operate to prevent haemorrhage.

Certain factors must be borne in mind concerning the causes of the bleeding, of which the presence of varicosities and the increased pressure within them are the most important. Thrombocytopenia and hypoprothrombinaemia should be considered as aggravating the bleeding. Erosions or ulcers of the oesophageal or gastric mucous membranes must necessarily be present before haemorrhage can occur. It is often found that a common cold or an acute specific fever precipitates a bleed, particularly in children. Peptic ulcers occur more frequently in association with portal hypertension than in the population at large.

The suppression of acute variceal haemorrhage is of vital importance, in that the immediate mortality in the cirrhotic patient is at least 30 per cent. Transfusion and sedation should be started immediately it is apparent that the cause of the alimentary haemorrhage is a matter of more serious importance than peptic ulceration. Pitressin may be given intravenously. If the haemorrhage does not stop soon, that is, within six hours, the Sengstaken tube should be passed forthwith (Sengstaken and Blakemore, 1950). The gastric balloon is inflated fully with water containing a radio-opaque solution and drawn back to rest at the cardia. The oesophageal balloon is inflated to two-thirds its full capacity. Aspiration on the gastric tube is maintained continuously, causing the stomach to contract on the gastric balloon and hold the tube in the correct position. The balloons are deflated 36 hrs. after the tube has been passed. All being well, the tube is withdrawn 24 hrs. later. From then on medical treatment is begun for anaemia and to build up the patient for a subsequent porta-caval anastomosis.

If bleeding recurs when the balloons are deflated or the tube removed, it is reinserted, the balloons reinflated and final preparations for immediate operation made. Rarely can an emergency porta-caval anastomosis be done safely. Usually the operation of choice is the Boerema-Crile transthoracic oesophagotomy and under-running of the bleeding varices.

It is wise to work out a programme of treatment for each patient with variceal haemorrhage on admission or on diagnosis. The timing of the application of the different stages in the treatment then becomes a matter of precision. The operating theatre staff can be warned in advance of the possibility of an exceptional operation at a particular time. The timing of the programme should be adhered to. In dealing with variceal haemorrhage, it is usually wise to assume that if there is doubt about whether or not the haemorrhage has stopped, it means that it is continuing and the programme should be adhered to, as planned.

Hypersplenism

A much enlarged, over-active and congested spleen requires to be removed, usually as a preliminary to spleno-renal anastomosis. Lesser degrees of hypersplenism tend to resolve after porta-caval anastomosis. Occasionally splenectomy is necessary after porta-caval anastomosis.

Ascites

The causes of ascites are as yet incompletely understood. A raised portal pressure and a reduction in the blood albumin increase the hydrostatic filtration pressure and reduce the osmotic pressure of the plasma respectively. Fibrosis or congestion of the portal tracts obstructs hepatic lymph flow. Alteration of the metabolic processes within the liver produces or fails to remove substances responsible for the retention of fluid, e.g. aldosterone. Operations designed to reduce portal pressure should only be done in patients whose livers function well enough to enable them to tolerate diversion of their portal blood.

Often ascites disappears under medical treatment and the patient is enabled to return to a fairly normal life. At present most workers would agree that such improved patients and certain cirrhotics, who have not had a haemorrhage nor developed ascites and who are able to remain at work, should not be operated on, but should remain under close medical supervision. This opinion may require to be modified when knowledge of the pathology of liver diseases has advanced sufficiently to reduce the risks of a prophylactic shunt operation, so that they are materially lower than the risks of a single haemorrhage.

Other Pathological Conditions

When related to portal hypertension, certain of these conditions require to be dealt with from time to time, e.g. the relief of obstructive jaundice; the removal of the pericardium in constrictive pericarditis. Yet other operations may need to be done on patients with portal hypertension such as the removal of an extrinsic cause, e.g. hypernephroma; or to relieve a complication such as a duodenal ulcer. The surgeon undertaking such operations should, if possible, be familiar with the special problems raised by the portal hypertension and its effects.

Methods of Surgical Treatment

It is, therefore, clear that no single operation is suitable for all cases of portal hypertension. The most effective procedure may prove to be impossible or may fail. Sufficient time has not yet elapsed for the value of the different operations to be fully assessed. The surgeon must, on occasions, be prepared to regard the patient as a problem which may require a number of different tactical approaches before the correct solution is found. This applies particularly to the patients with extra-hepatic portal obstruction. In general, however, it may be stated:

(i) That if the raised portal pressure *per se* is the cause of the symptoms, then reduction of this by an adequate portal-to-systemic venous anastomosis is undoubtedly a most successful method of restoring the patient to a normal state of health and preventing further haemorrhages.

(ii) That if the elevated portal pressure is associated with a markedly enlarged and over-active spleen, splenectomy should be done as part of the planned treatment.

(iii) That haemorrhage can be stopped for a time by interrupting the flow of blood from the portal bed to the bleeding segment. This

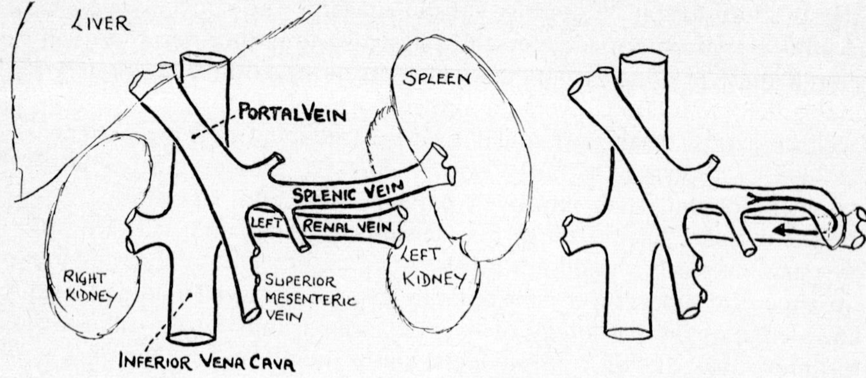

(*a*). Diagram of the normal anatomy.   (*b*). Spleno-renal anastomosis (end-to-side).

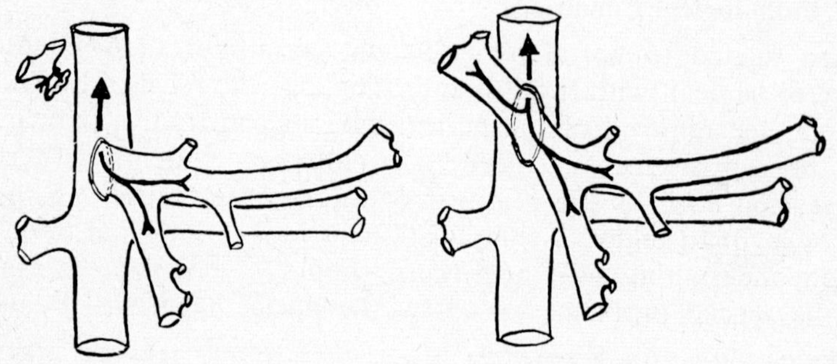

(*c*). Porta-caval anastomosis (end-to-side).   (*d*). Porta-caval anastomosis (in continuity).

FIG. 8.4

operation is usually reserved for patients who have no portal channel of sufficient size for the construction of an efficient shunt, but may also be of value as an emergency measure to stop uncontrollable bleeding.

(iv) That if only a segment of the portal bed is in a hypertensive state, as in splenic vein thrombosis, splenectomy alone or combined with proximal gastric resection may remove the hypertensive area and effect a clinical cure.

No attempt will be made here to give details of surgical techniques. However, certain considerations require to be borne in mind in comparing the different operative procedures.

Portal-to-Systemic Venous Anastomoses

Porta-caval shunt (Fig. 8.4). The portal vein and the inferior vena cava are both large veins which are easily handled. They are strong and hold stitches well. A large shunt can be unhurriedly constructed. The direction of flow in the portal vein is not reversed. The stoma is unlikely to thrombose (Hunt, 1965). It is an operation which is suitable for most patients with hepatic cirrhosis of mild and intermediate degree. Moderately enlarged spleens shrink and become less active after successful porta-caval anastomosis. The spleen should be preserved when there is no thrombocytopenia, because of the increased risk of thrombosis after splenectomy in such cases.

It is usually best to make the shunt by end-to-side anastomosis (Fig. 8.4) (Welch, 1947). Sometimes, however, the portal vein and inferior vena cava can be joined "in continuity" (Fig. 8.4) (Hunt, 1953), side-to-side or as a double-barrelled shunt (McDermott, 1960), thus allowing reflux of blood from the liver.

The results of porta-caval anastomosis are excellent in suitable cases.

Spleno-renal shunt (Fig. 8.4) (Linton *et al.*, 1948) is indicated in extra-hepatic portal obstruction when it is likely that the splenic vein is the only portal venous channel which can be utilized. It should also be done for cirrhotic patients when the portal vein is thrombosed, and when the spleen is very large and over-active and has led to such a degree of hypersplenism that it is necessary to regard splenectomy as the first step in any major operation. Platelets return in fair numbers to the circulation very soon after the spleen has been removed. An alternative approach to this group is to remove the spleen and later do a porta-caval anastomosis (Rousselot, 1949; Stock, 1952).

Other portal-to-systemic venous anastomoses may be necessary when neither the portal nor the splenic vein is available. Marion has devised the operation of side-to-end mesenterico-caval anastomosis (see Marion *et al.*, Voorhees *et al.*, and Clatworthy). This necessitates complete division of the inferior vena cava or, better, both common iliac veins, utilizing the right for the anastomosis and closing the stump of the left. It should not be done in the older patient who will develop peripheral oedema.

Porta-Asygos Interruption

The alternative to diversion of portal blood from the bleeding segment is division of the portal vessels below the dangerous area, at and above the cardia. This latter type of operation can take many forms, e.g. gastro-oesophageal resection (Phemister and Humphreys, 1947); transthoracic oesophageal transection (Milnes Walker, 1964); subdiaphragmatic gastric transection (Tanner, 1950). The purpose of these operations is to prevent high pressure portal blood from reaching the lower end of the oesophagus. Theoretically the most logical of such operations is that in which all vascular communications to the proximal half of the stomach and distal few inches of oesophagus are severed, sparing only safe venous communications to the abdominal parietes. The diaphragm must be incised and detached entirely from the alimentary canal, because the veins of the proximal stomach, spleen, diaphragm and oesophagus communicate freely. The stomach is then divided just below the cardia to complete the interruption between portal and azygos veins and re-anastomosed after careful ligature of the submucous gastric veins. The vagus nerves should be severed and pyloroplasty done in the hope that this may reduce the risks of peptic erosions and ulcerations. The diaphragm is repaired. It is not yet known how long these operations remain effective in preventing haemorrhage. The portal congestion persists unaffected, with its attendant troubles such as ascites and the risk of thrombosis.

The interruption operation is clearly indicated:

(i) When there is no available portal venous channel for a shunt;

(ii) When it is imperative that bleeding should be prevented in a child whose veins are too small for the construction of a spleno-renal anastomosis that will carry him through life;

(iii) As an emergency operation to stop uncontrollable haemorrhage in the case of cirrhotic patients. Some less extensive modification of the interruption operation may be sufficient in this last group of patients, such as the operation devised by Boerema and George Crile Junior. Distal oesophagotomy is done by a transthoracic approach through the bed of the 8th left rib and the varices are sutured under direct vision. The incision can be carried down into the abdomen by division of the diaphragm, if it is found that the bleeding is coming from the stomach.

Splenectomy was, until the pioneer work of Whipple and Blakemore, regarded as the standard operation for Banti's syndrome. It is now recognized that removal of the spleen should be reserved for the relief of hypersplenism, as a preliminary to a portal-to-systemic venous anastomosis, or when a venogram demonstrates clearly that splenic vein thrombosis is the only abnormality of the portal venous tree.

Transposition of the spleen into the thorax has been shown to develop a collateral circulation to by-pass the portal obstruction (Nylander and Turunen, 1955).

Injection of oesophageal varices with sclerosing solutions (Crafoord and Frenckner, 1939) is a useful palliative to reduce the size of varices. Repeated many times it may be of great value, especially in extrahepatic obstruction.

Many other operations require to be mentioned but cannot be recommended. They *are* all intended to relieve ascites, but the little benefit that may on occasions be derived from them is transient. The list includes the Talma Morison omentopexy, the peritoneal button operation, peritoneum-to-saphenous-vein anastomosis and peritoneum-to-renal-pelvis anastomosis, modifications of the Spitz-Holter valve, ileo-entectropy, hepatic arterial ligature.

Anaesthesia

It is only with the aid of expert anaesthesia that major operations are successfully done on cases of portal hypertension. The agents should be selected so that adequate relaxation is maintained with the very minimum of hepato-toxic drugs. The patient must be kept fully oxygenated throughout the operation and during the phase of recovery. It is not the author's custom to utilize hypothermia or hypotension.

Post-Operative Care

The principles of post-operative treatment are:
(i) To prevent infection.
(ii) To retain full nutrition, by intravenous therapy in the first place and then by mouth.
(iii) To observe closely for complications such as paralytic ileus and mesenteric thrombosis and to treat them with all available means as early as possible. Portal-systemic encephalopathy and hepatic coma are best treated along the lines suggested by Prof. Sherlock and her colleagues. Protein is eliminated from the diet, vitamins are given in abundance. Neomycin in sufficiently large doses to eliminate the ammonia-producing organisms from the bowel (Dawson *et al.*, 1957), and constipation is relieved by bowel washouts and laxatives. Occasionally chronic portal-systemic encephalopathy can be improved by the operation of subtotal colectomy (Atkinson and Goligher, 1960) or colonic exclusion (McDermott *et al.*, 1962).

Results of Surgical Treatment

(1) *Congenital extra-hepatic portal obstruction* carries a good prognosis provided a large enough shunt can be well constructed. Circumstances are unfavourable in a number of these cases, the mechanical difficulties forestalling all but the most painstaking or ingenious of operations. On the whole the results are disappointing though the patients may survive for many years.

(2) The outlook in cases of *cirrhosis of mild and moderate extent* is very favourable. A good shunt (using the portal or the splenic vein) can almost always be constructed. The operative mortality should not exceed 4 per cent. The great majority of these patients do not bleed again and are enabled to return to normal, vigorous lives (Hunt, 1965). The five-year survival rate is over 50 per cent.

(3) *Advanced cirrhosis* still presents a gloomy picture. Some patients deteriorate so rapidly that the opportunity for surgical intervention never occurs. In numbers these are about balanced by those that improve under medical treatment so that operation becomes, for the time being, unnecessary. Of the remainder, the majority are grossly ascitic and some also suffer from repeated haemorrhages. The return of nearly one-third of this group of bed-ridden patients to active, useful lives is fair compensation for many months of most carefully supervised medical treatment preceding an operation of increased hazard. Their only hope of reasonable life, rather than restricted and limited survival, lies in operative treatment, so that risks are justified. Surgery is used in an attempt to break the vicious circle of decline. Continued functional recovery of the liver depends on the persistence of medical treatment.

References

ATKINSON, M. and GOLIGHER, J. C. (1960). *Lancet*, **1**, 461.

BAYLY, J. H. (1964). *Amer. J. Gastroenterology*, **41**, 235.

BLAKEMORE, A. H. (1952). *Surg. Gynec. Obstet.*, **94**, 443.

BLAKEMORE, A. H. and LORD, J. W. (jun.) (1945). *Ann. Surg.*, **122**, 476.

BOEREMA, I. (1949). *Arch. Chir. Nederland*, **1**, 253.

BUTLER, H. (1951). *Thorax*, **6**, 276.

CLATWORTHY, H. W. (1956). Address at meeting of Association of Paediatric Surgeons, London.

CRAFOORD, C. and FRENCKNER, P. (1939). *Acta. oto-laryng. Stockh.*, **27**, 422.

CRILE, G. (jun.), (1963). *Surg. Gynec. Obstet.*, **96**, 573.

DAWSON, A. M., McLAREN, J. and SHERLOCK, S. (1957). *Lancet*, **2**, 1263.

GRAY, H. K. (1951). *Ann. Roy. Coll. Surg. Engl.*, **8**, 354.

HUNT, A. H. (1952a). *Brit. Med. J.*, **2**, 4; (1952b). *Proc. Roy. Soc. Med.*, **45**, 722; (1953). "Portal Hypertension" in "Abdominal Operations" (3rd edition), edited by Rodney Maingot. New York, Appleton-Century-Crofts; (1958). "Portal Hypertension". Edinburgh, Livingstone; (1965). *St. Bart's Hosp. J.*, Supplement No. 11, **69**, i-xv.

KELTY, R. H., BAGGENSTOSS, A. H. and BUTT, H. R. (1950). *Proc. Mayo Clin.*, **25**, 17.

LAVOIE, P., JACOB, M., LEDUC, J., LEGARE, A. and VIALLET, A. (1966). *Canad. J. Surg.*, **9**, 338.

LEGER, L. (1966). "Splenoportography". Springfield, Illinois, Charles C. Thomas.

LINTON, R. R., HARDY, I. B. (jun.) and VOLWILER, W. (1948). *Surg. Gynec. Obstet.*, **87**, 129.

McDERMOTT, W. V. (jun.) (1960). *Surg. Gynec. Obstet.*, **110**, 457.

McDERMOTT, W. V. (jun.), VICTOR, M. and WARREN POINT, W. (1962). *New Engl. J. Med.*, **267**, 850.

MARION, P., BOUCHET, A. and YON, M. (1960). *Ann. Chir. (Par.)*, **14**, 581.

NYLANDER, P. E. A. and TURUNEN, M. (1955). *Ann. Surg.*, **142**, 954.

PHEMISTER, D. B. and HUMPHREYS, E. M. (1947). *Ann. Surg.*, **126**, 397.

ROUSSELOT, L. M. (1949). *J. Amer. Med. Ass.*, **140**, 282.

SENGSTAKEN, R. W. and BLAKEMORE, A. H. (1950). *Ann. Surg.*, **131**, 781.

SHALDON, S. and SHERLOCK, S. (1962). *Lancet*, **1**, 63.

SHERLOCK, S. (1963). "Diseases of the Liver and Biliary System". 2nd edition. Blackwell Scientific Publications, Oxford.

STOCK, F. E. (1952). *Ann. Roy. Coll. Surg. Engl.*, **10**, 187.

TANNER, N. C. (1950). *Proc. Roy. Soc. Med.*, **43**, 150.

THOMPSON, W. P. (1940). *Ann. Intern. Med.*, **14**, 255.

VOORHEES, A. B. (jun.) and BLAKEMORE, A. H. (1963). *Surg.*, **54**, 559.

WALKER, R. M. (1952). *Lancet*, **1**, 729; (1959). "The Pathology and Management of Portal Hypertension". Edward Arnold, London; (1964). *Surg. Gynec. Obstet.*, **118**, 323; (1967) in Vol. XIX of the Colston Papers (Proceedings of the Nineteenth Symposium of the Colston Research Society). Butterworths Scientific Publications, London.

WALKER, R. M., SHALDON, C. and VOWLES, K. D. J. (1961). *Lancet*, **2**, 727.

WELCH, C. S. (1947). *Surg. Gynec. Obstet.*, **85**, 492; (1950). *New Engl. J. Med.*, **243**, 598.

WHIPPLE, A. O. (1945). *Ann. Surg.*, **122**, 449.

Chapter 9

CARCINOMA OF THE HYPOPHARYNX AND CERVICAL OESOPHAGUS

G. B. Ong

Although arising from specific areas, carcinoma of the hypopharynx and cervical oesophagus should be considered as one lesion both in its behaviour and treatment. There is no barrier to its extension from one to the other part of this region of the alimentary tract. Trotter (1929) classified carcinoma of the hypopharynx into the following groups:

(1) Superior group—growths arising from the epiglottis and the glosso-epiglottic fossa.

(2) Lateral group—growths from one of the following situations (*a*) the aryepiglottic fold, (*b*) pyriform fossa, (*c*) the lateral pharyngeal wall.

(3) Posterior group—consists of growths from the posterior pharyngeal wall and

(4) Inferior group—comprising growths from the postcricoid region.

To the last group should be added growths from the cervical oesophagus.

Incidence and Aetiology

With the exception of postcricoid carcinoma, growths in the hypopharynx and cervical oesophagus are much more common in males than females. Postcricoid carcinoma in women with the classical description of Plummer Vinson's syndrome has been reported as high as 90 per cent (Jacobsson, 1951). However not a single case of the above syndrome has been found in Chinese patients seen in Hong Kong.

Excessive use of alcohol has been found to carry a greater risk of developing carcinoma of the oesophagus, larynx and oral cavity (Wynder *et al.*, 1956, 1957, Schwartz, Denoix and Anguesa, 1957). Wynder and Bross 1961, basing on experimental work on mice concluded that alcohol renders the cells more susceptible to the carcinogens present in tobacco smoke. It is possible that users of both alcohol and tobacco may produce a state of chronic pharyngitis which may undergo malignant degeneration. Cases have been reported of carcinoma of the hypopharynx in whom irradiation of the neck had been carried out for benign lesions of the neck (Raven and Levison, 1954).

155

Pathology

Grossly the lesion may be:

(1) Proliferative in nature, giving a cauliflower appearance. It may fill the hypopharynx and cervical oesophagus and it is then not possible to separate the origin of the growth from one region to the other (Fig. 9.1). Pieces of the growth may break off from the main lesion and be regurgitated.

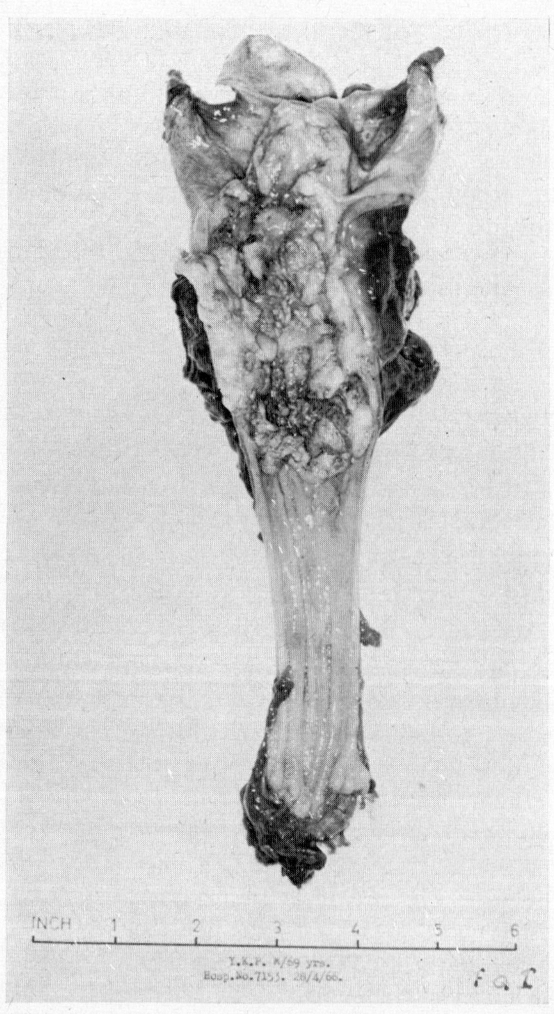

FIG. 9.1. Resected specimen of pharynx, larynx and oesophagus showing extensive proliferative growth of the hypopharynx.

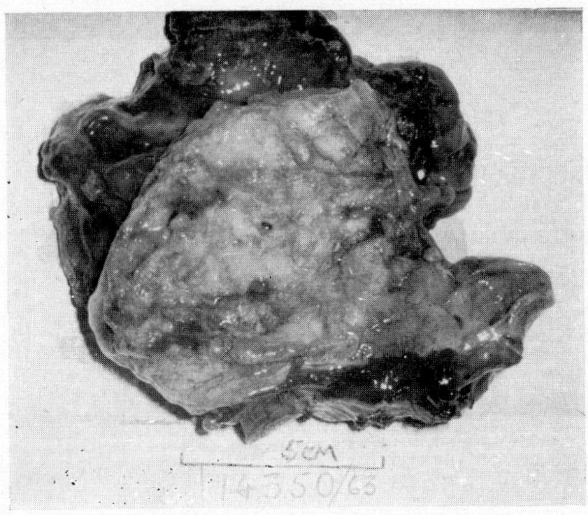

FIG. 9.2. Carcinoma of the hypopharynx showing a nodular growth. Resected specimen.

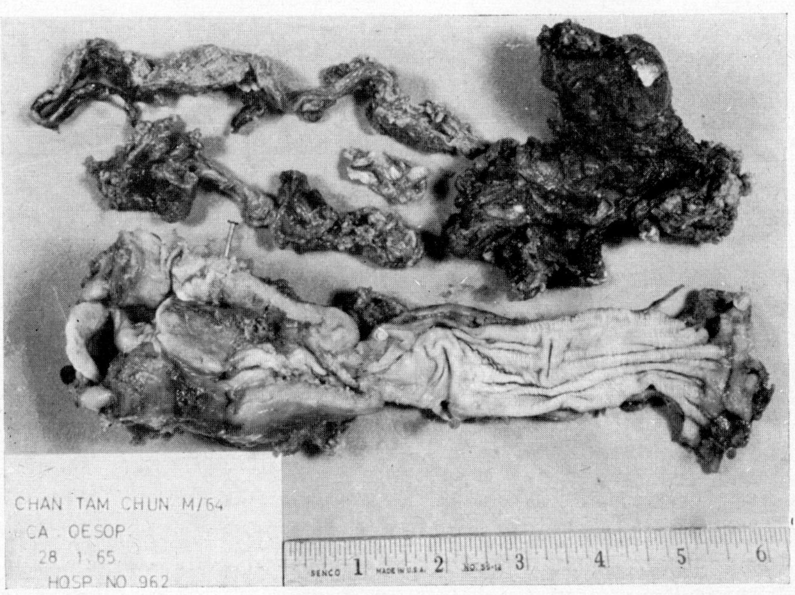

FIG. 9.3. Extensive carcinoma of the hypopharynx extending into the oesophagus.

(2) A malignant ulcer. It has an indurated base with heaped up edges. It is especially common in lesions of the pyriform sinus.

(3) A nodular tumour which protrudes into the lumen and may have superficial ulceration (Fig. 9.2). Sometimes it may be very extensive and fill the whole of the lumen and extend from the pharynx to the oesophagus. Once in the oesophagus it may then take an annular form. It infiltrates insiduously and when first seen may be very extensive (Fig. 9.3). Microscopically it is a squamous cell carcinoma with varying degree of keratinization. Sometimes it is composed of anaplastic cells which may be arranged in sheets with dark staining nucleus and showing active mitosis.

Spread

(1) Locally it spreads to the surrounding structures. The lesion tends to spread first circumferentially and then externally to involve the thyroid cartilage or trachea. Destruction of the thyroid cartilage and the posterior tracheal wall with the necrosis and secondary infection may lead to abscess formation or if into the trachea may end in severe aspiration pneumonia or lung abscess. It is not unusual for one or both lobes of the thyroid gland to be infiltrated by the growth and then the recurrent laryngeal nerve may be involved. Further extension of the growth may spread to the prevertebral fascia and muscles but this is not common except in very advanced stage of the disease.

(2) Lymphatics. Spread to the regional lymph nodes is frequent and extensive. From the regional lymph nodes it spreads to the deep cervical chain and then into the mediastinum. Occasionally the retropharyngeal nodes located near the base of the skull may be affected (Ballantyne, 1964). From the lymph nodes the carcinoma may invade the jugular vessels and then spread by blood stream may take place, or when extensive may cause sudden haemorrhage.

(3) Spreading by blood stream is not unusual. It may be by direct invasion of the growth into the jugular vessels or by secondaries in the lymph nodes. It spreads rapidly to the lungs and to other sites like liver and bones or even soft tissues including skin. This mode of spread is not unusual following successful treatment of the disease.

Clinical Features

When first seen the disease is usually in an advanced stage. Dysphagia is the usual complaint and aspiration pneumonitis or broncho-pneumonia is a fairly constant finding. With dysphagia there is evidence of marked loss of body weight. The loss of body weight is not only due to starvation but also to respiratory infection. When dysphagia is severe, the patient may be dehydrated and become moribund.

Careful interrogation will usually elicit a varying period of discomfort in the throat. Pain may be experienced and which is referred to the back of the ear. Abnormal irritating sensation in the pharynx induces the constant desire to swallow and clear the throat. Foul purulent material may be expectorated. Later change in the quality of phonation and even hoarseness may be experienced. Haemoptysis is unusual and

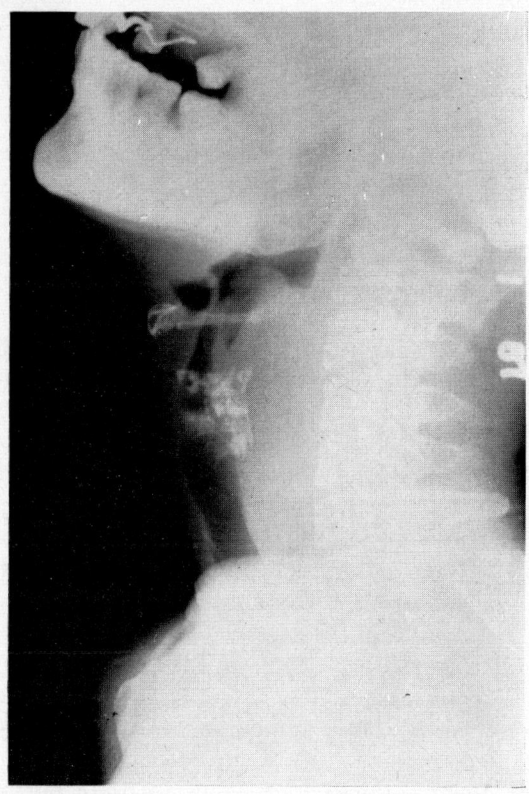

Fig. 9.4. Lateral X-ray of neck in a case of hypopharyngeal carcinoma showing the larynx and trachea being displaced forward.

when present may mean invasion and erosion of a vessel or the trachea. Dyspnoea and even asphyxiation may be a terminal event.

On examination, a forward bulging of the trachea or thyroid cartilage may be obvious. The alae of the thyroid cartilage may spread outwards. Cervical lymph adenopathy may be prominent. The lymph nodes are usually hard but very large ones undergoing necrosis may be soft. Rarely extensive lymph node involvement from a small primary growth in the hypopharynx may be a presenting symptom.

Diagnosis

When dysphagia is the presenting symptom, the diagnosis does not give rise to difficulty. In an elderly individual any appearance of persistent discomfort and pain in the throat is an indication to careful examination of the hypopharynx.

Lateral radiograph of the neck may show an increase of the space between the larynx or trachea and the vertebral bodies (Fig. 9.4). Barium swallow may not give positive information until the lesion is advanced. However, much information may be obtained with tomography (Ellis, 1966).

The most important aid to a correct diagnosis is direct endoscopy. This is carried out under anaesthesia. A Negus oesophagoscope is favoured. The hypopharynx and epilaryngeal regions can be examined in detail and any suspicious lesions biopsied with a punch forceps. It is important to take several specimens from edges of the suspicious lesion.

Treatment

Two methods of treatment are accepted viz: (1) Radiotherapy; (2) Surgery.

Both methods have their protagonists but the results are equally poor, although it was shown by the studies of Ormerod (1961) to be 30 per cent based on the five year cure rate.

Radiotherapy. This is given over a period of several weeks and a total dose of 5,000 to 8,000 rads is delivered either by means of a linear accelerator or Cobalt unit. While some five year cures are possible, ultimately most, if not all, of the cases would require surgery (Macbeth, 1963). This is our experience. Although, Ellis (1966) believed that with supervoltage X-ray machines, the condition of the tissue is without serious damage so as to make radical surgery possible, it is not our experience. Limited excision of the recurrent lesion is possible but with block dissection there is the serious danger of the skin to slough and expose the carotid artery. Split skin graft is not possible in such cases. The exposed artery will suddenly undergo necrosis resulting in fatal haemorrhage. However, radiotherapy is useful as an adjunct to surgery. A combined treatment may ultimately prove to be the best form of therapy. A smaller dose of 3 to 4,000 rads given over a short period and followed by surgery within a few weeks as practised by Nakayama (1959) for treatment of oesophageal cancer, should be given a trial in carcinoma of the hypopharynx and cervical oesophagus. It is perhaps wrong to wait for recurrence of the growth following radiotherapy, before surgery is resorted to.

Surgery. The aim of surgery in the treatment of hypopharyngeal and cervical oesophageal cancer is to cure the disease where possible. Failing to cure this condition, good palliation is often achieved. The constant aspiration of accumulated secretion with its accompanying paroxysm of cough is most distressing. As the growth progresses, infiltration in the larynx will give rise to respiratory stridor and asphyxiation. However, in whatever form of treatment employed, it must restore the ability to swallow freely and with each act of swallowing must also prevent the subject from choking. From the outset of surgical extirpation of the growth, the air passage becomes free. The ability to swallow depends on the appropriate method adopted in reconstructing the upper alimentary tract.

Preoperative Preparation

As these sufferers are usually in poor physical condition, a period of preoperative preparation is necessary. Special care is paid to the oral hygiene. Scaling of teeth and extraction of carious ones should be carried out. Anaemia is corrected and if there is evidence of respiratory infection appropriate antibiotics should be given. It has been customary in our patients undergoing radical surgery for carcinoma of the upper alimentary tract to have the bowels prepared with one of the non-absorbable sulphonamides and then neomycin on the day before the operation.

In cases who have complete dysphagia, intravenous drip may be necessary. Here gastrostomy is first performed for feeding and the definitive operation postponed until the general condition of the patient is fit enough to withstand major surgery. This period of delay for gastrostomy alimentation is well worthwhile for very often they do put on weight which is not possible where they are given only parenteral feeding.

Anaesthesia

General anaesthesia is as a rule given except in exceptional cases where the growth has extended to involve the larynx. This may hinder the anaesthetist's effort to pass the endotracheal tube. Here initial tracheostomy is carried out under local anaesthesia. The skin about 2 in. above the suprasternal notch is infiltrated with 2 per cent xylocaine and a transverse incision is made. After adequate exposure, the trachea is divided right across and dissected from the oesophagus. Constant suction is necessary to prevent blood from getting into the trachea. The lower divided tracheal end is then brought out through a separate circular incision on the skin above the suprasternal notch. The trachea is then stitched to the skin. A few drops of xylocaine into the trachea will prevent the bronchial irritation that will otherwise cause great discomfort. General anaesthesia is now induced with pentothal and a short cuffed-tube inserted. Further anaesthesia of gas and oxygen with relaxant is given through this tube.

The Operation

The operation area is now prepared from the neck to the abdomen. Many incisions have been advocated by various authors for exploration and excision of the growth. Ellis (1958) employed a horizontal H incision in his cases and he believed that in post irradiation cases there was a less likelihood of the reflected skin to slough. Macbeth (1963) on the other hand advocated the use of a median incision with lateral flaps and any defect afterwards is covered over by a Thiersch graft. A U-shaped incision was employed in our earlier cases. One limb of the incision extending from one mastoid process and coursing downwards across the middle of the anterior border of the sternomastoid muscle to about 1 in. of the suprasternal notch is made. The lower end of this incision is connected to a corresponding incision made from the other mastoid process. This incision has now been replaced by a long transverse incision made about the middle of the neck. The extent of this incision is carried as far posteriorly as possible and the upper flap is raised to the angle of the jaw and the lower one down to the clavicle. By raising these skin flaps there is sufficient exposure for radical excision and bilateral block dissection to be carried out. By dividing the investing fascia along the anterior border of the sterno-mastoid muscle, the carotid sheath is exposed and with lateral retraction, the hypopharynx and cervical oesophagus can be explored. This is repeated on the other side as well.

Extent of Resection

Attention is paid to infiltration of the growth into the prevertebral fascia. The upper and lower limit of the growth also can be easily palpated. Enlarged lymph nodes are noted on both sides of the neck. Should it be found to be resectable, a planned bilateral block dissection of neck with a pharyngo-laryngo-oesophagectomy is carried out. When the growth is small and situated in the postcricoid or upper cervical oesophagus, the temptation is to preserve the larynx. This should be resisted for despite the preservation of the recurrent laryngeal nerves, with each effort at swallowing choking takes place. This in itself will necessitate laryngectomy in order to restore the ability to deglutinate. Besides this drawback it is a compromise to cancer surgery and almost invariably will end in recurrence of the disease. If the thyroid is infiltrated, resection of the gland in continuity should be carried-out. However, if one lobe is free it is better to preserve a small portion of the gland together with at least one parathyroid. Nevertheless, attempt to preserve these glands at the expense of adequate surgery is not justified.

It has been our practice for some years to resect the hyoid bone together with the growth. This does facilitate the final construction of the pharynx for should it be decided to use a part of the gastrointestinal tract to restore the alimentary continuity the intact hyoid bone does interfere with a proper anastomosis. In resecting the upper part of the hypopharynx care must be taken not to damage the hypoglossal nerve. Damage to the hypoglossal nerve prevents movement of the tongue and thus hinders swallowing.

Block dissection in continuity with the growth should be carried out on the side of the lesion. It is our practice to dissect as much as possible the lymphatics on the opposite side of the growth as well. The internal jugular vein of the second side is however preserved. Division and removal of both internal jugular veins at one sitting will give rise to marked cyanosis, proptosis and oedema of the head and face. This may not subside for weeks and even months later may give rise to troublesome swelling.

Ellis (1959) does not believe in prophylactic block dissection of the neck and only does so when metastasis develops. Pickard (1965) on the other hand states that in view of the frequency of lymph node metastasis, block dissection should be carried out on the side of the lesion. We believe that when on clinical examination, the nodes are obviously metastatic, the chance of a cure is small. It is when the nodes are not palpable but only on microscopic examination are found to be positive, that there is a chance of cure.

Reconstruction of the Pharynx:

(1) **Skin reconstruction.** Reconstruction of the resected cervical oesophagus was first successfully carried out by Mikulicz in 1878 (Meade, 1961). However, it was Wookey (1940) who popularized the multi-staged reconstruction of the cervical oesophagus. A rectangular flap of skin together with the platysma is made and the upper and lower edges are anastomosed to the pharyngostome and oesophago-stome. The raw surface is covered by split skin graft. This leaves a lateral pharyngostome which is closed later. Various modifications of the operation is still being practised (Ellis, 1958; Macbeth, 1963 and Pickard, 1965). A one-staged attempt has been devised using skin graft tubes (Ellis, 1958), chest skin flap (Zehm, 1965) and tubular graft of penile skin (Kaplan and Markowicz, 1964).

The multi-staged reconstruction has a great draw back of lengthy procedures and hospitalization. Should the reconstruction at any stage be unsuccessful a delay of several months is not unusual. In a serious disease as carcinoma of the hypopharynx and cervical oesophagus, death from metastasis or recurrence may take place even before the final reconstruction is completed. Stricture and fistula formation at the sites of anastomosis is the other defect. Even the one-staged reconstruction with skin tubes is not free from this complication.

But it is a less severe operation and should not be entirely abandoned. If at the end of the extensive operation in the neck, the condition of the patient does not warrant further surgery, this method of reconstruction may be a way out of a difficult situation.

(2) **Reconstruction with anastomosis between the lower divided end of the oesophagus and the divided pharynx.**

Wooler (1952) and Jack (1955) described this method of reconstruction. A left thoracotomy with removal of the 8th rib is carried out. The oesophagus is mobilized, the diaphragm is then divided and the stomach freed as far as the pylorus. The upper thoracic oesophagus is next mobilized through a separate incision after resecting a segment of the fourth rib. The stomach is now anchored to the lower border of the aortic arch and the chest closed. The patient is now placed on his back and the pharyngo-laryngo-oesophagectomy carried out. The divided pharynx is anastomosed to the divided lower oesophagus. The blood supply to this segment of the oesophagus is from the oesophageal branches of the left gastric artery and must be very precarious. There must be a limit to the length of the lower oesophagus that can be utilized for anastomosis and it is doubtful if it can be longer than the fundus of the stomach. The operation itself is as severe as any other form of reconstruction that is currently being employed.

(3) **Pharyngo-gastric anastomosis:** The fundus of the stomach has been successfully anastomosed to the divided pharynx after pharyngo-laryngectomy (Ong and Lee, 1960; Le Quesne and Ranger, 1966). This is a useful method of reconstruction and one, if employed in a suitable case, should be a satisfactory procedure. The stomach, despite all that has been written of its acid producing properties and causing ulceration is a very convenient organ for upper alimentary tract reconstruction. The blood supply of the stomach after mobilization is from two sources namely the right gastric and the right gastro-epiploeic arteries. There are occasions when the anastomosis between the right and left gastro-epiploeic arteries may be deficient. However, when this is the case, the arcade formed by the right and left gastric arteries is exceptionally large. Despite deficient anastomosis of the right and left gastro-epiploeic arteries, the vascular arcade along the lesser curvature of the stomach does ensure adequate arterial supply to the fundus of the stomach. Le Quesne and Ranger (1966) believing that the intra-gastric circulation would improve if left for 10–14 days after mobilization of the stomach,

found that dense adhesion had formed round it. This staged procedure was suggested by Ivor Lewis (1946) in his operation for carcinoma of the middle third of the oesophagus in patients whose general condition was poor. This method of mobilizing the stomach and then leaving it in the abdomen, not only induces dense adhesion but also reduces its elasticity. This loss of elasticity will prevent it from reaching the neck.

This operation is severe. It involves extensive dissection in the neck and opening and closing the abdominal and thoracic cavities. However, with adequate preoperative preparation, it can be carried out even in

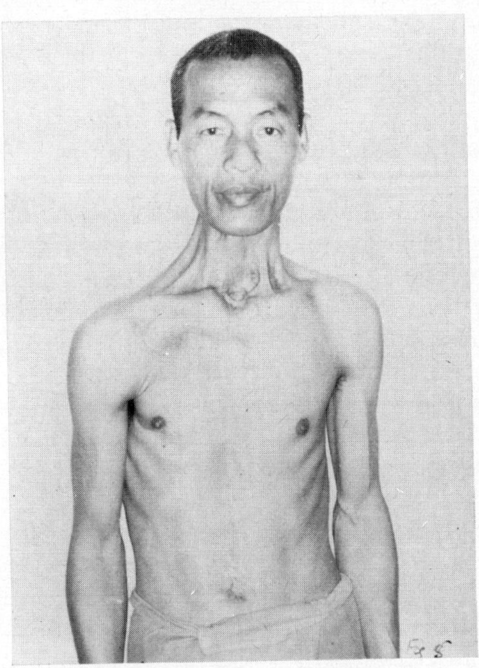

Fig. 9.5. Case of pharyngo-gastric anastomosis operated in January 1959 as he appears today, 8 years after the operation.

relatively poor risk patients. The operating time can be shortened by blind finger dissection of the oesophagus from above at the thoracic inlet and below from the abdomen. This dispenses with the opening and closing of the thoracic cavity. This method of dissecting the oesophagus was carried out by Turner (1936). In this dissection there may be difficulty in freeing the mid portion of the oesophagus due to the vagus nerves intertwining it. It can nevertheless be dissected out without too much disturbance to the patient.

Of all portions of the gastrointestinal tract the stomach has the best blood supply. It is supplied from two sources of blood namely the right gastric and right gastroepiploeic arteries. The fundus of the stomach which is normally richly supplied by the vasa brevia still has more than adequate blood as the whole of the submucosal layer is a lake of blood (Bentley and Barlow, 1952).

Although the stomach appears to be short it has great elasticity and stretches as far as the neck without difficulty. By gentle stretching, it can reach as far as the nasopharynx without any difficulty. In reconstruction of the pharynx, the shortest distance the stomach has to traverse is through the posterior mediastinum, that is, the route that the oesophagus takes. The subcutaneous ante-sternal route is the longest while the retrosternal, ante-mediastinal route is in the intermediate range.

The stomach provides an excellent suture material. This is improved by suturing it to the base of the tongue anteriorly and then posteriorly to the pharyngeal wall. It is best to remove the hyoid bone so as to facilitate suturing. No disability will result from its removal.

This method of reconstruction is a one-staged procedure and deglutition is restored within a short period and if the patient succumbs to the disease, he has been relieved of the major complaint of dysphagia within a very short time following the operation. A long term survival when it happens, is a tolerable one (Fig. 9.5).

(4) **Reconstruction by a reversed gastric tube** was successfully performed by Heimlich and Winfield (1955), and Heimlich (1966). This is a less severe operation.

The use of a gastric tube was first suggested by Meyers who in 1912 suggested that a Jianu gastrostomy be constructed from the stomach and anastomosed to the exteriorized segment of the oesophagus. A reversed gastric tube can be constructed from the greater curvature of the stomach. Starting from the pyloric end the tube is created over a large Malecot catheter. This tube can be made long enough for it to reach the pharynx for anastomosis. It derives its blood supply solely from the splenic artery through the arcade formed by the right and left gastro-epiploeic arteries (Fig. 9.6). In a small percentage of cases, this arcade is incomplete and in which case the pyloric end may not have sufficient blood supply to prevent avascular necrosis.

There is a danger of avascular perforation at the junction between the fundus of the stomach and the gastric tube. It is here that the blood supply normally comes from the vasa brevia and which after division may receive insufficient blood from the cardiac branches of the left gastric artery.

Anastomosis between the narrow pyloric end and the pharynx may present difficulty and leakage and stricture may develop. This tube will reach the pharynx with greater ease when the spleen is removed close to its hilum and the tail of the pancreas mobilized as far to the right as possible. Notwithstanding these disadvantages, this is a suitable operation in some cases and long term survival with good nutrition is possible (Fig. 9.7).

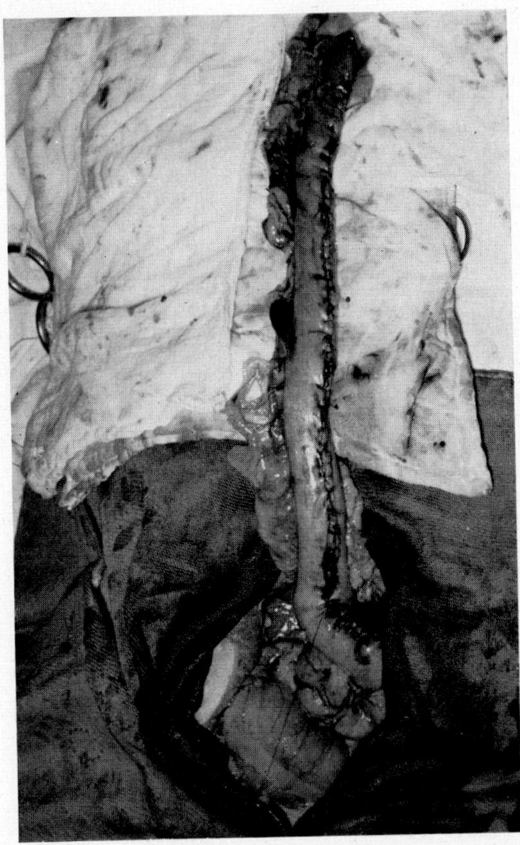

FIG. 9.6. Gastric tube has been made out of the greater curvature of the stomach. It could easily reach the neck for anastomosis to the pharynx.

(5) Use of the Colon for reconstruction. Kelling (1911) used the transverse colon to reconstruct the oesophagus through a subcutaneous tunnel and placed it in the isoperitaltic direction. Vulliet (1911) however, used it in the reverse direction. This old operation has been revived and is now extensively used for oesophagoplasty. The use of the transverse colon, when it is long, can be used for reconstruction of the pharynx. However, when it is short there may be difficulty in bringing it as high up as the pharynx. Orsini and Lemaire (1951) have used the left side of the large intestine for oesophagoplasty in mid thoracic lesions of the oesophagus. The descending colon is used to anastomose anti-peristaltically the divided oesophagus. The sigmoid as well as the left upper and lower colic vessels are divided. The left side of the transverse and descending colon is now supplied by the middle colic vessels. There is plenty of length for it to be brought up into the pharynx. This was successfully carried out by Goligher and Robin (1954) in a case of

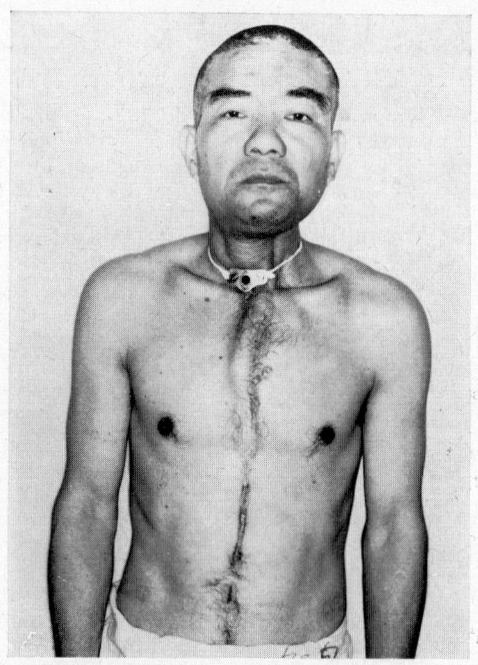

FIG. 9.7. Case of postcricoid carcinoma previously reported (Ong 1964) as he is today after more than 8 years since the operation.

postcricoid carcinoma that was subjected to pharyngo-laryngectomy. We have used this for lesions in middle third of the oesophagus but have not been satisfied with any antiperistaltic procedures. Gastrointestinal contents tend to be regurgitated and this causes constant discomfort and annoyance to the patients. It is possible this will adjust itself after a period of months and then the condition will become more tolerable.

The right side of the colon is currently the more popular colonic replacement of the oesophagus. Sherman, Mahoney, Dale and Stabins (1955), Nadal and Gustavson (1957), Battersby and Moore (1959) and Petrov (1959) have written much of their success in reconstructing the divided oesophagus.

The right side of the colon after preparation depends on its blood supply solely from the middle colic vessels. The right colic and ileocolic vessels are divided and the caecum or the terminal ileum may be used for anastomosis to the cervical oesophagus or pharynx. Its use is not without difficulties for in certain cases the right colic artery may be given off very close to the middle colic artery. When this happens, the anastomosis between the middle and right colic is exceptionally small and any division of the right colic artery will compromise the survival of the caecum, and ascending colon. If it is found that the right colic is the main artery to be preserved, additional length required for bringing the right side of the colon up to the pharynx, can be provided by the terminal ileum. It is our experience that when the vascular anastomosis between the middle and right colic arteries is deficient, the anastomosis between the former and the ileocolic is exceptionally good and a foot of the terminal ileum can be utilized with safety.

Besides the arterial insufficiency, venous inadequacy may be encountered. The middle colic vein may form a very small connecting channel with the right colic vein. Also at times the right colic vein may have a separate drainage into the right gastro-epiploeic vein. If this is the case it is most important not to ligate it. Failure to preserve this venous drainage will end in marked congestion of the colon and ascending colon. This will end in haemorrhage from the mucosa and gangrene of the loop.

Recently Brain and Reading (1966) used the right side of the colon in pharyngeal reconstruction and brought it up to the neck through a subcutaneous tunnel. This is a convenient route but if this method were employed additional length of the colon will be needed for it has to traverse a greater distance to reach the neck. The vascular pedicle should be placed behind the stomach and any kinking is to be avoided for a slightest kink will impede the venous return which may cause congestion and even gangrene. The caecum is anastomosed to the divided pharynx while the transverse colon is anastomosed to the body of the stomach.

The retrosternal route can be used also but in an obese individual the caecum may be bulky and then it may be difficult to advance it into the neck at the thoracic inlet. Should this be the case, it is wise to either abandon this method and use the subcutaneous route, or bring the colon into the neck through the posterior mediastinum. The retrosternal route gives a better cosmetic result and works well in suitable cases. In creating a retrosternal passage, it is most important not to tear the pleura to any large extent. This large tear in the pleura may go unnoticed and the colonic loop may then be displaced into the pleural cavity. The loop of colon may drop into the pleural cavity through this rent and marked distension of colon will take place. This distended loop of colon causes marked respiratory distress. It can be diagnosed by X-ray of the chest and when found should be relieved by aspirating the colon. Expansion of the lung and adhesion will prevent recurrence. Retrosternal route for reconstruction of the pharynx by colonic loop is a useful method.

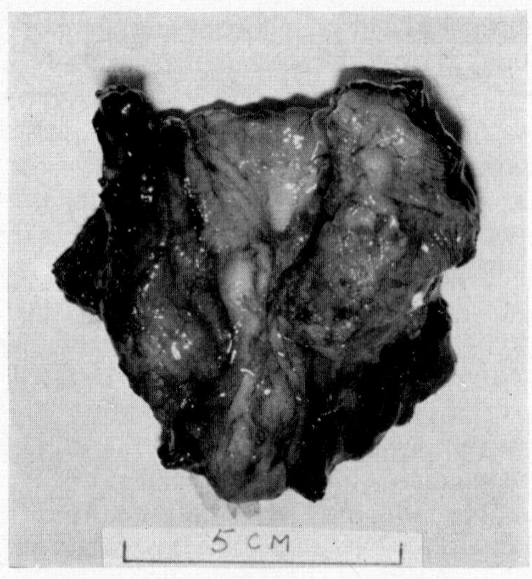

FIG. 9.8. Resected specimen of recurrent carcinoma of the hypopharynx.

The following case is a good example:

A male Chinese suffering from carcinoma of the epiglottis had laryngectomy carried out in 1961. Two years later he had a recurrence of the tumour which caused dysphagia. In 1963 he was operated on a second time and the pharynx including cervical oesophagus was excised. A retrosternal reconstruction with the right side of the colon was carried out. His convalescence was uneventful and was able to eat normally but finally succumbed to the disease 18 months later. (Figs. 9.8, 9.9 and 9.10.)

A convenient way of colonic replacement is through the posterior mediastinum. This has the advantage of the colon traversing the shortest route to the neck and the transverse colon can be anastomosed to the divided cardia while the caecum is anastomosed to the pharynx. Passage of food is not hindered in any way (Fig. 9.11).

(6) **Colonic graft.** With the development of fine vessel anastomosis, free grafts of segments of the gastrointestinal tract have been carried out. Seidenberg, Rosennak, Hurwitt and Som (1959) succeeded in grafting a

loop of jejunum to bridge the pharyngo-oesophageal gap after pharyngo-laryngectomy. Two years later Heibert and Cummings (1961) used the gastric antrum for the same purpose. In each instance the artery was anastomosed to the superior thyroid artery and the vein to its corresponding vein. The first to use the colon as a free graft was Eastcott (1964) who in 1954 on three cases, used the sigmoid colon as free graft.

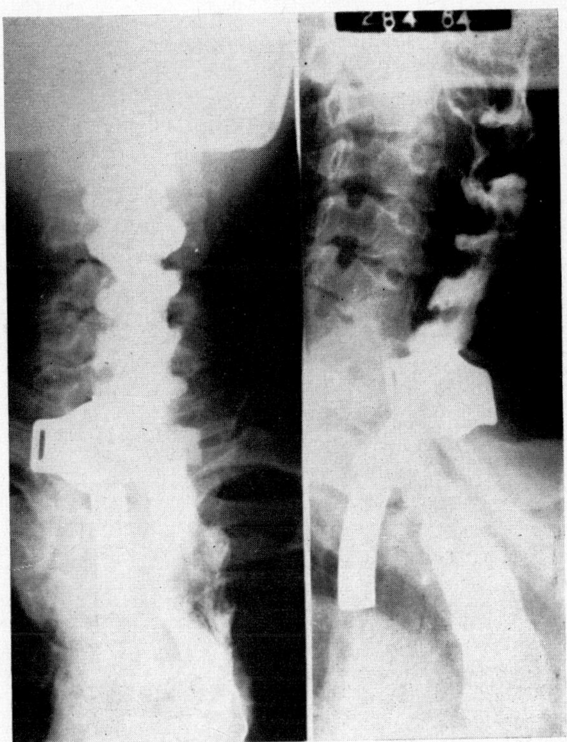

Fig. 9.9. Same case showing a barium swallow of the colonic-pharyngoplasty.

He anastomosed the inferior mesenteric artery to the external carotid artery and the vein to the lower end of the internal jugular vein. Nakayama (1962) succeeded in this form of reconstruction of the pharynx. He anastomosed the inferior mesenteric artery to the superior thyroid artery and the inferior mesenteric vein to the superior thyroid vein. He did this with the aid of his vascular stappler. Chrysopathis (1966) employing Nakayama's technique has had further success of this operation.

We have used transverse colonic graft for reconstruction of the pharynx but instead of using a stappler used direct suture anastomosis.

The patient was operated upon in 1963 for an advanced carcinoma of the hypopharynx. After pharyngo-laryngectomy with bilateral block dissection, a loop of the transverse colon was removed through a mid-line supra-umbilical incision. The loop of colon was placed in a separate trolley and there the middle colic was perfused with dextran in which 1,000 units per 500 ml. of heparin was instilled. Perfusion of the loop was kept on until the venous return was perfectly clear. The middle

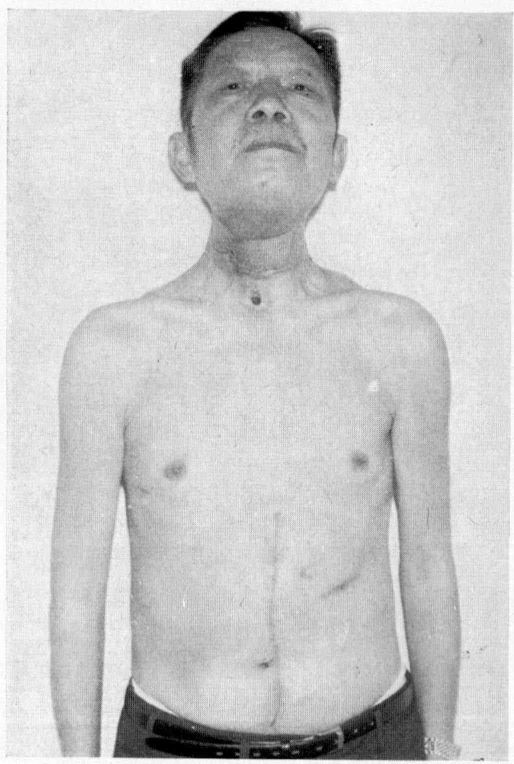

Fig. 9.10. The patient three months after the operation for a recurrent carcinoma of the hypopharynx.

colic artery was then sutured to the superior thyroid artery and the middle colic vein to the internal jugular vein. The proximal end of the colonic loop was then joined to the pharynx by a two layer suture and the distal end to the divided cervical oesophagus. At the completion of the operation, the colonic loop was healthy with peristalsis and the vessels were pulsating well. On the fourth day after operation the neck was found to be inflamed and by the end of the eighth day pus was oozing out from the suture line. It was therefore decided to excise the loop. This was done through the original incision and a drain was inserted into the neck.

Six weeks later the inflammation had subsided but a track had formed and which was draining saliva. Utilization of the skin for reconstruction

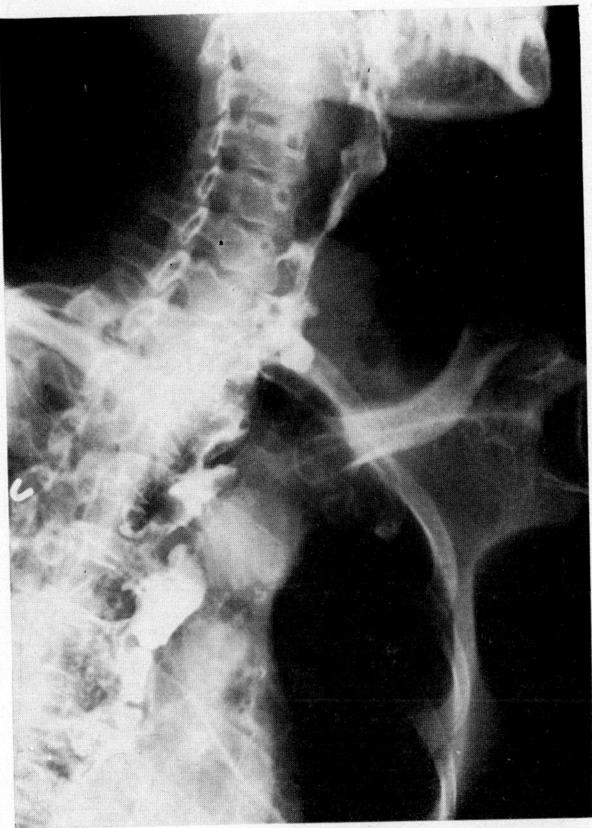

FIG. 9.11. Colonic replacement after laryngo-pharyngo-oesophagectomy in a case of hypopharyngeal carcinoma.

was not possible as it was unhealthy and the upper end of the oeso-phagus had completely closed. Several procedures were still available and which could be used for reconstruction:

(a) The left side of the colon could still be used. The right side could not be used as the middle colic artery had been severed.

(b) A reversed gastric tube could be made from the greater curvature of the stomach and the Heimlich-Winfield-Gauriliu procedure carried out or

(c) The jejunum could be utilized for reconstruction.

At laparotomy it was found that the jejunum was the most convenient organ to use in the reconstruction. Accordingly a long Roux loop was fashioned and one end was anastomosed to the pharynx while the other was joined to the stomach. This was done through a subcutaneous tunnel. Postoperative barium swallow showed it to be functioning well (Fig. 9.12).

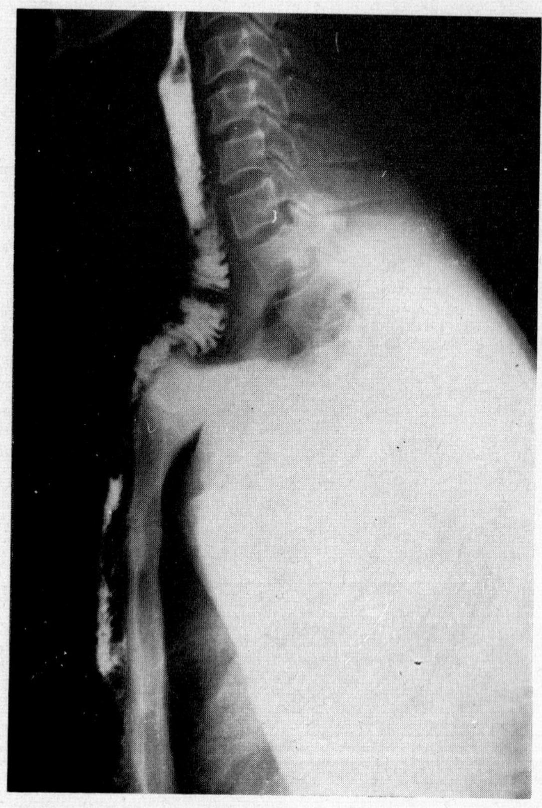

FIG. 9.12. Barium swallow of jejuno-pharyngeal reconstruction for carcinoma of the hypopharynx.

(7) **Use of the jejunum in the reconstruction of the pharynx.** Allison (1959) succeeded in fashioning a Roux loop and anastomosing one end to the base of the tongue and oropharynx. The other end was inserted into the stomach. The use of jejunum for replacing the oesophagus was first carried out by Roux in 1907. Robertson and Sargeant (1950) described the procedure in which they brought the jejunum to the neck through the anterior mediastinum. In most of these cases the jejunum was brought up as far as the neck where it was anastomosed to

the cervical oesophagus. However, there seems to be no difficulty in a
suitable case to stretch it higher to anastomose it to the pharynx.
Petrov (1959) found that he could advance the Roux loop by 10–20 cm.
into the neck if he were to free the mesentery from its attachment.
We have, however, not found this to be practicable.

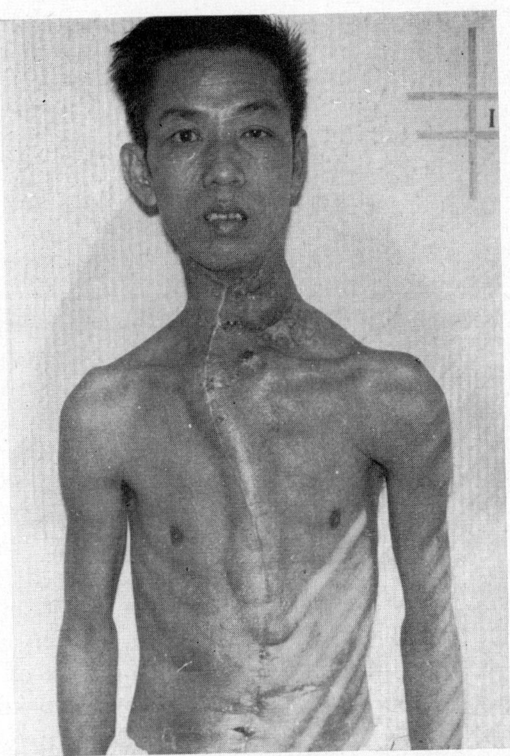

FIG. 9.13. Patient with carcinoma of the hypopharynx who had laryngo-pharyn-
gectomy and jejunal replacement. Note the long skin incision. See text.

The length of the loop depends on the length of the mesentery and
when the latter is long enough to reach the pharynx, in most instances,
there is a redundancy of the jejunum. Should anastomosis be carried
out as it is, there will be stasis in the jejunal loop. In order to avoid this
we have resected the excess of the small intestine by dividing the vasa
recti close to the anti-mesenteric border. This will shorten the loop
but will invariably straighten the intestine. Thus the undesirable side
effects of stasis is prevented.

The route, as in the case of the colon, by which the jejunum traverses
into the neck, is either subcutaneous, retrosternal or transthoracic.

But when it is brought up into the neck care must be taken that it does not undergo rotation with the mesentery as its axis. This is more likely to happen in the cases of the small intestine than in the colon. Rotation of the jejunum along its mesentery is liable to take place because of the redundancy of the loop. Cyanosis of the loop after being brought up into the neck is an indication that there is rotation and should be brought down into the abdomen again. This whole procedure of delivering it into the neck should be repeated until the displaced loop demonstrated a healthy pink colour. When the subcutaneous route is taken it is best to incise the skin throughout its length and after correctly placing the loop on the sternum, to stitch it over the intestine (Fig. 9.13).

Post-operative Care

Blood loss should be replaced and for the first two or three days before oral feeding is established intravenous fluids should be given. However, care must be taken not to overload these feeble individuals.

Care of the tracheostomy. The tracheostomy opening should be covered over by a layer of gauze kept moist with sterile saline. There is no necessity of inserting a tracheostomy tube until the wound has healed completely when a tracheostomy tube should be worn at night for at least six months. This will prevent stenosis of the trachestomy opening. Sputum tends to inspissate. A few drops of sterile saline instilled into the trachea before suction will facilitate evacuation.

Decompression of the gastrointestinal segment used for reconstruction is important. This is particularly so when the jejunum is used as distension of this loop may cause a delay in its recovery and sometimes may even compromise its blood supply. Aspiration of the displaced organ may be carried out with a nasal tube or in some patients with the aid of a gastrostomy tube.

Alimentation can be carried out when healing is proceeding well. Inspection of the suture line can be carried out by depressing the tongue or with the aid of a laryngoscope. If all goes well, fluids can usually be given about the third day and by the tenth postoperative, normal diet can usually be given.

Use of antibiotics. Post-operative antibiotics cover does not prevent wound infection but is most useful in avoiding respiratory infection. It is our practice to give penicillin and streptomycin for five days after the operation.

Prognosis

The advance made in recent years in surgical techniques has enabled more radical operations to be carried out in carcinoma of the hypopharynx and cervical oesophagus. In this, the development of modern anaesthesia, use of antibiotics to control infection and blood transfusion have greatly enhanced the safety of these major procedures.

Despite this improvement, the five year survival rate has not substantially improved (Macbeth, 1963; Ellis, 1966). From our own small series of 22 cases of postcricoid carcinoma only 2 survived for more than five years. Brain and Reading (1966) out of 16 cases had only 7 survivals and of these 3 were less than six months. One patient survived 4 years 3 months. Le Quesne and Ranger (1966) also had a similar result and only one case of their 10 cases operated upon was well after five years.

It would appear that on the average a five year survival of 10 per cent could be expected. Figures higher than this are exceptional but the rate may possibly be improved by carrying out surgery shortly after a course of radiotherapy. The current practice of operating only on recurrence after radiotherapy is not a good course to take. Operation should be carried out as soon as possible after an adequate dose of irradiation. The operation should be carried out before fibrosis has set in and a one-stage procedure should be adopted.

References

ALLISON, P. R. (1959). *Proc. R. Soc. Med.*, **52**, 176.

BALLANTYNE, A. J. (1964). *Am. J. Surg.*, **108**, 500.

BATTERSBY, J. S. and MOORE, T. C. (1959). *Surg., Gynec. Obstet.*, **109**, 207.

BENTLEY, F. H. and BARLOW, T. E. (1952). "The Vascular Anatomy of the Stomach"— Modern Trends in Gastroenterology, p. 309, edited by F. Avery Jones. London, Butterworths.

BRAIN, R. H. F. and READING, P. V. (1966). *Brit. J. Surg.*, **53**, 933.

CHRYSOSPATHIS, P. (1966), *Brit. J. Surg.*, **53**, 122.

EASTCOTT, H. H. G. (1964). *Lancet*, **2**, 1182.

ELLIS, MAXWELL (1958). "Pharyngo-laryngectomy", Operative Surgery, Vol. 8, p. 188 edited by Charles Rob and Rodney Smith. London, Butterworths.

ELLIS, MAXWELL (1959). *Proc. R. Soc. Med.*, **52**, 423.

ELLIS, MAXWELL (1966). "Clinical Surgery, Ear, Nose, Throat". Edited by Charles Rob and Rodney Smith, p. 220. London, Butterworths.

GOLIGHER, J. C. and ROBIN, I. G. (1954). *Brit. J. Surg.*, **42**, 283.

HEIMLICH, H. J. and WINFIELD, J. M. (1955). *Surgery*, **37**, 549.

HEIMLICH, H. J. (1966). *Brit. J. Surg.*, **53**, 913.

HEIBERT, C. A. and CUMMINGS, G. O., jun. (1961). *Ann. Surg.*, **15**, 103.

JACK, G. D. (1955). *Brit. J. Surg.*, **42**, 530.

JACOBSSON, F. (1951). *Acta Radiol.*, **35**, 1.

KAPLAN, I. and MARKOWICZ, H. (1964). *Brit. J. Plastic Surgery*, **17**, 314.

KELLING, G. (1911). *Zentbl. Chir.*, **30**, 1209.

LE QUESNE, L. P. and RANGER, D. (1966). *Brit. J. Surg.*, **53**, 105.

LEWIS, I. (1946). *Brit. J. Surg.*, **34**, 18.

MACBETH, R. (1963). *J. of the Royal College of Surgeons of Edinburgh*, **9**, 1.

MEADE, R. H. (1961). "A History of Thoracic Surgery", p. 659. Charles C. Thomas, Springfield, Illinois, U.S.A.

MEYERS, W. (1912). *J. Amer. Med. Assoc.*, **62**, 100.

NADAL, J. W. and GUSTAVSON, R. B. (1957). *Arch. Surg., Chicago*, **74**, 442.

NAKAYAMA, K. (1959). Personal Communication.

NAKAYAMA, K. (1962). *J. Int. Coll. Surg.*, **38**, 358.

ONG, G. B. and LEE, T. C. (1960). *Brit. J. Surg.*, **48**, 193.

ONG, G. B. (1964). *Brit. J. Surg.*, **51**, 53.

ORMEROD, F. C. (1961). Rep. 2 VIII Congress International Otorhino-laryngology Paris, 1961, 193.

ORSINI, P. and LEMAIRE, M. (1951). *J. Chir. Paris*, 67, 491.

PICKARD, B. H. (1965). "Benign and Malignant Tumours of the Larynx and Hypopharynx". Clinical Surgery, p. 91. Edited by Charles Rob and Rodney Smith. London, Butterworths.

PETROV, B. A. (1959). *Surgery*, **45**, 890.

RAVEN, R. and LEVISON, V. B. (1954), *Lancet*, **2**, 683.

ROBERTSON, R. and SARGEANT, T. R. (1950). *J. Thorac. Surg.*, **20**, 689.

ROUX, C. (1907). *Sem. mèdicale*, **27**, 37.

SCHWARTZ, D., DENOIX, P. F. and AUGUESA, G. (1957). *Bull., Ass. franc etude Cancer*, **44**, 336.

SEIDENBERG, B., ROSENNAK, S. S., HURWITT, E. S. and SOM, M. L. (1959). *Ann. Surg.*, **149**, 162.

SHERMAN, C. D., jun., MAHONEY, E. B., DALE, W. A. and STABINS, S. J. (1955). *Cancer*, **8**, 1198.

TROTTER, W. (1929). *Brit. J. Surg.*, **16**, 485.

TURNER, G. G. (1936). *Lancet i*, **67**, 130.

VULLIET, H. (1911). *Sem. mèdicale*, **31**, 529.

WOOKEY, H. (1940). *Brit. J. Surg.*, **27**, 696.

WOOLER, G. H. (1952). *Proc. R. Soc. Med.*, **45**, 264.

WYNDER, E. L., BROSS, I. J., and DAY, E. (1956). *J. Am. Med. Ass.*, **160**, 1384.

WYNDER, E. L., BROSS, I. J. and FELDMAN, R. M. (1957). *Cancer*, **10**, 1300.

WYNDER, E. L., BROSS, I. J. (1961). *Cancer*, **14**, 389.

ZEHM, S. (1965). *J. Laryn.*, **79**, 237.

CHAPTER 10

CONGENITAL URINARY OBSTRUCTION

D. INNES WILLIAMS

In spite of the many advances in the medical management of renal failure, the surgical relief of urinary obstruction provides, for the appropriate case, the best opportunity for obtaining a permanent improvement in renal function. This opportunity will be lost, however, if the disease process is already too far advanced by the time the patient presents for surgery, and in congenital obstruction this has all too frequently occurred. As in acquired disease the renal destruction may have reached an irreversible stage but in the congenital group there is in addition the danger that secondary changes in the urinary passages above the obstruction may also be irreversible. The grossly dilated, inert and tortuous ureter can never again function properly even if the renal tissue above it is adequately preserved. There is thus in children a pressing need for early diagnosis and for surgery which takes into account not only the relief of obstruction but the effects which that obstruction has already produced on the urinary tract motility.

Urinary obstruction may occur in very many forms and at various levels in the urinary tract. A complete review would be beyond the scope of this article but certain common abnormalities are picked out for discussion.

Pelvi-Ureteric Obstruction

Hydronephrosis due to pelvi-ureteric obstruction is the best known of all the congenital obstructive lesions since it often presents in adult life. It is, however, generally accepted that almost all these cases have a basic defect of structure or function in the segment of ureter immediately below the renal pelvis with, in addition, such factors as kinks, high insertion or overlying vessels. The time to check this defect should clearly be in childhood and diagnostic measures should be geared to detect the lesion before there is serious dilatation of the renal pelvis. It is common to find in well established cases of hydronephrosis during later childhood or adolescence a history of unexplained attacks of vomiting in infancy, followed in childhood by sporadic severe loin pain, perhaps so infrequent that they have not been investigated.

Sometimes, however, a pyelogram has been performed but pronounced normal, for at this stage the obstruction is intermittent and in states of dehydration with low urinary output no dilatation of the renal pelvis will be seen. Most intravenous pyelograms are, in fact, performed in the state of dehydration but a high dose pyelogram with a fluid load which results in a diuresis will show up the relative obstruction of the pelvi-ureteric junction and consequent hydronephrosis. It must therefore be emphasized that early cases will inevitably be missed unless high dose diuresis pyelograms are employed in all suspect cases.

The very earliest cases available for surgery should be those discovered at birth or soon after but in fact the neonatal hydronephroses form a separate group with several points of difference from those presenting later in childhood. In the neonate a renal enlargement is the most common presentation because the renal pelvis itself is enormously ballooned leaving the kidney as a small cap on one side. Bilateral disease is much more common at this stage than later in life and in some unilateral cases the contralateral kidney is cystic and non-functioning. In this group, therefore, the incidence of renal failure is high and the mortality by no means negligible although the simple ballooned renal pelvis is well worth treating by pyeloplasty (Williams and Karlaftis, 1966).

Techniques

The operative techniques of pyeloplasty hardly require further comment. The Anderson-Hynes operation (Fig. 10.1) is probably the

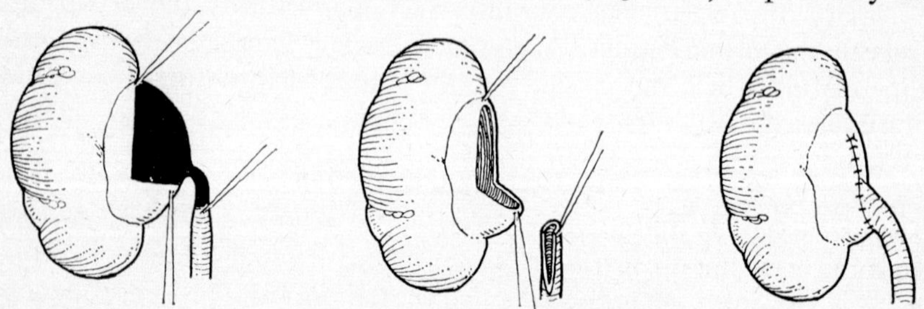

FIG. 10.1. The Anderson-Hynes pyeloplasty.

one most frequently performed in this country, though the Culp procedure is equally suited to many. The Foley Y-V. Plasty is well adapted to the ureter with a high implantation into the pelvis and the Davis intubated ureterotomy should be reserved for cases with a long strictured segment to the upper ureter. All these techniques, when carefully performed, are capable of giving good functional results although sometimes the radiological appearances are disappointing. Failures are often due to the operation being performed for a kidney already too severely damaged by dilatation or, more particularly, by complicating urinary infections and pyelonephritis.

Obstructive Mega-Ureter

The lesion which is responsible for congenital obstruction at the lower end of the ureter has much in common with the pelvi-ureteric obstruction producing hydronephrosis. There is an abrupt termination to the dilatation at, or a few centimetres above, the bladder; the terminal ureter is normal or narrow but will almost always accept the ureteric catheter with ease. The precise cause of the obstruction is unknown. Mega-ureter is much less common than hydronephrosis and is more likely to present in childhood. There is a considerable male predominance. Spasms of abdominal pain may be the initial complaint but recurrent urinary infection is very much more frequent than in cases with the higher level of obstruction. The diagnosis is usually adequately established by intravenous pyelogram provided a large dose of opaque medium is given and late films are taken. It may well be two or three hours before the dilated ureter fills and the lower end can be defined. Micturating cystograms are essential to differentiate this type of dilatation of the ureters from those with reflux or those in which a small saccule adjacent to the ureteric orifice produces a local obstruction to the ureter.

Treatment

The treatment of this type of obstruction consists essentially of excising the narrow segment of the ureter and re-implanting the cut

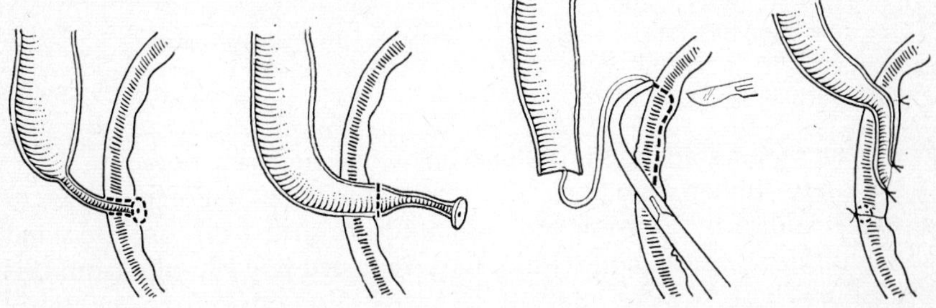

FIG.10.2. Reflux preventing re-implantation of the ureter.

end into the bladder. If, however, a direct wide anastomosis is made the consequent vesico-ureteric reflux will cause as much trouble as the obstruction, infection and progressive pyelonephritis are likely to follow. Provided the ureter is not too enormously dilated a reflux-preventing re-implantation can be made by a number of methods, most simply perhaps by the Politano-Leadbetter technique illustrated in Fig. 10.2. With a good re-implantation very satisfactory long term results may be anticipated with significant improvement in ureteric dilatation if not an entire return to normal (Fig. 10.3).

The difficulties encountered in these cases are, however, with the very gross dilatations where a valvular junction between ureter and bladder is hard to construct and the motility of the ureteric muscle

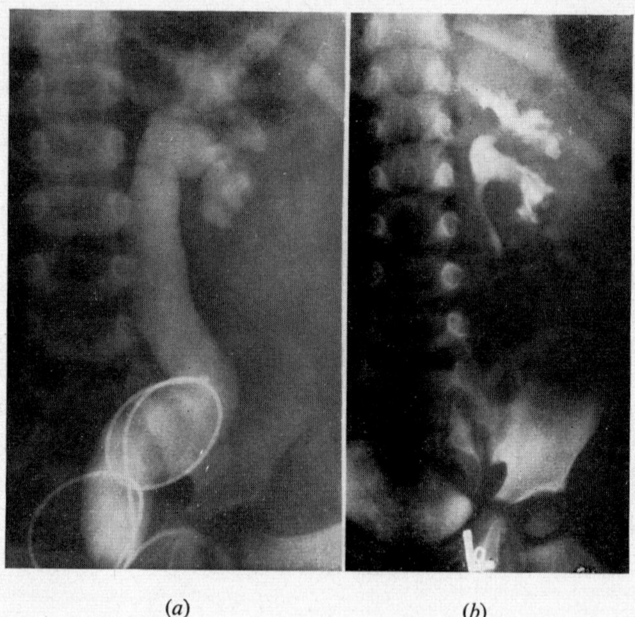

(a)   (b)

Fig. 10.3. Mega-ureter. (a) Pre-operative retrograde pyelogram.
(b) Post-operative intravenous pyelogram.

has been impaired to such an extent that active emptying does not occur. A very large ureter which has active muscle may be "tailored" down to a small calibre by excision of a longitudinal strip from one side and some authors, e.g. Bishoff, (1957) have reported good results from this procedure. It is, however, difficult to excise a long strip from the ureter without damaging the longitudinal blood supply and often the "tailored" segments become avascular and rigid. To overcome this other surgeons have attempted to replace a ureter by an isolated segment of ileum anastomosed to the bladder at the lower end. In children, however, isolated segments of ileum, even when draining freely on to the surface, are apt to become elongated and dilated and where they are anastomosed to the bladder such dilatation may be extreme, producing a vast reservoir of infected urine. Clearly in the face of such difficulties a nephro-ureterectomy is the appropriate treatment for an advanced unilateral case but in bilateral disease if a satisfactory junction cannot be established with the bladder, then the ureters must be drained on to the surface. With the long and tortuous ureters involved, a cutaneous ureterostomy is easily performed, both ureters may be brought around the peritoneum to open as a double-barrelled stoma in the mid-line of the lower anterior abdominal wall or one ureter may be led retro-peritoneally to join its fellow and brought to the surface in the iliac fossa at the site ordinarily selected for an ileostomy. Many good results may be obtained in this way, but no position of the stoma gives completely unimpeded flow through the ureter and if the musculature is inert cutaneous ureterostomies may require a period of indwelling catheter drainage before they are satisfactory.

In some cases it has been demonstrated that after a period of six to twelve months of cutaneous ureterostomy drainage the motility of the ureter has returned, the calibre has narrowed somewhat and re-implantation is then possible. Such a fortunate outcome is, however, unusual. In the long run cutaneous ureterostomies may be troublesome and become stenosed so that ileal conduit ureterostomy is preferred by many. If a long ileal segment is selected to drain urine directly from the renal pelves to the skin it can overcome the problem of an aperistaltic ureter. A long segment of ileum has, however, the disadvantage of exposing a large reabsorptive area and with damaged kidneys there is likely to be a severe bio-chemical imbalance as a result.

Ectopic Ureterocele

Ectopic ureterocele is an anomaly which has received less attention in the text-books than it deserves, being a relatively common cause of severe obstruction and sepsis in children. It almost always involves a duplex kidney and ureter, the ureter from the upper pole ending ectopically in the urethra a little below the bladder neck, but the terminal course of this ureter lies beneath the mucosa of the trigone where it is grossly dilated resembling the cystic dilatation of a ureterocele (Fig. 10.4). The upper pole ureter is dilated throughout its length and the segment of the kidney is hydronephrotic, but the presence of the ureterocele at the bladder neck obstructs the outflow from the bladder producing residual urine and dilatation of the other ureters: in addition the openings of these ureters may be distorted by the ureterocele and consequently allow reflux which persists after surgery to relieve the obstructive effect and maintains a chronic pyuria.

Ectopic ureterocele may present in a variety of ways; recurrent attack of pyuria with fever being the commonest. Retention of urine may occur, particularly in infants and in the female this may be associated with prolapse of the ureterocele through the urethral meatus. Severe attacks of abdominal pain are produced in a few by kinking and exacerbation of the obstruction in the ureterocele bearing ureter. The diagnosis is most easily made from intravenous pyelograms. The segment of the kidney from which the involved ureter arises has seldom sufficient concentrating ability to be opacified, but results in a

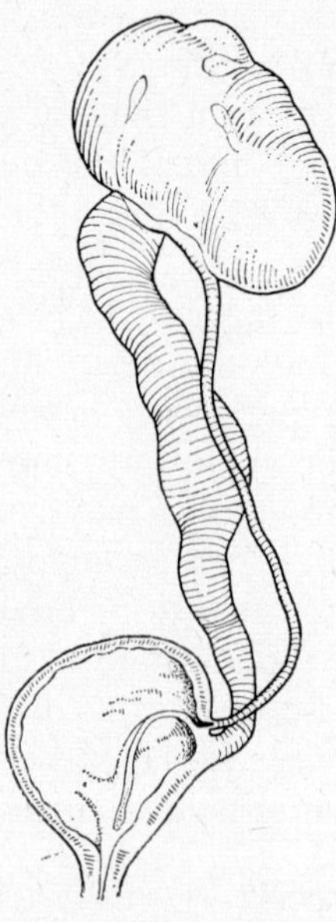

Fig. 10.4. Diagram to show the anatomy of a typical ectopic ureterocele.

characteristic displacement of the lower pole. The ureterocele itself shows as a filling defect in the bladder. Urethroscopy and cystoscopy confirm the diagnosis.

Relief of the bladder outflow obstruction may be obtained by opening the bladder and "uncapping" the ureterocele, ensuring that no flaps of mucosa are left to interfere with the bladder neck. This measure alone is, however, seldom sufficient, it will always leave a free reflux into the involved upper pole ureter which is dilated and functionally impaired. In these circumstances persistent pyuria is inevitable. The associated renal segment is very seldom worth preserving and a hemi-nephrectomy with ureterectomy is therefore appropriate. In the very few cases in which, because of overall renal failure, the upper pole must be preserved, an anastomosis between the upper ureter and the lower renal pelvis is the best treatment which allows excision of the greater part of this dilated ureter. It has already been mentioned, however, that the lower pole ureter itself, because of distortion of its lower end, may allow reflux and in a proportion of ureterocele cases re-implantation of this ureter by a reflux-preventing method is required.

Ectopic ureterocele, therefore, provides a further example of the way in which a congenital obstruction requires not only removal of the primary cause but appropriate treatment for the secondary effects on the urinary tract.

Posterior Urethral Valves

Valvular folds in the posterior urethra of the male infant are responsible for some of the most severe congenital obstructions to bladder outflow and a discussion of this lesion will illustrate the effects produced in a greater or lesser degree by all such obstructions.

Urine is produced by the foetal kidney at a very early age, probably by the 35 mm. stage. The urine is normally passed out into the amniotic fluid, swallowed and reabsorbed. Urine formation, therefore, plays no part in the maintenance of the bio-chemical equilibrium of the foetus but its complete absence as, in total obstruction, leads to oligo-hydramnios and to pressure deformities of the limbs. If the urine flow is partially obstructed the volume of amniotic fluid is not affected, secretion continues but the urinary tract exhibits all the changes customarily associated with later acquired obstructions but in a very advanced form, detrusor hypertrophy, with sacculation of the bladder, hydro-ureter and hydro-nephrosis. In addition the continued development of the later generations of nephrons is interfered with and cystic changes are produced in the kidney.

In severe examples of urethral valves, therefore, the kidneys are already irreversibly damaged at birth. The newborn infant appears normal for the first few days but suffers a rapidly progressive uraemia, manifested by vomiting, loss of weight, abdominal distension, dehydration and acidosis, accompanied by a distended overflowing bladder. The less severe the damage the later will the first signs appear, perhaps with renal failure, perhaps with acute urinary infection with difficult micturition or overflow incontinence.

A recent review of cases at Great Ormond Street (Williams and Eckstein, 1965) showed that nearly half the cases presented during the first three months of life and that during this early period the mortality approached 50 per cent: for the cases presenting later it was 12 per cent. The problem to be solved is therefore that presented by the uraemic infant, it is comparable in some respects with the uraemic prostatic, but the differences are worth examination. As in the elderly, the infant is extremely susceptible to a complicating infection, which is often the immediate cause of death. Whereas, however, in the prostatic we may think in terms of getting the patient fit for prostatectomy and then maintaining sterility until he resumes normal micturition, in urethral valves the removal of the obstruction is a relatively minor matter but the secondary changes in the urinary tract are such that even after operation there is still a great danger of continuing and fatal infection. Fig. 10.5 illustrates the extraordinary changes in the ureter which result from urethral valvular obstruction: drainage from these

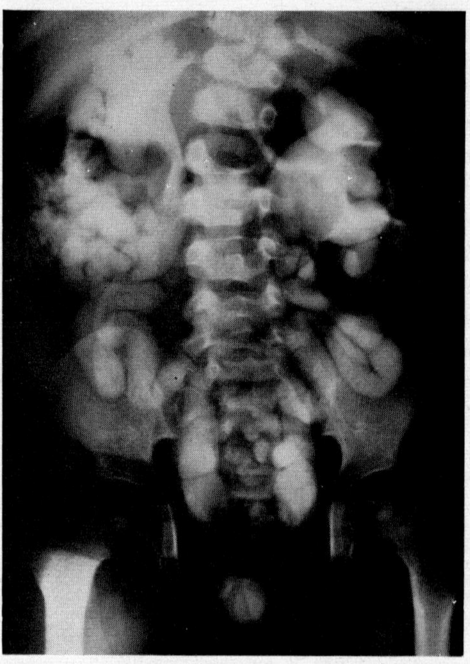

Fig. 10.5. I.V.P. showing tortuous ureters in a case of posterior urethral valves.

ureters is always poor and is made worse if the bladder is allowed to contract around an indwelling catheter since the bulk of the bladder muscle then constricts the intramural segments. It is the sacculated bladder, the dilated, obstructed or refluxing ureters and the dysplastic kidneys which make a successful outcome in these cases so difficult to achieve. Once infection is established in such a urinary tract it may be rapidly fatal or slowly destructive and in these circumstances free drainage of the upper urinary tract provides the only hope for survival.

In the older child without renal failure the diagnosis of urethral valve is suspected from the clinical signs of outflow obstruction and is confirmed by the micturating cysto-urethrography (Fig. 10.6). Transurethral resection removes the valvular fold and with careful control of sepsis a good result can be anticipated. In the uraemic infant a much more careful assessment is required and the programme varied according to particular circumstances. When the urine is sterile and the general condition is satisfactory, even though the blood urea may be well over 150 mg. per 100 ml., immediate preparation for operation should be made and no instrument passed until the child is brought to the operating theatre. Under anaesthetic a cysto-urethrogram is performed with expression of the bladder contents to demonstrate the presence of valves: the infants resectoscope is then introduced through a perineal

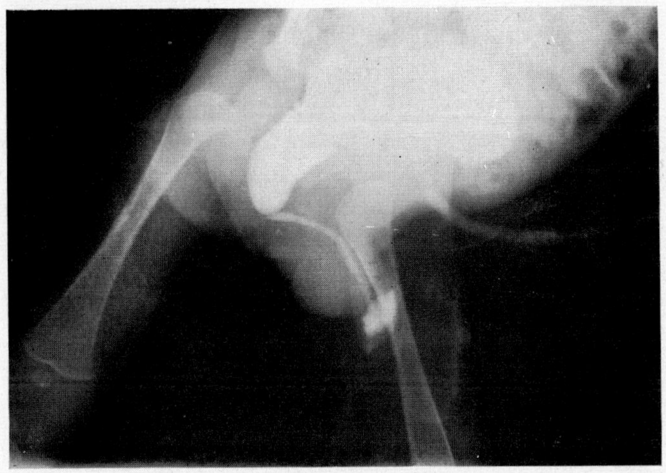

FIG. 10.6. Expression cystogram showing obstructive valves in the posterior urethra.

urethrostomy and post-operative drainage maintained by a 12 or 14 F self-retaining catheter passed through the same opening.

If the child's general condition seems precarious bio-chemical correction by peritoneal dialysis is probably the best measure. Catheter drainage alone is dangerous since the small calibre catheter which can be passed through the infant's urethra seldom gives free drainage for more than a few hours and inevitably introduces infection. A suprapubic cystostomy empties the bladder contents more effectively but allows contraction of the thickened bladder wall, thereby compressing the ureters. If, therefore, the urinary tract requires drainage for more than twelve hours, and a severe infection on admission is the usual and urgent indication for the procedure, then it must be by nephrostomy or ureterostomy.

Bilateral nephrostomy is easily performed and can be effective in infancy but maintenance of the tubes *in situ* for more than a few weeks is sometimes difficult and the presence of indwelling catheter itself maintains some infection. Nephrostomy drainage is therefore suitable for children with acute infection where the urinary tract is not too severely damaged and in whom early restoration of function can be anticipated.

Ureterostomy, on the other hand, provides the most effective drainage where this is required for a long period and indeed some cases require permanent ureterostomies if the child is to survive. The procedure for terminal cutaneous ureterostomy has already been mentioned, an alternative for the urethral valve case is provided by the loop ureterostomy, analagous to the loop colostomy, which leaves the ureter in continuity over a skin bridge. This is suitable for drainage for some months and is relatively easy to reconstitute if renal and ureteric function have improved. The loop is excised and the cut ends of the ureter anastomosed. It is, however, essential that reflux should be eliminated if this has been present, and for refluxing ureters, a terminal ureterostomy, subsequently re-implanted into the bladder, is preferred. These complex measures are required on a relatively few cases: they have been emphasized, however, to underline the differences between congenital and acquired lower urinary tract obstruction.

References

ANDERSON, J. C. and HYNES, W. (1949). *Brit. J. Urol.*, **21**, 209.
BISCHOFF, P. (1957). *Brit. J. Urol.*, **29**, 416.
CULP, O. S. and DE WEERD, J. H. (1951). *Proc. Mayo Clinic*, **26**, 483.
FOLEY, F. E. B. (1937). *J. Urol.*, **38**, 643.
POLITANO, V. A. and LEADBETTER, W. F. (1958). *J. Urol.*, **79**, 932.
WILLIAMS, D. I. and ECKSTEIN, H. B. (1965). *J. Urol.*, **93**, 236.
WILLIAMS, D. I. and KARLAFTIS, C. M. (1966). *Brit. J. Urol.*, **38**, 138.
WILLIAMS, D. I. and WOODARD, J. R. (1964). *J. Urol.*, **92**, 635.

Chapter 11

NEONATAL INTESTINAL OBSTRUCTION

A. W. Wilkinson

During the last 10 or 15 years there has been a good deal of progress in the understanding and management of intestinal obstruction in the newly born child. As the overall mortality for all types of lesion has diminished critical analysis of the results has shown where improvement may still be made, as well as the benefits of new forms of treatment and the disadvantages of some of the old practices.

Diagnosis

The importance of a full and accurate history of the clinical disturbance remains as great as ever. The history will in many cases give a good indication of the level of obstruction and sometimes the precise diagnosis, for example the observation of bubbling frothy saliva in oesophageal atresia, bile stained vomiting in obstruction below the Ampulla of Vater and the early alteration in the nature and frequency of the stools in Hirschsprung's disease. There is no doubt that often much too little attention is paid to the account of the illness. It is still not uncommon for newly born babies to vomit bile stained fluid repeatedly for a week or more before the suspicion of intestinal obstruction is aroused; it cannot be too strongly or too often emphasized that while most babies vomit occasionally, one who vomits repeatedly, especially if the vomit is bile stained, must be assumed to have an intestinal obstruction and be referred to a surgeon.

In the neonate, as in older patients, the degree of distension of the abdomen with fluid and gas depends on the level of the obstruction as well as on its duration. In meconium obstruction and in Hirschsprung's disease abdominal distension may be so marked at the time of birth as to hinder the delivery of the baby. The postnatal accumulation of swallowed air and fluid and of intestinal secretions merely aggravates existing abdominal distension. There may also be notable abdominal distension associated with rectal atresia in the absence of a fistula. In atresia of the small intestine there is seldom much distension of the belly at birth but in ileal atresia this may soon appear. Distension is seldom if ever obvious in duodenal atresia except between the costal margins. The scaphoid abdomen associated with a large diaphragmatic hernia is as characteristic a sign as the great distension found in colonic obstructions.

Because of the much greater importance of the diaphragmatic part of respiration in the neonate, abdominal distension which is severe enough to interfere with the free movement of the diaphragm will have a marked effect on respiratory exchange. This leads sooner or later to the failure of the baby to excrete carbon dioxide adequately and to a respiratory acidosis. It then depends on the type of fluid which is being lost by vomiting or into the lumen of the obstructed intestine what kind of total disturbance in acid base equilibrium will result.

Diagnosis of the existence as well as the level of obstruction is greatly assisted by, if indeed it does not depend on, the appearances seen in an anteroposterior radiograph of the abdomen taken with the baby in the upright position. This simple procedure, which is often not used until a late stage, is usually all that is needed to provide the indication for an exploratory laparotomy, and further radiological investigation with radio-opaque medium is seldom needed. Perhaps only in Hirschsprung's disease is it necessary or justifiable to employ a barium enema. Even in oesophageal atresia there is no real need to outline the proximal segment with radio-opaque material. Obstruction is indicated by the presence of fluid levels of which the site and size may be characteristic in particular kinds of obstruction, for example the "double bubble" of duodenal atresia. In lower obstructions there may be many fluid levels each with a superimposed gas shadow which should show variations in size consistent with the different degrees of distension of the intestinal loops. In obstruction due to the inspissated meconium associated with mucoviscidosis ("meconium ileus") fluid levels are less common, if they are seen at all, because the material inside the intestine is too thick and viscid to form fluid levels in the lower reaches of the obstructed bowel. Abdominal distension may be very severe in meconium obstruction as in Hirschsprung's disease and these two forms of obstruction have several other features in common which may increase the difficulties of distinguishing between them; in both the average birth weight is within the normal range (Holsclaw et al., 1965; Fraser and Wilkinson, 1967). The X-ray appearances of the abdomen in Hirschsprung's disease may be confusing and un-characteristic, there may not be any fluid levels but the loops of distended intestine may be very large.

In volvulus of the midgut although the radiological appearances of the abdomen are sometimes quite characteristic more often they give little direct help; this in its own way may be suggestive of the diagnosis. It is important to remember that abdominal distension with vomiting, sometimes of bile stained fluid, and delay in passing meconium may

occur in premature babies born after complicated deliveries. The
upright radiograph of the abdomen may show gas shadows but without
fluid levels. This disturbance may occur also in association with severe
infection in the early neonatal period and after head injury or severe
anoxia. The confusion of this clinical situation is made worse by the fact
that some babies with this sort of disturbance may improve soon after

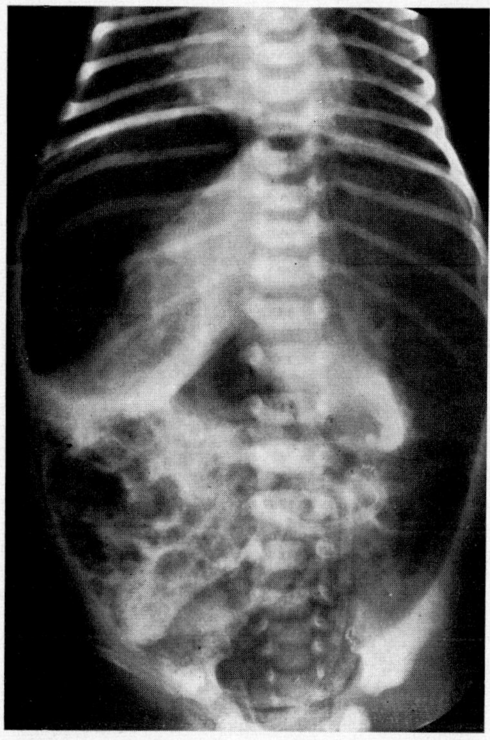

Fig. 11.1. X-ray in the upright position of neonate with spontaneous gangrene
and perforation of the small intestine with extensive escape of gas in the
peritoneal cavity showing large collections of gas beneath the diaphragm and
thick peritoneal exudate amongst the loops of intestine.

the passage of firm and rather pale abnormal meconium (meconium
plug syndrome). In others at laparotomy a similar piece of meconium
is found apparently obstructing the bowel whereas in another nothing
to explain the distension can be found. Hirschsprung's disease can
usually be largely excluded by X-ray examination after a barium enema,
provided the child is fit for this and the bowel has not previously been
washed out. There is however no question that when real doubt exists
whether there is an organic obstruction or not the safest course is to

open the abdomen, rather than to continue to try to treat an organic obstruction by conservative measures. Provided the diaphragm and part at least of the lung fields are always included in any film of the abdomen, diaphragmatic hernia should not usually be difficult to recognize. If the possibility is remembered congenital cysts of the lung should not be confused with diaphragmatic hernia in the neonate. The so-called "saddle bag" appearance (Parrish *et al.*, 1964) (Fig. 11.1) is characteristic when perforation of the intestine has been followed by the escape of a lot of gas from the bowel. The perforation may be due to tension gangrene of the wall of the caecum or colon in Hirschsprung's disease or to so-called "spontaneous gangrene of the newborn" at any or several levels in the small or large intestine.

Most normal babies usually pass normal meconium within 24 hrs. of birth. It is still not generally recognized that normal meconium may be passed on several occasions during the first 48 hrs. after birth by a baby who has intestinal obstruction due to atresia of the small intestine; this is undoubtedly liable to mislead if the coincident repeated bilious vomiting is not given its full significance. It is now generally accepted that atresias of the small intestine are most probably due to a vascular accident during gestation and that at the time this occurs the intestine contains meconium above and below the level of the occlusion. Not all the material in the distal segment of intestine may have been passed before birth and its subsequent appearance on the napkins may lead to the wrong assumption that the bowel is normal. Clinicians in general still fail to take enough interest in the detailed personal examination of vomitus and faeces. It is equally important to recognize the abnormal meconium which may be seen in meconium obstruction (or "ileus") and in Hirschsprung's disease. On rectal examination in the former the anal canal and rectum feel normal but there is no normal meconium, only perhaps some dry and pale gray clay-like material. In the latter unless the rectum has already been examined the anal canal and rectum may be tight, and withdrawal of the finger may be followed by the explosive expulsion of gas and offensive smelling pale khaki coloured fluid.

Acid-base Disturbances

Disturbances of acid base equilibrium are common and may be complicated in babies with intestinal obstruction. Their course can now be followed readily since the introduction of the micro-Astrup technique of blood gas analysis (Siggaard Andersen *et al.*, 1960) and the modification of the Astrup nomogram (Siggaard Andersen, 1962). It is now possible to separate rapidly and easily the respiratory and metabolic components of acid base equilibrium in the blood. pH is measured on arterialized capillary blood from a heel stab which is then equilibrated with mixtures of oxygen and carbon dioxide of known composition. Although both respiratory and metabolic components are measured in addition to pH the metabolic component is the most important and is expressed as base excess. A positive base excess indicates a deficit of fixed acid or metabolic alkalosis and a negative base excess a deficit of base or an excess of fixed acid, metabolic acidosis. Because compensation is usually good pH alone is not of much help. The aetiology of any disturbance of acid base equilibrium in a neonate should always be carefully studied and the contributions and primacy of the respiratory and metabolic components assessed before any treatment is applied. Although the compensatory capacity of the neonate may be less than that of an adult it appears to be adequate for most circumstances.

Most neonates with obstruction of the alimentary tract are subjected to a degree of starvation which is enough to cause acidosis but it must be remembered that this will be rapidly corrected when the baby is fed with milk. In oesophageal atresia acidosis due to starvation is aggravated by hypoxia due to inhalation of mucus or to pneumonia. Although a severe negative base excess can be temporarily corrected by the administration of T.H.A.M., treatment should rather be directed to the correction of hypoxia and starvation. The benefits of early feeding with milk after operation are well known but it remains uncertain whether there is any disadvantage in allowing the bio-chemical disturbance of the blood to disappear spontaneously. In duodenal atresia acidosis due to starvation is obscured by the much more marked alkalosis due to the loss of hydrogen ion in the fluid vomited or aspirated from the distended stomach and proximal duodenum. The value of an indwelling fine portex tube passed across the duodeno-jejunostomy into the distal limb of the jejunostomy (Ehrenpreis and Sandblom, 1949) is twofold. First, further extrarenal losses of fluid and especially of hydrogen ion can be prevented by injection of the fluid sucked from the stomach into the jejunum beyond the duodenal obstruction, and secondly, full strength milk feeds can be administered from 24 hrs. after operation.

In more distal obstructions the acid base disturbance, due to the vomiting of gastrointestinal secretions, is complicated by interference with respiratory exchange by gross abdominal distension which hinders diaphragmatic movement. Here also early operative treatment may be critical. In addition to relief of the obstruction the proximal intestine should be sucked empty of accumulated gas and fluid. This improves both intestinal and respiratory function. The secondary effects of negative base excess on cardiac function may be exaggerated in patients with cardiovascular anomalies and more attention should be given to this aspect of treatment both before and after operation.

Pre- and Post-operative Treatment and Surgical Technique

Broadly speaking there are two attitudes to the pre-operative treatment of the baby with acute intestinal obstruction. Some clinicians believe that before operation an attempt should be made to replace by intravenous infusion the fluid which has been lost by vomiting or in other ways. These clinicians estimate the losses of body fluid from the loss of weight which has occurred from birth until the time of admission. In replacement allowance is also made for the insensible loss of water vapour through the skin and expired air and for an arbitrary volume of urine based on the intake and output of a normal child of the same age. These estimates would probably be more physiological if they made more allowance for the large difference in composition and caloric content of the replacements compared with human breast milk. Others hold on the contrary that such replacements are not necessary unless the blood volume has been reduced, in which case it should be restored to an adequate level by the transfusion of blood before the operation is begun. While the truth probably lies somewhere between these two extremes no one now doubts that before any operation on a neonate begins, blood should be available for transfusion to replace losses during operation which exceed 10 ml. The widespread use of non-explosive anaesthetic agents in neonatal surgery allows the surgeon to use diathermy and to reduce the loss of blood during thoracotomy or laparotomy to only 5 or 10 ml. and thus to avoid the need for transfusion in most patients. Until recently it was thought to be essential that a needle or cannula should be placed in a sufficiently large vein to enable the anaesthetist to inject his drugs and blood if this should be necessary. For abdominal operations during the first two or three weeks of life the umbilical vein offers a very convenient means of rapid blood replacement (Wilkinson, 1963). This vein is divided in making the transverse laparotomy incision and will accommodate a larger cannula than any vein in the limbs. The need to withdraw the cannula towards the end of the operation means that replacement transfusion must be completed during the operation and if further intravenous therapy is judged to be necessary another vein must be used. The umbilical vein can also be used for rapid transfusion or infusion before operation; the vein is exposed by a short transverse incision in the line of the laparotomy incision and lifted out of its bed in the falciform ligament.

There are also divergent views about postoperative treatment which have an important influence and effect on the technical procedures which are adopted for the relief of intestinal obstruction. The free use of intravenous fluid therapy based on arbitrary estimates of "normal" requirements, with the associated delay in the return of intestinal motility and absorptive capacity to normal, and the larger extrarenal losses of minerals and water in the more prolonged periods of gastric aspiration, is slowly giving way to a more rational approach to the homeostatic and nutritional problems of the neonate after laparotomy or thoracotomy.

The capacity of the human neonate to tolerate deprivation of water and food for several days, provided there are no large extrarenal losses, is widely recognized and respected. Some degree of starvation for up to four days after birth is common for normal neonates (Wilkinson, Stevens and Hughes, 1962) and may be extended for several days after operation without great harm. The dependence of normal metabolic development and homeostasis on the establishment of an adequate intake of milk has been repeatedly emphasized by McCance and Widdowson (1961). Moreover the neonate is not able to deal with large loads of water or mineral salts either by mouth or by infusion with the same speed or efficiency as an older child or adult and is thus much more vulnerable to the injudicious or excessive administration of solutions by intravenous infusion. A week after birth the normal infant may be consuming about 400 ml. of milk containing about 7 g. of protein, 7–8 m.Eq. potassium and 5–6 m.Eq. sodium, and will absorb about 85 per cent of this intake from the bowel and retain about 65 per cent for incorporation in new tissue. Only the equivalent of about 20 per cent of this intake requires to be excreted in the urine and renal capacity of the neonate is related to this low normal excretory requirement. It is too often forgotten that when parenteral therapy is planned on the basis of a normal intake of milk much less of the parenteral intake can be incorporated in new tissue because it contains so incompletely the normal constituents of protoplasm. Whereas about 65 per cent of the water content of a daily intake of 400 ml. of milk will be included in the water of new tissue and only 20 per cent will require to be excreted, when 400 ml. of water is infused as saline or glucose or other solutions about 60 per cent or more must be excreted after the normal requirements for insensible water loss and urine formation have been satisfied.

The appreciation of the importance of starting feeds as soon as possible after operation has led to several important modifications in post-operative treatment. In oesophageal atresia for example some surgeons pass a fine soft Portex tube through the nose and down the oesophagus across the anastomosis into the stomach and feed the child through this tube from about 24 hrs. after operation (Hughes *et al.*, 1965). Others use a gastrostomy for feeding. In duodenal atresia a modification of the method suggested by Ehrenpreis and Sandblom (1949) may be used. In this a fine Portex tube is passed through the abdominal wall into the stomach by the side of a gastrostomy tube and then on across the pylorus, through the dilated proximal portion of duodenum, across the anastomosis made between the obstructed duodenum and the first loop of jejunum into the distal limb of the jejunal loop (Wilkinson *et al.*, 1965) (Fig. 11.2). By injecting all the fluid which is aspirated from the stomach into the jejunum in this way extrarenal losses of gastric and duodenal secretions are completely avoided. In

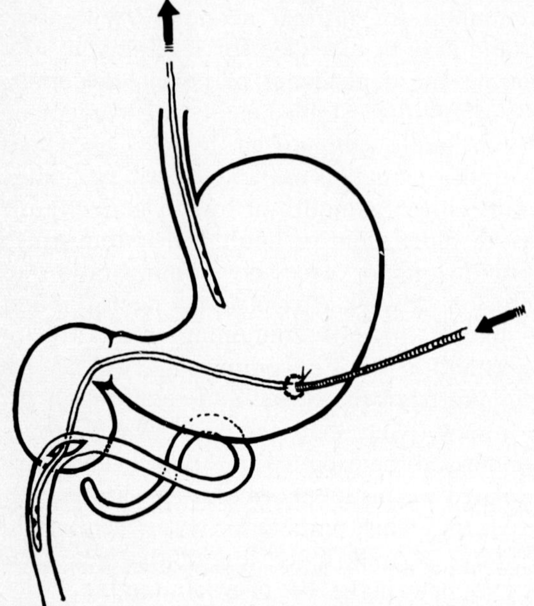

FIG. 11.2. Arrangement of tubes for gastric aspiration and jejunal feeding in duodenal atresia.

addition milk feeds can be started within 24 hrs. of operation by direct injection into the jejunum. When this method is used parenteral therapy is unnecessary. The large quantities of sodium which can be lost when the aspirated gastric and duodenal secretions are thrown away are clearly shown in Fig. 11.3. In ten days such losses may be equal to the total initial extracellular sodium content of the baby and the need to replace by infusion is obvious, a need which can be completely avoided by the method described.

The same principles of avoiding extra-renal fluid losses by the instillation of fluid sucked out of the stomach into the bowel below the level of obstruction, combined with the early institution of full strength milk feeds, is now also applied to obstructions of the jejunum and ileum. This is made possible by the use of the Bishop-Koop type of

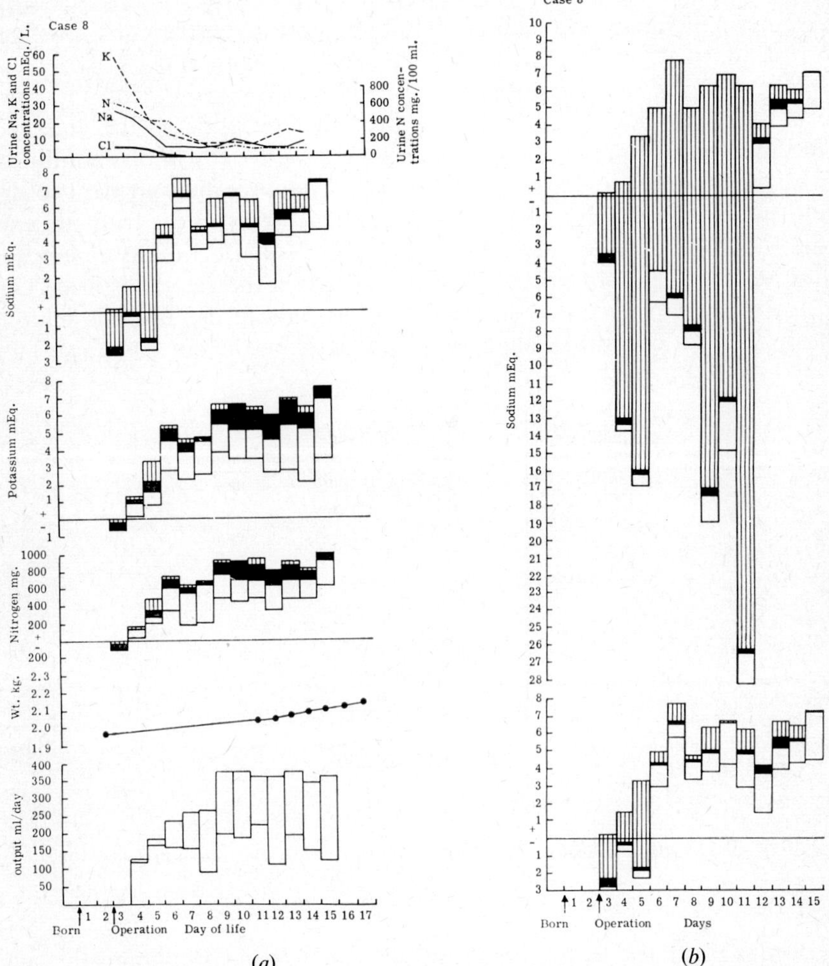

FIG. 11.3(*a*). Metabolic balance study of baby with duodenal atresia treated by duodeno-jejunostomy and jejunal tube to show prevention of extrarenal losses by the replacement of fluid aspirated from stomach into jejunum and the rapid achievement of positive balance for nitrogen and potassium as soon as feeding through the jejunal tube was begun. Vertical lines indicate losses by aspiration, in this case due to the retention of aliquot of aspirated fluid for chemical analysis; black areas losses in faeces; clear areas losses in urine. The intake is plotted up from the base line and the output down from the top of the intake. (With kind permission of the Editor of the British Journal of Surgery.)

FIG. 11.3(*b*). Sodium balance as in Fig. 3(*a*) above plotted to show the quantities of sodium which would have been lost if replacement of the fluid aspirated from the stomach had not been reinjected through the jejunal tube.

end-to-side enterostomy (Bishop and Koop, 1957). In dealing with atresia of the jejunum or ileum the dilated and hypertrophied terminal 6 to 8 in. of the proximal blind segment of intestine must be resected. In the past the usual method of restoring continuity of the intestine was to anastomose the end of the proximal intestine to the end and anti-mesenteric border of the distal segment. In a baby in bad condition it is often quicker to anastomose the end of the proximal segment to the anti-mesenteric border of the distal segment about 3 in. from its end and then bring out the proximal end of this distal portion as an enterostomy. (Fig. 11.4.) In obstruction due to atresia the gastric aspirate can be instilled into the enterostomy as well as milk feeds. There is seldom more than an occasional slight loss of fluid from the enterostomy. This

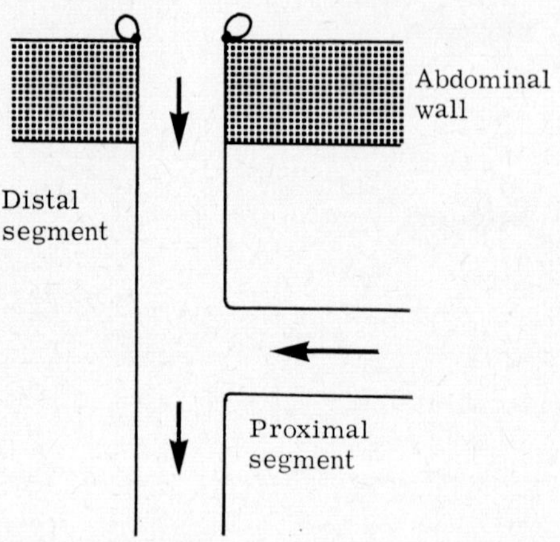

Fig. 11.4. End-to-side type of enteroanastomosis with distal terminal ileostomy (Bishop and Koop 1957).

procedure which was originally devised for use in meconium obstruction has been used successfully for obstruction due to atresia even in the upper loops of jejunum.

When the Bishop-Koop enterostomy is used for meconium obstruction it is no longer necessary to clear the inspissated meconium from more than 3 or 4 ins. of the distal contracted segment of ileum, but the dilated proximal segment should of course be resected until bowel of more normal size is obtained for anastomosis to the distal ileum. Pancreatic extract should be instilled into the enterostomy as well as given by mouth or stomach tube. Meconium obstruction is only one manifestation of the triad of mucoviscidosis but the use of the end-to-side anastomosis with terminal ileostomy has made it possible to avoid completely post-operative parenteral therapy, with a consequent diminution in pulmonary complications and a reduction in the immediate mortality rate to about 30 per cent.

Diaphragmatic Hernia

The Perinatal Mortality Survey (1962) showed that many babies with congenital diaphragmatic hernias died soon after delivery. It was hoped that earlier recognition and surgical treatment of the herniation, combined with the insufflation of oxygen through an intratracheal catheter during transfer to a surgical unit, would result in a higher survival rate. This hope has been only partially realized because it is now recognized that the respiratory difficulties which are such an important factor in these deaths may be due at least partly to the poorly developed state of the lung on the affected side; this is probably secondary to the presence of a large part of the intestine and abdominal viscera in the chest for some time before birth. Snyder and Greaney (1965) found that the weight of the lungs of neonates who died of diaphragmatic hernia was only 70 per cent of that of normal neonates equivalent to a reduction in respiratory capacity of about 40 per cent. Even when operative reduction of the hernia is expeditious and abdominal distension is not an important factor because the intestine has not had time to fill with swallowed air, persistent pulmonary insufficiency may be so severe as to prevent survival.

A transverse upper abdominal incision provides the most convenient way of reducing the contents of the hernia and the best access for repair of the diaphragm. It also allows the creation of extra space by wide mobilization of the abdominal skin for the formation of a temporary ventral hernia should the capacity of the abdomen itself be too small to accept all the contents of the hernia. When the intestine is distended with gas and fluid it should always be sucked out at operation to reduce tension after closure of the abdomen. Before the last stitch in the diaphragmatic repair is tied, as much as possible of the air in the pleural cavity should be aspirated by a catheter passed up from the abdomen. Opinion is divided on whether post-operative drainage of the pleural cavity is always necessary. Sometimes however there is a sudden deterioration in the condition of the child towards the end of the operation and following an earlier improvement in colour and cardiac and respiratory function after reduction of the contents of the hernia. This may be due to a spontaneous pneumothorax on the opposite side of the chest the cause of which remains uncertain. This should be treated immediately by aspiration of the air from the pleural cavity and the establishment of sealed drainage; in this situation it is desirable to put a similar drain into the other pleural cavity as well.

Exomphalos and Gastroschisis

Exomphalos or omphalocoele continues to tax the pediatric surgeon and, in spite of various forms of treatment, to carry an overall mortality rate of about 40 per cent. The mortality rate is highest, about 80 per cent, when the sac is very large or is ruptured during or soon after delivery, when the baby is small or when there are associated severe anomalies. It was hoped that conservative treatment for example by repeatedly painting the wall of the sac with mercurochrome or some similar solution would reduce the mortality rate; unfortunately this has not been very successful, partly because it involves a long stay of 8 to 10 weeks in hospital with the inseparable risks of infection. Operation is essential when the sac has a narrow neck and contains liver or when it is suspected that the intestine contained in the sac is atretic. With a wide rather hemispherical defect it is sometimes possible to cut the skin away from the margins of the sac which is left intact. The skin is then widely freed on all sides except over the costal margins and its edges sewn together over the fundus of the intact sac. The remaining muscular defect of the anterior abdominal wall is dealt with when the child is several years old.

Gastroschisis is often mistaken for a ruptured exomphalos. In gastroschisis there is a circular defect of the anterior abdominal wall usually immediately to the right of a normal umbilical cord. There is seldom any sign of a hernial sac and through the defect most of the alimentary tract prolapses in utero. The baby is born with a matted mass of intestine protruding at the side of the umbilical cord. This should be covered at once with some kind of protective dressing; gauze soaked in 0·9 per cent saline is probably the best form of cover provided cooling of the baby by evaporation of water from the gauze is prevented by an outer cover of some impermeable material such as plastic sheeting. At operation it is seldom possible to separate the matted loops of intestine nor does this seem to be necessary. The opening in the abdominal wall should be enlarged by transverse incision on either side which should divide all layers of the abdominal wall including the whole width of the rectus muscles. The skin and subcutaneous tissue should be widely raised by dissection with the cutting diathermy from the surface of the external oblique aponeurosis and the skin then closed over the bowel and the enlarged defect in the muscle layers. The wide division of the muscles is necessary to prevent such a large increase in intra-abdominal tension that diaphragmatic excursion is hindered and gaseous respiratory exchange is reduced. When after two or more years the time comes to repair the muscular defect the capacity of the abdomen should first be increased by repeated distension with oxygen injected into the peritoneal cavity.

Stenosis and Atresia of the Colon

Atresia of the colon is one of the rarest anomalies of the intestine and probably occurs only about once in every 15,000 births. Peck, Lynn and Harris (1963) found only 36 reported cases and added 2 of their own. The transverse and pelvic parts are most commonly affected and there may be extensive loss of the bowel most probably because of intrauterine volvulus. Colonic atresia presents as a low intestinal obstruction and at laparotomy is usually readily recognized. It may be associated with absence or atresia of the rectum and extroversion of the bladder. Colonic atresia can be satisfactorily relieved by colostomy and restoration of continuity of the bowel can be delayed until the child is older. When the ileocaecal valve is competent there is a risk of perforation of the caecum and X-ray examination after a barium enema is liable to give misleading evidence of the nature of the obstruction.

Colostomy in Infancy

The commonest indication for colostomy in infancy is low intestinal obstruction due to a congenital anorectal anomaly or Hirschsprung's disease. Such colostomies are usually closed after the definitive operation on the primary lesion, which is now commonly delayed until the child is about a year old. Only rarely when there are gross abnormalities of the central nervous and urinary systems as well as of the alimentary tract is a colostomy likely to be permanent and the temporary nature of the colostomy should always be explained to parents.

For anorectal anomalies the colostomy should be made in the right half of the transverse colon since this allows a good deal more freedom to mobilize the rectum at the definitive abdominoperineal operation than a pelvic colostomy; this is the best site also in Hirschsprung's disease provided the aganglionic segment does not extend above this level. Prolapse of the colostomy is much commoner in infants than in adults and to prevent this the colon proximal to the opening should be sewn to the anterior abdominal wall. The best access for laparotomy in the newly born child is through a long transverse incision just above the umbilicus. The colon should be drawn out through the right half of such an incision and emptied of gas and fluid by suction through a wide-bored needle inserted at the apex of the loop. The posterior layer of the rectus sheath is closed in the left half of the incision, and then as the continuous catgut stitch is continued across the right half of the incision each bite includes the wall of the distal limb of the colon for an inch or so and the stitch is tied. The limbs of the colon loop are then sewn to the posterior rectus sheath with interrupted stitches, care being taken to close off the space between the limbs and the mesocolon. The rest of the deep layer of the wound is then closed with a continuous stitch, which also includes each time a bite of the transverse colon.

The faeces which are discharged from a right transverse colostomy during the first year of life are usually loose, contain much intestinal secretion and are highly irritant to the skin of the abdominal wall. To prevent excoriation the skin should be liberally smeared with a protective barrier cream or with karaya gum. When excoriation is extensive the child should be nursed face downwards on a frame so that the faeces fall clear away from the abdominal wall and the skin should be treated with a mixture of eggwhite and brandy. Bleeding from the mucosa of the colostomy is difficult to prevent even with lint smeared with ointment or with gauze impregnated with soft paraffin. Every infant with a colostomy should have the haemoglobin concentration of the peripheral blood measured every month, most will develop a secondary anaemia for which iron supplements should be prescribed. Stenosis or retraction of the colostomy can usually be avoided if the bowel is decompressed before the loop is drawn out at the original operation. Closure of the colostomy after the definitive operation will be accompanied by much bleeding which can be almost completely avoided by using diathermy for the dissection of the colon loop out of the abdominal wall; but blood for transfusion should always be available.

Spontaneous Gangrene of the Intestine

This term should be applied only to perforation of the bowel soon after birth when at laparotomy no evidence of intestinal obstruction can be found. In this condition patches of gangrene appear in the wall of the intestines, rarely there is only one patch and sometimes only a small segment of the colon or small intestine is affected but it may occur anywhere from the cardiac end of the stomach to the rectum. There is usually a history of a vague but progressive illness of several days duration, accompanied by increasing abdominal distension and vomiting of bile stained fluid. The baby is usually brought to hospital ill with a distended abdomen and there may be oedema of the anterior abdominal wall. There may be tenderness suggestive of peritonitis and sometimes a vague mass may be felt in the abdomen. The appearances on radiological examination of the abdomen in the erect position depend on the stage the disease has reached. In the early form small bubbles of gas may be seen in the wall of the intestine or there may be a mottled effect in a localized area. A little later one or more loops of intestine may be outlined by gas on both sides of the intestinal wall. When the bowel has perforated there may be obvious accumulations of gas in the peritoneal cavity but not always under the diaphragm. In the most severe form the liver hangs limply down from the central part of the diaphragm and is outlined by large gas shadows ("saddle bag" sign, Parrish *et al.*, 1964) (Fig. 11.1) and there is separation of the gas shadows in the intestine by the purulent exudate which lies amongst the intestines.

The mild and solitary forms of this disease may resolve spontaneously but uncertainty about what may happen usually leads to laparotomy. This should be preceded by transfusion with enough compatible whole blood to ensure a satisfactory circulating blood volume; the abdomen should be opened through a long transverse incision above the umbilicus from one costal margin to the other. There may be only one or more red or purplish patches on or near the antimesenteric border of the intestine or the wall may show darker more advanced areas. In some places there may be complete gangrene with wide holes in the bowel wall, with greyish brown ragged necrotic sloughing edges, and much faecal or meconium stained purulent exudate and inflammatory fluid. For the more advanced lesions resection of the affected segment of bowel is the only satisfactory treatment and it is probably the best course also even in the milder types. Even when all the affected intestine is removed further gangrenous areas may appear in parts of the bowel which appeared normal at the time of operation.

The cause of these lesions is unknown and although various explanations have been proposed such as anaerobic infection of the intestinal wall, antigenic reaction and embolization none will fit the situation satisfactorily. Culture of the peritoneal fluid and exudate has produced the wide range of organismal growth which might be expected. Some surgeons have reported associated septicaemias, others have failed to grow anything in blood cultures (Scott, 1963; Thelander, 1939). The vessels in the mesenteries and intestinal walls do not show any typical characteristics. Prompt laparotomy and resection of the affected portion of bowel combined with adequate blood transfusion is now usually associated with a mortality of 50 to 75 per cent. Fonkalsrud and Clatworthy (1965) found that neonatal perforations of the rectum and colon were accidental in one sixth of their cases. The causes included damage by rectal thermometers, probing of the rectum with stiff catheters and enemas given to constipated infants and they recommended that catheters and thermometers should be clearly marked at 2 cm. from their tips and should not be inserted further than this. Perforation of the rectum has also been reported after washouts for Hirschsprung's disease (Fraser and Wilkinson, 1967) and dilatation of congenital anorectal stenosis. (Cozzi and Wilkinson, 1968).

Massive Intestinal Resection

The removal of more than 75 per cent of the small intestine from a neonate is occasionally necessary because of infarction of a volvulus of the midgut or of bowel in an exomphalos or gastroschisis. Multiple atresias of the small intestine also may so reduce the length of the small intestine that only a small part can be preserved. Various estimates have been made of the amount of intestine which is necessary for survival but the newly born baby certainly needs more than an older child or adult because of the much larger nutritional requirements for growth. The length of the normal human intestine at birth is uncertain but is probably in the region of 300 to 350 cm. and at least 10 to 15 per cent (35 to 40 cm.) seems to be necessary for survival (Wilkinson, Hughes and Toms, 1963); a few adults however have survived after resection of the whole of the jejunum and ileum and half of the colon. It is now evident that the type of residual bowel is as important as its length and that ileum is of more use than a similar length of jejunum. The ileocaecal valve should always be preserved if possible with as much of the terminal ileum as can be saved. The length of the remaining small intestine should always be measured with a metal ruler at the operation. It seems likely that if in the human neonate there is more than 70 cm. of small intestine the ultimate prognosis is good but that there will be some difficulty in the early weeks. The lower limit for survival seems to be about 20 to 30 cm. but even when 50 cm. remain many recurrent difficulties will be encountered during the first year.

Flint (1912) found that adult dogs would survive after he had removed half the small intestine but that there was hyperplasia and hypertrophy of the remaining intestine. However review of the clinical and experimental findings in a number of subsequent reports shows a good deal of variation. Althausen *et al.* (1950) agreed in general with Flint but Clatworthy *et al.* (1952) did not find any evidence of growth in length above that to be normally expected even though the intestines of their puppies increased in diameter and thickness. Loran *et al.* (1956) found that dilatation followed excision of as little as 10 per cent of the small intestine of rats but Booth and Mollin (1965) found that dilatation of the adult rat's intestine appeared to be directly related to the length of intestine resected and did not occur with simple transection and reanastomosis at any level. When the distal ileum was resected barium passed through the intestine two or three times as fast as in the normal. The suggestion that reversal of a short segment at the distal end of the residual small intestine would delay emptying and thus promote absorption from the intestine (Hammer *et al.*, 1955, 1959; Stahlgren *et al.*, 1962) has seldom been adopted; it is difficult to judge how long a segment should be reversed, too little is ineffective and too much would cause sufficient obstruction to interfere with absorption. However Venables *et al.* (1967) have recently described the remarkable improvement which followed the reversal of a 3 in. segment of terminal jejunum 2 in. above the jejunocolic anastomosis in a patient from whom all but 4 ft. of upper jejunum, the whole ileum and right half of colon had previously been resected. Budding and Smith (1967) showed that after extensive small bowel resection transit time could also be increased by the construction of recirculating loops of the remaining intestine but that such procedures were associated with their own mortality and complications and doubt if they would be justified in practice unless dietary and other measures had failed.

When most of the small intestine has been removed the main nutritional problem arises from the very rapid passage of food through the short length of intestine which remains. Digestion is limited both by the reduced quantity of intestinal secretions and the short time for which food is exposed to them in the intestine. Absorption is limited by the smaller surface of mucosa which is available and the reduced time for which the partially digested food is in contact with the mucosa. One result is that much partially digested food reaches the large bowel where it may have an irritant effect on the mucosa thus accelerating its passage through the colon; in addition the putrefaction of food, especially starch, in the colon produces irritant materials and an unusual quantity of gas which also accelerate transit of the contents. The rapid passage of fatty acids into the colon is particularly irritating as the result of the great reduction in pH which this causes. The problem of maintaining nutrition at a level high enough to satisfy both the daily requirements for maintenance of ordinary metabolism as well as those of growth is considerable. This problem can be solved by first providing an intake of food which has been made as ready for absorption as possible by careful choice of its constituents and predigestion and secondly by slowing its passage through the short length of small intestine.

The irritant action of fat is well known. Weckesser *et al.* (1949) showed that when fat intake was doubled the resulting increase in the loss of fat and protein in the faeces was so large that only 25 per cent of the increased intake of calories was absorbed and the total calorie intake fell. When the carbohydrate intake was doubled however the total calorie absorption was increased. The adverse effect of animal fat is so marked after large resections of small intestine that it should be excluded from the diet as completely as possible. Recent work (Winawer *et al.*, 1966) has shown that medium chain triglycerides offer an excellent alternative to other sources of fat as a supply of calories and should be substituted gram for gram for milk fat.

In the neonate feeds should be based on reconstituted dried skimmed milk which should be made up in less water than usual and predigested with Benger's food or some similar preparation. Carbohydrate should be added as glucose and may also be used as a substitute for animal fat on an equicaloric basis. Some children may tolerate olive oil better than medium chain triglycerides or a large increase in glucose. There seems to be little advantage in using diluted milk feeds even in the early stages since bulky feeds increase the volume of fluid within the intestine and the rate of transit. It is usually better to use more concentrated feeds than usual and further to thicken them with arrowroot.

The oral consumption of glucose solutions and saline also increases the rate of transit through the intestine. The faeces should be collected and their daily volume measured. Transit time from mouth to anus should be measured with a suitable marker such as carmine but this may sometimes be so diluted as to be barely recognizable.

From time to time bursts of frequent liquid stools will cause such large extrarenal losses of minerals and water that replacement by intravenous infusion becomes essential. Suitable quantities of 0·9 per cent saline, Darrows solution and sodium lactate solution should then be given, with 6 per cent glucose solution in addition as a source of free water. The parenteral administration of fat emulsions is of very limited value since the volume of fluid which must be given to provide an adequate number of calories is usually more than these small and often emaciated babies can tolerate. The prolonged use of fat emulsions may lead to disturbances of blood coagulation and the appearance of widespread petechial haemorrhages. Similarly the limit of tolerance of amino acid preparations, even when their calorie content is increased by the addition of alcohol and fructose, is soon reached in the infant and the available veins are thrombosed by chemical thrombophlabitis.

It is now more generally realized that when repeated losses of intestinal secretions in loose stools are replaced by intravenous infusion of various sodium and potassium salts, but the intake of food is inadequate, and its digestion and absorption are deficient, there is a constant risk of magnesium deficiency. This should be suspected when in such circumstances the child fails to improve and lies listless, apparently half asleep, with flaccid limbs and refuses to take feeds. The serum magnesium concentration will be of little help in such a child. The best indication that magnesium deficiency exists is to collect the urine for 24 hr. and to compare its magnesium content with that of a 24 hr. output of urine after the administration of a large supplementary dose of a magnesium salt, preferably by intravenous infusion. In the subject with a normal content of magnesium the equivalent of 90 per cent of the supplementary magnesium will be excreted in the urine within 24 hr. but in the deficient subject 40–80 per cent of the dose will be retained (Thoren, 1963). Booth *et al.* (1963) recommended the use of 0·5 m.Eq. magnesium per kg. body weight per day as magnesium chloride, but Fletcher *et al.* (1960) used magnesium hydroxide. In magnesium deficient patients there is usually a prompt reduction in the volume and number of stools which are passed as well as a marked clinical improvement. The supplement should be continued for at least two weeks if the deficit is to be adequately replaced.

Other deficiencies may follow intestinal resection. Folic acid and iron absorption may be affected when all of the jejunum is removed, but it is not now so certain that resection of the ileocaecal valve and terminal ileum causes vitamin B_{12} deficiency. There is still too little knowledge of function after even very extensive intestinal ablation for dogmatic statements to be made about its effects. The small intestine appears to have a large reserve of function, provided the food and products of digestion can be kept in contact with the mucous membrane for long enough. Careful follow-up and repeated study of the patient are essential if deficiencies are to be recognized. It is as well however to provide supplements of the fat soluble vitamins A, D and K whenever there is steatorrhoea.

One of the most important precautions however is to warn the parents and their general practitioner of the great danger associated with even apparently minor alimentary infections, which in the child with an unusually short intestine may cause severe diarrhoea with rapid large losses of secretion. Such losses may be so large that the child is reduced to a grave state of collapse within a few hours. They should be advised to take the child to hospital without delay, preferably the one in which the child is already known so that intravenous therapy may be promptly started and the losses of intestinal fluid replaced.

Mortality

There has been an encouraging reduction in overall mortality rate in most types of neonatal intestinal obstruction. Amongst the factors which have contributed to this improvement are wider interest in and much greater knowledge of the causes and clinical features of these congenital anomalies. The ensuing improvement in diagnosis has led to more being recognized at an earlier stage. Nearly half the babies who require emergency surgical treatment within a few days of birth have more than one anomaly or some important complication of the primary lesion or have been prematurely born. In order to get a truer appreciation of the prognosis it is now customary to classify these patients according to risk in the manner first used for oesophageal atresia by Waterston *et al.* (1962) (Table I). The classification is based primarily on weight at birth which is then loaded by the coexistence of another anomaly or a complication. In accordance with international convention (United Nations, 1955) a baby who weighs $5\frac{1}{2}$ lb. or more at birth is arbitrarily regarded as mature and in the absence of another significant anomaly or complication is regarded as being a good risk and is placed in Group A. Babies who weigh $5\frac{1}{2}$ lb. or more are downgraded to Group B or Group C according to the severity of the associated anomaly or complication. Babies are also put into Group B or C on weight alone if they weigh 4 to $5\frac{1}{2}$ lb. or less than 4 lb. respectively and Group B babies by weight may be downgraded if they have an associated anomaly or complication.

TABLE I. *Classification into three risk groups according to weight at birth and presence of another anomaly*

RISK GROUP A = Over 2·5 kg. ($5\frac{1}{2}$ lbs.) birth weight, no other anomalies or complications.

RISK GROUP B = 1·8–2·5 kg. (4–$5\frac{1}{2}$ lbs.) birth weight, no other complications or anomalies
    OR Group A with moderately severe anomaly or complication

RISK GROUP C = Less than 1·8 kg. (4 lbs.) birth weight
    OR Group B with moderately severe anomaly or complication
    OR Group A with severe anomaly or complication.

In Table II this method of classification has been applied to three series of patients who were treated at the Hospital for Sick Children, Great Ormond Street. It shows clearly how widely the mortality rate varies between the three risk groups. The low mortality in Group A for oesophageal, duodenal and rectal atresia implies that the method of treatment which was used is satisfactory. It is obvious that for the poorer risk babies there is a lot of scope for improvement. Unfortunately the most important factors which influence the prognosis adversely are small birth weight and other associated severe congenital anomalies. Holder *et al.* (1962) found that improvement in the mortality of oesophageal atresia could be achieved by dividing the operative treatment into stages and Gross (1964) and Koop and Hamilton (1965) have also claimed improvements after staging treatment in a similar way. Cozzi and Wilkinson (1967) reported a recent improvement in the results of the treatment of Group C babies but this was due to more babies surviving primary anastomosis and not to any reduction in mortality which could be attributed to the staged treatment. It may be that better understanding of the care of the small premature baby will do more to reduce mortality rate than division of the operation into stages.

For anorectal anomalies there was not much difference in mortality between Groups A and B and even in Group C the mortality rate was lower than either oesophageal or duodenal atresias. Yet the mortality rate for neonatal colostomy is 25 per cent although that for the delayed abdomino-perineal operation done at the age of one year was only just over 2 per cent. The most important lethal factors were low birth weight and severe associated anomalies. The amount of improvement that can be achieved by staging treatment in this way is still limited by very low birth weight and by the severity of the associated anomalies, especially those of the cardiovascular system.

TABLE II. *Classification of risks and mortality rates for various neonatal surgical emergencies*

Group	Oesophageal atresia (1959–67) (1)			Duodenal obstruction (1951–64) (2)			Rectal atresia (1958–67) (4)		
	No. of patients	Deaths	%	No. of patients	Deaths	%	No. of patients	Deaths	%
A	30	0	0	58	5	8·6	26	1	3·8
B	28	8	28	37	13	35	27	1	3·7
C	35	26	74	37	29	78	38	21	55
Totals	93	34	36·1	132	47	35·6	91	23	25

To show the mortality rate in three groups of congenital anomalies of the alimentary tract classified by weight and associated anomalies:

Oesophageal atresia, Cozzi and Wilkinson, 1967.
Duodenal obstruction, Young and Wilkinson, 1966.
Rectal atresia, Cozzi and Wilkinson, 1968.

This method of classification is less applicable to the form of obstruction due to inspissated meconium ("meconium ileus"), which is part of the triad of mucoviscidosis, and to Hirschsprung's disease. In both these types of neonatal intestinal obstruction birth weight lies in the same range as that found in normal babies (Holsclaw *et al.*, 1966; Fraser and Wilkinson, 1967) and associated congenital abnormalities are rare. Yet in both diseases the mortality rate of surgical relief of the obstruction is in the region of 33 per cent in spite of early recognition of the disease and admission to hospital. This persisting high mortality is due in mucoviscidosis mainly to pulmonary complications, the factor which is the most important determinant of the prognosis throughout the lifetime of the survivors. In Hirschsprung's disease the most important factors are delay in diagnosis and complications of the surgical treatment; so-called enterocolitis is the most severe complication either before or after colostomy or resection of the aganglionic bowel in the majority of the series of cases which have been reported in the last ten years and its aetiology and nature are still not understood. However, Ehrenpreis has recently emphasized that enterocolitis has not been a fatal complication in Sweden and supposes that if it occurs there it is in a less virulent form than in other countries.

In the series of 132 duodenal obstructions reported by Young and Wilkinson (1966) the mortality rate was twice as high in babies born after a complicated pregnancy as in those born of a normal gestation. There is at present no satisfactory explanation for this because it is impossible to decide whether the pregnancy was complicated by the presence of a baby with an abnormality which may have interfered with the normal circulation of amniotic fluid, or whether perhaps a more important factor was the effect on the body composition of the baby of both the duodenal obstruction and the associated disturbance of pregnancy.

The type of obstruction also has an important bearing on the outcome. Intrinsic duodenal obstruction is due to atresia begun before birth and is persistent; more than half the babies with this type of lesion weighed less than $5\frac{1}{2}$ lb. at birth and 44 per cent died and when another serious abnormality existed the mortality rate was 91 per cent. Extrinsic obstruction is most often due to malfixation and volvulus of the midgut and is usually intermittent; only 12 per cent of babies with extrinsic obstruction weighed less than $5\frac{1}{2}$ lb. at birth, only 9 per cent died and the mortality rate was only 30 per cent when there was some other severe anomaly.

Acknowledgment

I am indebted to the Editor of the *British Journal of Surgery* for permission to reproduce Figures 2, 3(*a*) and 3(*b*).

References

BISHOP, H. C. and KOOP, C. E. (1957). *Ann. Surg.*, **145**, 410.

BOOTH, C. C., HANNA, S., BABOURIS, N. and MACINTYRE, I. (1963). *Brit. Med. J.*, **2**, 141.

BOOTH, C. C. and MOLLIN, D. L. (1959). *Lancet*, *i*, **18**.

BUDDING, J. and SMITH, C. C. (1967). *Surg. Gynecol. and Obst.*, **125**, 243.

BUTLER, N. R. and BONHAM, D. G. (1963). Perinatal Mortality. The first report of the 1958 British Perinatal Mortality Survey under the auspices of the National Birthday Trust Foundation, Edinburgh and London, Livingstone.

CLATWORTHY, H. W., SALEEBY, R. and LOVINGOOD, C. (1952). *Surgery*, St. Louis, **32**, 341.

COZZI, F. and WILKINSON, A. W. (1967). *Lancet*, *ii*, 1222. (1968). *Brit. Med. J.*, **1**, 144.

EHRENPREIS, T. and SANDBLOM, P. (1949). *Acta. Paediat.*, Stockh., **38**, 109.

FLETCHER, R. F., HENLY, A. A., SAMMONS, H. G. and SQUIRE, J. R. (1960). *Lancet*, *i*, 522.

FLINT, J. M. (1912). *Johns Hopkins Hosp. Bull.*, **23**, 127.

FORKALSRUD, E. W. and CLATWORTHY, H. W. (1965). *New Engl. J. Med.*, **277**, 10.

FRASER, G. C. and WILKINSON, A. W. (1967). *Brit. Med. J.*, **3**, 7.

HAMMER, J. M., SEAY, P. H., JOHNSTON, R. L., HILL, E. J., PRUST, F. H. and CAMPBELL, R. J. (1959). *Arch. Surg., Chicago,* **79,** 537.

HOLDER, T. M., McDONALD, V. G. and WOOLLEY, M. M. (1962). *J. Thoracic and Cardiovas. Surg.,* **44,** 344.

HOLSCLAW, D. S., ECKSTEIN, H. B. and NIXON, H. H. (1965). *Amer. J. Dis. Child.,* **109,** 101.

HUGHES, E. A., STEVENS, L. M., TOMS, D. A. and WILKINSON, A. W. (1965). *Brit. J. Surg.,* **52,** 403.

KOOP, C. E. and HAMILTON, J. P. (1965). *Ann. Surg.,* **162,** 389.

LORAN, M. R., ALTHAUSEN, T. L. and IRVINE, E. (1956). *Gastroenterol,* **31,** 717.

McCANCE, R. A. and WIDDOWSON, E. (1961). *Brit. Med. Bull.,* **17,** 132.

PARRISH, R. A., SHERMAN, R. T. and WILSON, H. (1964). *Ann. Surg.,* **159,** 244.

PECK, D. A., LYNN, H. B. and HARRIS, L. E. (1963). *Arch. Surg., Chicago,* **87,** 428.

SCOTT, J. E. S. (1963). *Arch. Dis. Childh.,* **38,** 120.

SIGGAARD ANDERSEN, O. (1962). *Scand. J. Clin. Lab. Invest.,* **14,** 598.

SIGGAARD ANDERSEN, O., ENGEL, K., JORGENSEN, K. and ASTRUP, P. (1960). *Scand. J. Clin. Lab. Invest.,* **12,** 172.

SNYDER, W. H. and GREANEY, E. M. (1965). *Surgery, St. Louis,* **57,** 576.

STALGREN, L. H., UMANA, G., ROY, R. and DONELLY, J. (1962). *Ann. Surg.,* **156,** 483.

THELANDER, H. E. (1939). *Amer. J. Dis. Childh.,* **58,** 371.

THOREN, L. (1963). *Acta. Chir. Scand. Supp.* **1306,** 1.

UNITED NATIONS (1955). "Handbook of Vital Statistical Methods". Series F, no. 7, New York.

VENABLES, C. W., ELLIS, H. and SMITH, A. D. M. (1966). *Lancet,* **2,** 1390.

WATERSTON, D. J., BONHAM CARTER, R. E. and ABERDEEN, E. (1962). *Lancet,* **1,** 819.

WECKESSER, E. E., CHINN, A. B., SCOTT, M. W. and PRICE, J. W. (1949). *Amer. J. Surg.,* **78,** 706.

WILKINSON, A. W. (1963). *Lancet,* **1,** 86.

WILKINSON, A. W., STEVENS, L. H. and HUGHES, E. A. (1962). *Lancet,* **1,** 983.

WILKINSON, A. W., HUGHES, E. A. and TOMS, D. A. (1963). *Brit. J. Surg.,* **50,** 715.

WILKINSON, A. W., HUGHES, E. A. and STEVENS, L. H. (1965). *Brit. J. Surg.,* **52,** 410.

WINAWER, S. J., BROITMAN, S. A., WOLOCHOW, D. A., OSBORNE, M. P. and ZAWCHECK, N. (1966). *New Engl. J. Med.,* **274,** 72.

YOUNG, D. G. and WILKINSON, A. W. (1966). *Lancet,* **2,** 18.

Chapter 12

THE SURGICAL TREATMENT OF DUODENAL ULCER

A. W. Kay

A review of the historical background to the surgical treatment of duodenal ulcer reveals that, after a spell of popularity, each operation advocated has been found deficient in some respect. Today, vagotomy is in vogue.

The safety of surgery, and in particular of vagotomy, has tended to broaden the indications for operation in patients with duodenal ulcer.

The place of gastric secretion studies before and after operation, the choice of drainage operation to be used with vagotomy, and the relative merits of truncal and selective vagotomy are matters of topical interest.

In recent years, endeavour has been directed to securing information which will allow surgical treatment to be planned for the needs of the individual patient with duodenal ulcer.

Interest continues on the endocrine aspects of peptic ulcer disease.

Historical Landmarks

The surgical treatment of duodenal ulcer had its origins over eighty years ago. For most of this time the various operations devised were based on empirical reasoning and it is only in the past quarter century that a sound physiological approach to management has evolved.

Gastrojejunostomy

Wölfler, in 1881, reasoning that diversion of gastric contents into the jejunum would shield a duodenal ulcer from the mechanical trauma of food, introduced gastrojejunostomy. This proved to be a successful operation as far as the duodenal ulcer was concerned but the almost invariable healing of the primary lesion was followed at a later date by the occurrence of jejunal or stomal ulceration in almost half of the patients so treated.

Gastrojejunostomy, now abandoned as being a totally inadequate attack on the problem of duodenal ulcer, served to demonstrate the important fact that ulcer is not merely a local disease dependent solely upon an area of decreased mucosal resistance but that other general and at that time unknown factors were involved.

Antral Exclusion

Gastrojejunostomy as performed before the turn of the century seems to have been associated frequently with cyclical vomiting and symptoms resulting from difficulty in gastric emptying. This led von Eiselsberg in 1895 to advocate transection of the stomach through the antrum, with closure of the distal pouch and restoration of gastro-intestinal continuity by anastomosis of the proximal cut end of stomach to the first loop of jejunum. This operation proved to be even more disastrous than gastrojejunostomy in that it gave an even higher incidence of recurrent ulceration.

The experimental studies of Dragstedt and his colleagues (1951) and more recent clinical observations (Kay, 1956 and Gillespie, 1959) have provided the explanation; the reflux of food and of alkaline juices from the afferent loop into the excluded antrum stimulates the release of gastrin from its mucosa and leads to the hypersecretion of acid by the proximal stomach.

Partial Gastrectomy with Gastrojejunal Anastomosis

Polya, in 1911, under the mistaken idea that the pyloric antrum actually secretes hydrochloric acid advised resection of the distal portion of the stomach with gastrojejunal reconstitution. The incidence of recurrent ulceration was markedly reduced after this operation and when it was appreciated that hydrochloric acid was secreted from the mucosa of the gastric body, more extensive gastric resections were performed. This double physiological blow of removing the hormone-secreting antrum and excising part of the acid secreting gastric mucosa reduced the incidence of recurrent ulceration to the low level of 1–3 per cent.

While diminution in the digestive function of the stomach does not seem to be of paramount importance, loss of its storage function may have troublesome repercussions. Some 10 per cent of patients suffer such symptoms as bilious vomiting, faintness and sweating, abdominal discomfort after meals, diarrhoea, loss of weight, and symptoms of anaemia after gastrectomy. It can now be said that the more radical the gastric resection the more certain is the solution of the ulcer problem but the greater is the physiological defect created.

Partial Gastrectomy with Gastroduodenal Anastomosis

It was rightly considered that a gastroduodenal reconstruction, by permitting better mixing of food with digestive juices, would reduce the incidence of post-gastrectomy symptoms but careful follow-up has shown this operation to be attended by a higher incidence of recurrent ulceration. Furthermore, duodenal ulceration reappears in a significant proportion of patients having a conversion from Polya to Billroth I for post-gastrectomy symptoms, despite complete freedom from ulcer trouble for several years after the initial operation.

Surgical practice has thus drawn attention to some peculiarity of the duodenal bulb. Whether this is due to excessive vulnerability or, more likely, because it plays an important role in regulating gastric secretion and emptying, is a subject worthy of further study.

Vagotomy

In 1943, based on the concept that the hypersecretion of acid in duodenal ulcer is primarily due to vagal drive, Dragstedt and Owens introduced supradiaphragmatic vagotomy of the stomach.

In a series of careful secretory and clinical studies Dragstedt himself showed that vagotomy as a sole procedure, while profoundly reducing acid secretion, was frequently followed by symptoms directly attributable to gastric retention such as bloating and foul eructations after food, and that the antral stimulation caused by the retention occasionally led to hypersecretion of acid of humoral origin and to the development of a gastric ulcer.

Vagotomy with Antrectomy

Their armamentarium strengthened by the firm knowledge that complete vagotomy would markedly reduce the acid output of the stomach, surgeons now sought to devise procedures which would eliminate these disadvantages and Farmer and Smithwich (1952) were early advocates of limited gastric resection with vagotomy. The theoretical advantages claimed for this procedure are that it ablates both the vagal and hormonal drives to acid secretion and at the same time preserves the greater part of the gastric reservoir. In practice, this operation has an almost unique record for preventing recurrent ulcer but, not surprisingly, retains a similar operative risk to partial gastrectomy and carries the chance of both post-gastrectomy symptoms and the sequelae of vagotomy.

Vagotomy with Drainage

In an attempt to rehabilitate the usefulness of simple vagotomy and to eliminate its motility disturbances and associated symptoms gastrojejunostomy, and later pyloroplasty, have been added. This has proved to be an exceptionally safe, simple and reliable procedure for the majority of duodenal ulcer patients. Transabdominal truncal vagotomy with a drainage procedure is currently in vogue in this country.

Note on Controlled Trials in Ulcer Surgery

The current popularity of vagotomy with a drainage operation, which has not yet been subjected to the same lengthy and critical follow-up as has gastrectomy, may well be evanescent. Furthermore a comparison of the results of partial gastrectomy in the 1940's with those of vagotomy in the 1960's is unacceptable. It is only by means of carefully controlled trials that an unbiased assessment of the value of various operations to the ulcer patient can be made.

The plan of the current Leeds-York trial provides a model for the acceptable comparison of surgical operations in the treatment of duodenal ulcer (Goligher, 1966). In this trial three operations have been judged: Vagotomy and Gastrojejunostomy, Vagotomy and Antrectomy, and Subtotal Gastrectomy of the polya type with removal of the ulcer. Patients requiring emergency surgery were excluded from the trial. An "escape clause" was also included so that patients who for various reasons (poor general condition, pulmonary tuberculosis, etc.) were unsuitable for gastrectomy were excluded. Again, at the time of operation those in whom for technical reasons any of the three procedures seemed unjustified were also excluded. In those who remained, the particular procedure to be performed was determined by random selection. The assessment of results has been done yearly by a small panel who are not allowed to know which operation has been performed until they have recorded their comments and verdict.

It is of interest that the most recently reported results (all patients have now been followed for at least three years and many for four, five or even six years) show that the differences in the results between individual operative procedures are marginal but, perhaps surprisingly, they presently tend to favour subtotal gastrectomy. Despite this Goligher and his associates, mainly on the basis of the higher mortality (although zero in their own series of 634 patients!) and known deterioration of results with the passage of the years, question if gastrectomy can any longer be justified as the routine surgical treatment for all cases of duodenal ulceration.

Indications for Operations

The traditional view that surgery should be advised only after a patient has had the benefit of a lengthy course of medical treatment is no longer tenable. Not so many years ago elective surgery was a major factor in the mortality from duodenal ulcer; today, however, advances in anaesthesia and in supportive therapy have made surgery safer and there is no longer any need for a medical advisor to protect his patient from the surgeon. It is now generally accepted that conservative management including lengthy bedrest, dietary measures and the use of antacids will regularly relieve symptoms but cannot be relied upon to effect healing of the ulcer or to prevent recurrence.

Failure to control symptoms by conservative measures is the usual indication for surgical treatment, and loss of work, loss of sleep through nocturnal pain, back pain and recurring episodes of bleeding are helpful pointers in making a decision to operate. Surgical treatment is necessary when pyloric stenosis supervenes, for acute perforation, and occasionally for massive or continuing haemorrhage.

Formerly, partly on account of the operative risk involved but largely in anticipation of nutritional disturbances, surgeons hesitated to advise gastrectomy in young patients with duodenal ulcer. Today, recurring severe symptoms over a period of three years would be a sufficient basis for the recommendation of the simpler and safer procedure of vagotomy with drainage, although it should be noted that the picture of possible late effects of this operation is incomplete.

Because of its current popularity, the remainder of this review will be concerned largely with the use of vagotomy as surgical treatment for duodenal ulcer.

Gastric Secretion Tests before Vagotomy

The introduction of reliable and repeatable tests of gastric acid secretion some fifteen years ago has led to a rapidly increasing literature on the acid secretory pattern in duodenal ulcer patients. The use of these tests in planning surgical treatment has been advocated and so it is important to know if this is an essential step in management. In the present state of our knowledge it would be right to say that there is not yet a clear indication for the routine use of, for example, the augmented histamine test in patients with long-standing proven chronic duodenal ulceration.

This assertion should not be taken to underrate the vast and continuing contributions accruing from the regular use of such tests, both before and after operation, by surgeons particularly interested in elucidating unsolved problems of human gastric physiology or in studying the effect of various surgical procedures on gastric secretion. Thus studies of this kind have shown that a complete section of the vagus nerves will reduce the maximal acid output of the stomach in response to the augmented histamine test by some 65–70 per cent. Again, an attempt by Gillespie and Kay (1961) to determine pre-operatively the likely effect of surgical section of the vagus nerves has led to the concept that a minority of patients with duodenal ulcer may have acid hypersecretion predominantly of antral origin and, if this is confirmed, these patients would seem to merit antrectomy at the time of nerve section. Furthermore, the routine use of a maximal histamine test, which provides values for basal secretion and "maximal acid output", is probably the most certain means of identifying the patient with a Zollinger-Ellison syndrome in whom basal approximates to maximal secretion (p. 329). This test may also be of value in the investigation of the patient suspected of having a duodenal ulcer although radiological support is lacking: the finding of complete achlorhydria excludes the diagnosis of duodenal ulcer; the presence of acid in any specimen throughout the test makes the diagnosis of peptic ulceration possible; an acid output of more than 20 m.Eq. in the peak half hour after histamine is strongly suggestive of duodenal ulceration. Finally, recent attempts to select surgical treatment to meet the requirements of the individual patient with duodenal ulcer have been based largely on the results of acid secretion tests performed before operation (p. 217).

Gastric Secretion Tests after Vagotomy

An aim of any operation for chronic duodenal ulcer is to reduce the amount of acid produced by the stomach sufficiently to allow the ulcer to heal and to prevent recurrent ulceration. Although it could be claimed that a disappointing reduction in acid secretion is unlikely to induce the surgeon to re-operate immediately, the reduction in acid output effected by vagotomy is a matter of great interest and importance to all surgeons performing the operation, and this for several reasons. Firstly, a surgeon should gain evidence of his own ability to perform complete section of the vagus nerves in a high proportion of his patients. Secondly, incomplete vagotomy is known to be the commonest cause of recurrent ulcer after this operation and it is useful to know that an individual patient requires particularly close observation at the out-patient clinic. Thirdly, at subsequent follow-up of patients who have had vagotomy with drainage it is important to know if we are assessing the results of complete vagotomy with a drainage procedure or merely the results of the drainage operation alone.

Since its introduction by Hollander almost a quarter of a century ago, the insulin test has gained general acceptance as the best available method for the determination of completeness of vagal nerve section. It is based on the fact that insulin-induced hypoglycaemia regularly evokes gastric acid secretion when vagal pathways to the stomach are intact, but fails to do so after their complete division. According to Hollander a positive insulin test (incomplete vagotomy) has been taken as one in which there is an increase in acid concentration of at least 20 m.Eq./L. upon basal levels within two hours after giving an intravenous injection of 20 units of soluble insulin; a rise of 10 m.Eq./L.

is acceptable when the basal secretion is anacid. A lesser response is interpreted as a negative insulin test (complete vagotomy) provided the blood sugar has fallen below 45 mg./100 ml.

A review of several reported series of post-vagotomy insulin tests interpreted according to these rigid criteria showed that over 30 per cent of patients have a positive response and would seem to have had an incomplete vagotomy (Ross and Kay, 1964). If this is a true reflection of the surgeon's ability to perform complete nerve section, the long-term recurrent ulcer rate is likely to be prohibitive and to provide a strong argument against the routine use of the operation.

On the basis of a detailed analysis of the results of insulin tests in a consecutive series of 100 patients, Ross and Kay proposed an alternative method of interpreting the test and postulated an arbitrary grouping according to the timing of a positive response. It was suggested that positive responses occurring within 45 min. (early positive) reflect incomplete vagotomy, whereas responses between 45 and 120 min. (late positive) indicate "adequate vagotomy". This work has already stimulated further studies on the interpretation of the insulin test and the results of these and of their application to patients after vagotomy will be critical to the continued acceptance of vagotomy as a routine procedure.

While the reduction in the augmented histamine response after vagotomy cannot be expected to give reliable evidence of completeness of nerve section, a reduction of between 65 and 70 per cent is usually found in patients with a negative insulin test; in the absence of an insulin test this finding would be reassuring. A further reason for performing an augmented histamine test before and ten days after operation is that it provides a baseline reduction for future reference, and, in this way, Bell (1964) has been able to show that the reduction in gastric acid secretion effected immediately by complete vagotomy persists for at least three years and, in all probability, permanently.

Total or Selective Vagotomy?

Selective vagotomy has been promoted on theoretical, clinico-physiological, and technical grounds. Total (truncal) vagotomy divides all vagal fibres passing to the stomach, liver, pancreas, gall bladder, all of the small intestine, and the proximal part of the colon. If complete gastric vagotomy can be achieved safely and reliably without denervation of other organs, commonsense and surgical principles demand that this should be our objective. Although selective vagotomy has been in use for many years (Franksson, 1948), it is only now that acceptable data has become available from carefully performed maximal histamine and Hollander insulin tests on comparable groups of patients undergoing selective and truncal vagotomy which has shown that selective vagotomy is as effective as truncal vagotomy in reducing the level of gastric acid secretion (Bank *et al.*, 1966). With this new evidence it can now be claimed that selective vagotomy denervates the stomach as completely as does total vagotomy.

Advocation of selective vagotomy on clinico-physiological grounds is less secure. Vagotomy has been criticized as leading to an allegedly high incidence of diarrhoea although recent careful reviews have indicated that the true incidence of this complaint in troublesome form is of the order of 5 per cent (Cox and Bond, 1963). While this complication of vagotomy has been greatly exaggerated a real problem exists and it has been suggested that selective vagotomy provides its solution. This presupposes a fuller understanding of the pathogenesis of the diarrhoea.

Infective enteritis, denervation of the small intestine, pancreas and biliary tract, the drainage procedure used in association with vagotomy, and steatorrhoea have all been implicated, singly or in combination, as the cause of post-vagotomy diarrhoea. Each of these mooted mechanisms has been studied in some detail by various workers and the subject has recently been reviewed by Kay (1966) who came to the conclusion that the precise cause of diarrhoea after vagotomy is not yet known and that there is no reason to expect that selective vagotomy is likely to prove superior to total vagotomy in its prevention. Factual support for this view has been given by the recently reported findings of Bank *et al.* (1966) on a series of 160 patients, 77 after selective and 83 after total vagotomy. The incidence of persistent diarrhoea after the selective operation was 2·6 per cent and after total vagotomy 3·6 per cent. These findings confirm the invalidity of earlier reports on the supposed high incidence of this complication of vagotomy, and fail to show a significant difference between selective and truncal nerve section in causing diarrhoea.

Proponents of selective vagotomy claim that the more meticulous dissection required for its performance ensures a greater certainty of gastric vagal denervation than is usually accomplished by the standard truncal vagotomy. This assertion is not supported by the studies of Bank and his colleagues. In any event most methods of selective vagotomy involve a meticulous and time-consuming technique and have not commended themselves to the majority of surgeons.

Recently, however, Tanner (1966) has described a method of selective gastric vagotomy which is relatively simple in its performance. In effect an elliptical gastric circumcision is made from the incisura cardiaca on the left to the point just below the division of the left gastric vessels on the right, dividing the descending branch of this vessel. By elevating an encircling flap to a level 3–4 cm. above the cardia a gastric vagotomy is effected without exposing either main vagal trunk. If this operation proves to be a simple, safe and reliable method of performing selective vagotomy as judged by Hollander insulin testing, a controlled randomized trial of the two types of vagotomy would be called for.

Choice of Drainage Operation

Debate continues on the relative merits of gastrojejunstomy and pyloroplasty as the drainage procedure to be used with vagotomy, some surgeons acclaiming pyloroplasty, others gastrojejunostomy, while a few have found reason to change allegiance.

On physiological grounds pyloroplasty would seem to be the least disturbing of the drainage operations as it permits the antrum to remain in the acid stream thus preserving the acid inhibitory mechanism, and it also allows satisfactory mixing of food with digestive juices. It must be conceded however that experience to date has shown the reduction of acid secretion and the rise in faecal fat excretion after vagotomy to vary but little with the type of drainage operation. On surgical grounds, pyloro-duodenotomy should be regarded as an essential manoeuvre when a visible or palpable duodenal ulcer cannot be detected at operation as this will frequently reveal the ulcer causing symptoms; the pyloroplasty is then completed by transverse closure and vagotomy added. Again, pyloroplasty avoids the risk of the "blind loop" syndrome. Several cases of diarrhoea from this cause had been reported following vagotomy with gastrojejunostomy. These have responded to neomycin and subsequent operation has revealed an unexpectedly long afferent loop: pyloroplasty has usually been effective in relieving symptoms in these patients (Kay, 1966). Finally, pyloroplasty prevents the problems arising from the misplaced gastrojejunostomy.

A controlled trial of the two drainage procedures using random selection was begun in the author's department two years ago and the results should, in time, provide the factual information which is lacking at present. All that can be said now is that there is no significant difference in the acid reduction achieved by each operation (provided the vagotomy is complete), and that the early postoperative course is similar in both. Comment on the incidence of recurrent ulceration, nutritional disturbances, diarrhoea and mechanical symptoms is not justified meantime.

Types of Pyloroplasty

Gastric retention with vomiting is thought by some to be a major disadvantage of pyloroplasty and gastrojejunostomy has been preferred on this account. However, it now seems likely that the occurrence of this sequel is dependent largely on the technique of performing pyloroplasty. Thus, taking the extreme example, pyloromyotomy has been shown to provide inadequate drainage (Hopton and Torrance, 1966). Personal experience over the past eight years with a 2 in. incision through the pyloric antrum extending for a further 1 in. into the duodenum followed by transverse closure in one layer using interrupted catgut sutures has been entirely satisfactory. The Finney type of pyloroplasty is recommended by many and unquestionably provides good gastric drainage, but if vagotomy has been incomplete and is followed by recurrent ulceration, the ulcer may be situated close to the duodenal ampulla and pose a major problem in surgical management particularly if this is called for to control massive haemorrhage.

Vagotomy and Pyloroplasty for Bleeding Duodenal Ulcer

During the past twenty years, prompted largely by the improved mortality rates associated with elective subtotal gastric resection, more and more surgeons applied this operation to the bleeding duodenal ulcer and there can be little doubt that many needless resections have been performed. Recently there has been a trend towards a more conservative operative approach.

Encouraged by the success of pyloroplasty and vagotomy in the treatment of duodenal ulcer, Weinberg (1949) inaugurated a plan for direct ligation of the bleeding vessel combined with a Heineke-Mikulicz type of pyloroplasty and vagotomy. This form of management has gained in popularity and from their review of cumulative data Farris and Smith (1963) believe that this approach offers the safest and simplest procedure available for the management of these patients. They consider that the occurrence of haemorrhage from an ulcer should not alter the fundamental concept of treatment, namely, to correct the acid hypersecretion of vagal origin. It is probably true to say that this direct attack on the bleeding point gives less certain control of haemorrhage than does gastric resection with excision of the ulcer, and patients treated by vagotomy and under-running of the artery merit the closest observation in the early postoperative period. In the event of any major recurrence of bleeding the surgeon should not hesitate to perform antrectomy with excision of the ulcer as soon as blood loss has been replaced.

Vagotomy and Drainage for the Perforated Duodenal Ulcer

Simple closure of the perforated ulcer is simple and safe under widely varying circumstances, has a mortality rate lower than either non-operative management or definitive surgery, achieves permanent control of symptoms in about one-third of patients so treated, and avoids surgery of unnecessary magnitude in more than half. This form of management is advocated for the great majority of patients with acute perforated duodenal ulcer. There is however a growing experience of the management of this condition by vagotomy and pyloroplasty as an emergency procedure. Where the perforation is small and induration around the ulcer is minimal, pyloroplasty of the Heineke-Mikulicz type itself deals with the perforation and vagotomy is added; for perforation of a massive and callous ulcer simple closure of the perforation in the usual way followed by vagotomy with posterior gastro-jejunostomy is recommended.

Routine use of this form of definitive surgery is not advised and, where indicated, should be practised only by surgeons experienced in the performance of vagotomy. In selecting patients it is probably wise to exclude patients over the age of 55, those in whom the perforation is of more than 12 hr. duration, where excessive peritoneal spill has occurred, where shock persisted for some hours after perforation, and patients with severe systemic disease.

Selective Surgical Management in Duodenal Ulcer

Since Wölfler introduced gastrojejunostomy surgical endeavour has been directed largely towards the quest for an ideal operation for use in the management of all patients with chronic duodenal ulcer. This quest cannot be said to have been entirely successful and there is now little reason to believe that it is attainable.

In the present decade we have seen the first serious attempts to select surgical treatment to meet the requirements of the individual patient with duodenal ulcer. The results of current trials (Bruce *et al.*, 1959; Johnson and Orr, 1954) are awaited with interest but, as the main aim of both has been the avoidance of recurrent ulceration rather than the prevention of the other sequelae of gastric surgery, it seems unlikely that either will provide the ultimate policy of selective surgery. However some principles which merit consideration in formulating such policy have been established.

Account must be taken of mortality, recurrent ulceration and post-operative sequelae associated with the various acceptable operations. Pre-operative acid secretion studies will help to exclude the few patients with Zollinger-Ellison syndrome. Refinement of the medical vagotomy test may lead to the identification of a minority group of ulcer patients who require limited gastrectomy as part of their surgical treatment. Defects of intestinal absorption should be recognized as they may be aggravated by operation on the gastrointestinal tract. It is not yet certain if patients with a tendency to diarrhoea before vagotomy are particularly liable to this complication as a sequel of the operation.

Finally, reports from Scandinavian centres describe tests which may permit identification of patients particularly liable to develop dumping symptoms after gastric surgery.

The application to patients with duodenal ulcer of modern techniques in collecting, processing and analyzing data will greatly assist the acquisition of information essential to the formulation of a sound policy of selective therapy.

The Endocrine System and Duodenal Ulcer

In recent years there has been a growing awareness of the relationship between hormonal imbalance on the one hand and acid-pepsin production and peptic ulcer on the other. Many cases of polyendocrine adenomatosis associated with ulcer have been reported. Murphy and his colleagues (1960) and Mieher and his associates (1962) have presented excellent reviews of the historical background.

The precise mechanism by which the ulcer diathesis is promulgated in polyendocrine adenomatosis is not yet clear but studies of malfunction of the individually involved endocrine glands have offered a rare and potentially rewarding opportunity for endocrinologist and gastroenterologist alike.

Pituitary adenomata, without obvious disease of other endocrine glands, are associated with the ulcer diathesis less frequently than would be expected in the general population and so the relationship between the conditions is likely to be coincidental. On the other hand, pituitary adenomata in polyendocrine disease are frequently associated with peptic ulcer, have a male to female incidence ratio of 2:1, and have an established familial occurrence rate. It has also been noted that there is an increase in the pituitary basophilic cells in the Zollinger-Ellison syndrome but the significance of this is not yet clear.

The relationship of the adrenal gland, and more specifically of the adrenal cortex, to peptic ulcer has not been completely clarified despite an immense amount of study. While no final conclusions can be drawn at this time, it seems unlikely that disordered adrenal function is a major factor in the ulcer diathesis noted either with the Zollinger-Ellison syndrome or with polyendocrine adenomatosis.

There is no well documented evidence that gastric secretion is abnormal in clinical hyperparathyroidism and no consistent influence on gastric secretion has been demonstrated following administration of parathormone in man. Approximately 7–10 per cent of patients with parathyroid adenomata not associated with polyendocrine adenomatosis have a concurrent ulcer diathesis, and it seems likely that association is coincidental. On the other hand, in the presence of polyendocrine disease there is a frequent association of peptic ulcer with parathyroid adenomas (in one series of 34 patients with polyendocrine adenomatosis and peptic ulcer, 31 had parathyroid adenomas), but all available evidence leads to the conclusion that the ulcer diathesis is not dependent on a direct hormonal influence of the parathyroid glands.

Insulin-producing islet cell tumours of the pancreas, though causing hypoglycaemia which might be expected to increase vagally mediated gastric secretion, are rarely associated with peptic ulcer disease.

The non-insulin-producing islet cell tumours of the pancreas on the other hand give rise to a clinical syndrome characterized by ulcer disease, marked gastric acid hypersecretion, diarrhoea, and hypokalaemia (Zollinger-Ellison syndrome). The tumour is situated in the body or tail of the pancreas in 60 to 70 per cent of patients; multicentric islet cell tumours have been demonstrated in about 30 per cent of patients. The incidence of malignancy in these lesions has varied from 33–75 per cent. The cell type has been demonstrated as non-Beta and Gregory and his colleagues (1960) have isolated a hormone from the tumour and found it to be indistinguishable from gastrin as produced by antral mucosa. So far the hormone has not been detected in extracts of normal pancreatic tissue.

It has now been established that gastric acid hypersecretion in such patients continues after division of the vagus nerves, even when this is combined with excision of the antrum. Thus, normally acceptable surgical treatment of the duodenal ulcer is inadequate. The pancreas must be explored thoroughly and treatment directed towards removal of the pancreatic tumour; if the tumour cannot be found, or if multicentric tumours are present, total gastrectomy is advised.

On the basis of available evidence the present view is that the ulcer diathesis associated with polyendocrine adenomatosis derives primarily from the excessive hormonal secretions of the non-Beta cell tumour of the pancreas. It is therefore suggested that the finding of ulcer associated with any endocrine tumour of the pituitary, pancreas, parathyroids or the adrenals should be an indication to obtain a detailed family history and to initiate investigations for the appropriate detection of polyendocrine disease.

Further work is required to determine whether the Zollinger-Ellison syndrome is merely one mode of expression of polyendocrine adenomatosis or whether it can occur as an independent entity. Finally, every opportunity should be taken to make an exhaustive investigation of patients with the Zollinger-Ellison syndrome presenting with diarrhoea in the absence of peptic ulceration and without acid hypersecretion; it is not yet known if a hormone other than gastrin is the responsible agent.

References

BANK, S., MARKS, I. N., LOUW, J. H. (1966). Gastric Secretory patterns after vagotomy. *Lancet*, **2**, 548.

BELL, P. R. F. (1964). The long term effect of vagotomy on the maximal acid response to histamine in man. *Gastroenterology*, **46**, 387.

BRUCE, J., CARD, W. I., MARKS, I. N. and SIRCUS, W. (1959). *J. Roy. Coll. Surg.*, Edinburgh, **4**, 85.

COX, A. G. and BOND, M. R. (1964). Bowel habit after vagotomy and gastrojejunostomy. *Brit. Med. J.*, **1**, 460.

DRAGSTEDT, L. R. and OWENS, F. M. (1943). Supradiaphragmatic section of the vagus nerves in treatment of duodenal ulcer. *Proc. Soc. Exper. Biol. and Med.*, **53**, 152.

DRAGSTEDT, L. R., OBERHELMAN, H. A. and SMITH, C. A. (1951). Experimental hyperfunction of the gastric antrum with ulcer formation. *Ann. Surg.*, **134**, 332.

FARMER, D. A. and SMITHWICK, R. N. (1952). Hemigastrectomy combined with resection of the vagus nerves. *New Eng. J. Med.*, **247**, 1017.

FARRIS, J. M. and SMITH, G. K. (1963). Vagotomy and pyloroplasty for bleeding duodenal ulcer. *Amer. J. Surg.* (Symposium on ulcer.)

FRANKSSON, C. (1948). Selective vagotomy for peptic ulcer. *Acta. Chir. Scand.*, **96**, 409.

GILLESPIE, I. E. (1959). Influence of antral pH on gastric acid secretion in man. *Gastroenterology*, **37**, 164.

GILLESPIE, I. E. and KAY, A. W. (1961). Effect of medical and surgical vagotomy on the augmented histamine test in man. *Brit. Med. J.*, **1**, 1560.

GOLIGHER, J. C., PULVERTAFT, C. N. and FRANZ, R. C. (1966). "A comparison of surgical methods in the treatment of duodenal ulcer. Postgraduate Gastroenterology". Edited by T. J. Thomson and I. E. Gillespie, Bailliere, Tindall and Cassell, London.

GREGORY, R. A., TRACEY, Hilda J., FRENCH, J. M. and SIRCUS, W. (1960). Extraction of a gastrin-like substance from a pancreatic tumour in a case of Zollinger-Ellison syndrome. *Lancet*, **1**, 1045.

HOLLANDER, F. (1946). The insulin test for the presence of intact nerve fibres after vagal operations for peptic ulcer. *Gastroenterology*, **7**, 607.

HOPTON, D. S. and TORRANCE, H. B. (1966). Vagotomy and pyloromyotomy in the treatment of duodenal ulcer. *Brit. J. Surg.*, **53**, 757.

JOHNSON, H. D. and ORR, I. M. (1954). *Surg. Gyn. Obst.*, **98**, 425.

KAY, A. W. (1953). Effect of large doses of histamine on gastric secretion of hydrochloric acid: an augmented histamine test. *Brit. Med. J.*, **2**, 77.

KAY, A. W. (1956). Hemigastric exclusion in the treatment of duodenal ulcer. *J. Roy. Coll. Surg. of Edinburgh*, **2**, 54.

KAY, A. W. (1966). Whither duodenal ulcer surgery? *Amer. Surg.*, **32**, 579.

MIEHER, W. C., HARTSOCK, R. J., GEOKAS, M. C., BALLARD, H. S. and FRAME, B. (1962). Peptic ulcer and the manifestation of familial polyendocrine disease. *J.A.M.A.*, **179**, 854.

MURPHY, R. T., GOODSITT, E., MORALES, H. and BILTON, J. L. (1960). Peptic ulceration with associated endocrine tumours: collective review. *Amer. J. Surg.*, **100**, 764.

ROSS, B. and KAY, A. W. (1964). The insulin test after vagotomy. *Gastroenterology*, **46**, 379.

TANNER, N. C. (1966). A technique of selective vagotomy. *Brit. J. Surg.*, **53**, 185.

WESTLAND, J. C., MOVIS, H. J. and WEINBERG, J. A. (1958). Emergency surgical treatment of severely bleeding duodenal ulcer. *Surgery*, **43**, 897.

CHAPTER 13

ULCERATIVE COLITIS

BRYAN BROOKE

Diagnosis

Throughout the last decade more general recognition has been given to the fact that Crohn's disease can affect the large intestine and affect it alone thus simulating ulcerative colitis. This would be of little consequence but for the fact that the natural history of the two diseases and their prognoses differ. Were they similar in these respects surgical treatment would be the same for both. But ulcerative colitis is a primary disorder of the large intestine affecting the terminal ileum only when the ileo-caecal valve becomes incompetent; whereas Crohn's disease is a disorder of the alimentary tract in general. Removal of the large intestine therefore cures ulcerative colitis. But for Crohn's disease there can be no sure extirpation since removal of a lesion at any site is followed sooner or later by recurrence, commonly in adjacent areas less commonly at remote sites. In cases of Crohn's disease presenting with colitis recurrences appear later in the small intestine; right-sided colitis displays an inevitable tendency to spread distally until even the rectum is involved.

These differences between the two disorders create the need for a different strategy of surgical approach and require that the diagnosis be clearly made. For ulcerative colitis large bowel excision is an effectively gratifying measure. For Crohn's disease surgery is never final and is only undertaken when disability due to diarrhoea, malnutrition or complications demand the removal of the obvious lesion. Surgery is therefore piecemeal and operation becomes a necessity at repeated intervals over periods of variable duration. Moreover conservation must be the keystone since as much intestine as possible has to be preserved to reduce to a minimum the effects of malabsorption due to the disease itself compounded with the loss of small intestine by resection. It is clearly an advantage to conserve anal function as long as possible and to discard this only when rectal and anal disease has caused such disability as to warrant the removal of those organs.

The diagnosis of Crohn's disease of the large intestine is simple when colitis is found radiologically in conjunction with the typical small bowel lesion, when such rare complications as perineal ulceration make the true cause of the colitis evident, or when the area of inflammation is clearly localized, as in regional or right-sided colitis. It is when colitis presents *de novo* and alone that the diagnosis may be missed or, if considered, difficult to confirm. To some the proof lies in obtaining histological evidence of a granuloma—a non-caseating follicular system usually containing giant cells—either by biopsy from an anal fistula or the rectum or from an operation specimen itself. Proof this certainly is, but its absence does not exclude the diagnosis, which then must be made from a conjunction of clinical and radiological evidence. Anal fistulation, particularly multiple, may provide a clue since this is unusual in ulcerative colitis.

It is seldom that frequency of motions is so great in the exacerbations of Crohn's colitis as in ulcerative colitis when the rate may rise to twenty or more in 24 hrs. The large intestine shows a flexibility of its wall in Crohn's disease so that the initial films of a barium enema reveal considerable contrast in size of lumen and in mucosal appearance from the evacuation films; whereas lumen size and mucosal appearances tend to differ little between the two particularly in the chronic case of ulcerative colitis. Sometimes the increased thickness of the intestinal wall in Crohn's disease, which is absent in ulcerative colitis, can be discerned in the X-ray through the pseudospiculation projected by barium deposited between oedematous mucosal folds.

Finally the macroscopic appearances of the operation specimen may assist. Crohn's ulceration tends to be linear and serpiginous in disposition with intact though often oedematous mucosa intervening-sometimes resembling the cobblestones traditionally seen in the ileum. At those sites where ulceration has occurred in ulcerative colitis it affects all the circumference so that epithelium is lost all round the lumen though at superficial glance the irregularity of the depth of the ulceration may at first be misleading; furthermore deeper ulceration is often trilinear lying opposite the taeniae coli in ulcerative colitis. Oddly, internal fistulae do not appear to occur from the large bowel in Crohn's colitis though on occasion a primary small bowel lesion may fistulate into the colon, particularly the sigmoid, and even start a site of secondary colitis there. Acute toxic dilatation is extremely rare in Crohn's colitis but when it occurs it may be impossible to differentiate from ulcerative colitis unless an ileal lesion is also present or subsequent histology presents the follicular pattern.

There is always a tendency to place too much diagnostic weight upon morbid histological appearances, to consider this to be the final court of appeal. This is not justified in the differentiation between Crohn's and ulcerative colitis when the sections fail to reveal the follicular systems. A positive result in this regard carries considerable weight though it must be borne in mind that the discovery of giant cells alone is not significant since these may be the result of foreign body implantation from the bowel content in areas of ulceration. The diagnosis of Crohn's colitis can only be made on a full assessment of clinical, radiological and histological evidence.

Indications for Operation

In many cases of ulcerative colitis the decision for surgery is dictated by progressive disability and the advent of complications. When persistent diarrhoea begins to limit the ability to work and participate in the enjoyment of life despite conservative treatment, or exacerbations recur at increasing frequency so that time is lost from work, removal of the large intestine must be considered. The development of arthritis or iritis provide more urgent indications since such complications tend to resolve rapidly if the colon is removed expeditiously before permanent damage to eye or joint occurs. There is some evidence to indicate that skin lesions such as erythema nodosum and pyoderma gangrenosum may sometimes develop due to treatment, the drug salazopyrine being suspect. Whether it is so or not the occurrence of skin lesions provides another indication for even when this may be iatrogenic in origin it must place a limitation on the conservative measures available. In most cases therefore the patient's disability provides the cardinal point of assessment. There are however two circumstances which still provide difficulty—when to operate for the acute severe disease and when to operate for cancer.

In the acute case a dilemma arises as to how long medical treatment should be maintained and when the moment for operation has arrived. Emphasis has been placed upon the development of acute toxic dilatation since this clearly represents irreversible damage to the colon wall. Destruction has by then progressed to such an extent that even if the acute phase passes operation will be necessary on grounds of disability and complications. A tendency has therefore developed to await for clinical signs of dilatation before deciding to operate. This is, however, a grave error since operative mortality at this stage is no better than 30–50 per cent (identical with the mortality of conservative therapy). This high mortality is in part due to serious liver damage associated with portal bacteraemia and the biochemical disturbances inherent in hypo-albuminaemia and sodium, potassium and water depletion; in part to the considerable technical difficulties encountered at operation when disintegration of the bowel wall has occurred.

The emphasis on toxic dilatation as a clinical signpost is inappropriate and its development should be regarded as indictment of failure of management. The need is to find a sign that ulceration has begun to penetrate the muscle wall beyond the muscularis mucosae and that the stage is set for disintegration. Neither clinical examination nor sigmoidoscopy can achieve this. It is however possible to ascertain the situation by straight X-ray of the abdomen; barium studies at this stage may not only be dangerous but are less revealing since they cause uncertainty by revealing ulceration of a lesser depth. When ulceration penetrates to this depth in the acute case it leaves islands of intervening mucosa of sufficient size to be visualized as soft tissue shadows against the relative radiolucency of the gas always present under these circumstances within the bowel lumen. These mucosal islands can be observed most frequently in the transverse colon, splenic flexure and descending or sigmoid areas; they appear berry-like in shape and 0·5–1·0 cm. in size and are sometimes numerous but at the important early stage only a few may be seen. Even when few have been revealed, examination of the operation specimen invariably shows deep penetrating ulceration usually over a wide area. This radiological sign provides an urgent indication since disintegration can progress apace even to free perforation within 12 hrs.; moreover portal bacteraemia is probable thus causing rapidly increasing liver damage and exacerbating disturbances of biochemistry and osmolarity due to disturbance of albumin synthesis.

Using this sign it has proved possible to reduce the mortality of the acute severe case to the elective operative mortality of 3 per cent. A straight X-ray of the abdomen should be taken at the outset in the severe case and the demonstration of mucosal islands calls for colectomy, with excision of the rectum at a later date. If no islands are seen it is safe to treat with steroids; should there be no favourable response within 48 hr. further straight X-rays should be taken and monitoring of the state of the bowel be continued in this way.

Carcinoma provides a greater difficulty since there is no clinical and often no radiological indication at a stage when it is still curable. Its incidence is thirty times higher in all parts of the large intestine in ulcerative colitis of 10 to 15 years duration than in those with a normal intestine; the mean age of development is 20 years earlier (47:67) and its development is clinically insidious since the onset of bloody diarrhoea is interpreted by the patient as a recurrence of the original disease. Moreover cancer develops in those cases which have been mild symptomatically because inflammation and ulceration has been confined to the mucosa; the more severe cases have come to surgery before 10 to 15 years. And so the further occurrence of bloody diarrhoea is neglected until pain ensues either because of pericolic or perirectal spread or rarely because of obstruction. At this stage the growth always proves to be inoperable in the curative sense. Nevertheless the author has several patients surviving 5 years or more after large bowel excision for cancer, some more than 10 and one past 15 years. This has only been achieved either in late cases ultimately operated upon because of gradual increasing disability when cancer was found in the specimen, or by the chance radiological or sigmoidoscopic demonstration of a stricture. In one case a pedunculated tumour projecting into the lumen was demonstrated radiologically. Only one conclusion can be drawn: longstanding disease in itself provides an indication for operation: that though its course may have been symptomatically mild, after ten years excision becomes necessary because of the hazard of carcinoma and this possibility should be put to the patient. The whole of the large intestine must be removed since cancer is as likely to arise in the rectum as elsewhere; cancer has proved fatal in two of the author's patients with retained rectums, one in circuit with an ileorectal anastomosis one not, and similar experience has been recorded in other series.

Management

Salazopyrine and corticosteroids have added considerably to the effectiveness of conservative treatment. Both can be effective in inducing a remission at the stage before the muscularis mucosae is breached and the remission may be prolonged though sometimes maintenance therapy is required. Where the barium enema reveals the telltale collar-stud projections from the lumen, indicating breach of the muscularis mucosae by crypt abscesses, improvement may still be obtained but full remission is unlikely to be obtained or if obtained to persist. To this extent barium studies give further weight to the clinical indications for operation. In brief, as with the straight X-ray appearances in the acute severe case, barium contrast provides clues to the degree of penetration in pathological terms and so provides evidence upon which a decision may be made as to the likelihood of clinical improvement being achieved by medical measures. Similarly on sigmoidoscopy crypt abscesses can sometimes be observed discharging in punctate fashion.

In the author's experience salazopyrine is particularly helpful for distal disease confined to rectum and sigmoid; proctosigmoiditis responds better to salazopyrine than steroids, particularly when these are given by enemata. Though in the hands of some hydrocortisone enemata appear to have an almost 100 per cent response even for more widespread disease this has not proved to be so in the author's practice. Moreover it has yet to be proved that cortisol has a topical effect; that it can induce improvement there is no doubt but this could be due simply to systemic effects since sufficient cortisol is absorbed into the portal system even to elevate systemic blood levels and after a three week course of enemata sufficient can be absorbed to depress the response to the A.C.T.H. test. It seems likely therefore that rectal administration in reality provides only an alternative route for absorption which is less effective than the oral one.

In the author's practice salazopyrine 4–6 g. daily is tried first for procto-sigmoiditis, turning to prednisone by mouth should this fail. For more widespread disease steroids provide the first choice starting with prednisone 30 mg. per day and doubling this in the absence of response. The dosage is arbitary and a matter of choice; in some centres considerably higher doses are used with disregard for the effects of hypercorticism. Should prednisone fail, a switch to A.C.T.H. can be effective. A return to prednisone has proved helpful after failure of A.C.T.H. There is no satisfactory explanation for the effects of such therapeutic changes; the regime in empirical.

Conservative treatment is particularly helpful to the surgeon early in the disease. It could be argued that once the mucosa has been seriously damaged removal of the bowel is inevitable and therefore operative cure should be undertaken sooner rather than later. But this is to ignore the human factor. Duodenal ulcer provides an analogous situation since there are those who, not without reason, regard the proved lesion to be irreversible and recommend surgery early, regardless of the fact that post-operative satisfaction and sense of well-being will be less if the contrasting period of pre-operative symptoms has been shortlived. So it is with ulcerative colitis. Though drug treatment can at best produce a remission it provides time for the patient to understand his disease and appreciate the situation this places him in. If an ileostomy is to be performed it will be less easily accepted if the disabilities of the disease have been brief and not severe. This is not to say that operation may not have to be undertaken during the first few weeks; if the disease is acute and severe this may be necessary on the grounds already discussed, or if no response follows steroid therapy. But under these circumstances diarrhoea, incapacity and the sense of illbeing are borne in upon the patient. In brief it is easier to persuade a patient to accept surgical action when it is clear that medical means have been tried and shown to fail to alter the course of the disorder.

When the patient who has received corticosteroids comes to operation the possibility of adrenal collapse must be borne in mind. This is not predictable on clinical grounds for it is not possible to foretell which patients will fail under the stress of operation. The adrenal response of a patient displaying the facies of hypercorticism may be normal and collapse can occur in the absence of such stigmata. For anyone who has received a full course of steroids within two years of operation it is advisable to test adrenal response either by the A.C.T.H. or pyrogen test. Should the response be depressed steroid cover can be provided by

50 mg. hydrocortisone with premedication, repeating the dose at the time of anaesthetic induction. When unsuspected adrenal collapse occurs during operation 100 mgm. hydrocortisone should be given at once intravenously but not before a sample of blood has been taken to ascertain the cortisol level and confirm the diagnosis, so that subsequent management may be facilitated. Hydrocortisone should then be administered slowly by means of intravenous infusion 100 mg. in 500 ml. of saline and set to run at the rate of one litre in the next twelve hours. Thereafter hydrocortisone may be given according to the need to maintain a normal blood pressure.

Which Operation?

The choice lies between total excision of the large intestine and incomplete excision with ileorectal anastomosis. Cure can only be obtained by total excision since retention of the rectum can lead to exacerbations of the disease, its complications and to cancer; cure therefore necessitates an artificial stoma. Circumstances arise when less than cure must be accepted either because an ileostomy is not acceptable, or cannot be managed either because of the inability of the patient to do so or because the milieu in which he lives does not provide the necessary facilities to enable him to manage the adherent bag. So much is common ground; controversy has arisen regarding ileorectal anastomosis as the operation of first choice. The protagonists of ileorectal anastomosis take the not unreasonable view that retention of anal function is preferable to an artificial stoma. This can, however, be a mistaken view since an efficient stoma carries no disability whereas patients with an ileorectal anastomosis at best have two loose motions a day, commonly four, sometimes more. Not infrequently precipitancy adds to their disability as occasionally does perineal excoriation. The real criticism of an ileostomy lies in the need to maintain its efficiency since an inefficient stoma gives rise to considerable disability. Operative revision is required for a proportion of all ileostomies: due to failure of attachment of the mesentery across the iliac fossa causing recession of the stoma until it is flush with the skin which then becomes excoriated through leakage and so unseating the bag: to prolapse from the same cause: to skin-level fistula from chaffing against the flange of the bag usually through improper siting of the stoma, with effects similar to recession: rarely, since eversion of the stoma, to stenosis. With increasing experience the revision rate has fallen. In the author's series of 112 ileostomies instituted in the years 1948–55 24 (21·5 per cent) required revision, from then to 1963 of 232 10 (4·3 per cent) needed further operation, while of the 148 performed in the five year period 1960–64 only 3 (2 per cent) came to revision. No mortality was incurred and though 4 patients needed more than one revision no multiple revisions occurred after 1958.

In summary, cure can only be obtained by total excision of colon and rectum; this now carries a 2 per cent possibility of further operation to maintain the efficiency of the stoma. Those who regard ileorectal anastomosis as preferable must consider the morbidity and mortality due to failure to eradicate the disease and the disabilities associated with anal preservation.

Results

Elective procedures to remove the large intestine carry an operative mortality of 3 per cent or less; this rises to 30 per cent in acute severe disease but, as previously stated, this figure is capable of reduction. Regarding late results a comparison with untreated cases is instructive. Ulcerative colitis untreated by surgery carries an increasing mortality, 40 per cent in a series followed to 20 years, 50 per cent after 25 years. In the author's series of 442 cases surgically treated and followed to 18 years the cumulative total mortality including operation, its late complications and unrelated deaths, was 25 per cent. Excluding deaths from operative causes and those known to have died of cancer the observed deaths after operation was no greater than expected in a similar population for age and sex—18 expected, 19 observed out of 358 patients. It is notable that of the 39 late deaths 15 were due to cancer, 7 to liver failure, 2 to intestinal obstruction, the remaining 15 patients dying of incidental disease. These figures serve to emphasize the importance of the indications for operation in the longstanding and the acute presentations. While the reasoning regarding cancer is self-evident, liver failure ultimately causing the death of 7 patients almost certainly arose in severe disease which was allowed to persist too long before operative relief.

As regards morbidity, the results following removal of the whole of the large intestine reveal restoration to a normal state of nutrition, weight being gained in all cases. Anaemia, universally present at the time of operation, has been overcome in all except those patients with cirrhosis, women with iron deficiency states of gynaecological origin and the geriatric case taking an inadequate diet. Impotence has been a sequel in approximately 10 per cent of men, the evidence in these cases indicating damage to the presacral nerve, the parasympathetic nerves deep in the pelvis or both. This is clearly due to technical failure and should be avoidable; it was notable that it occurred in those patients in whom the pelvic dissection of the combined operation fell to relatively inexperienced hands. The fault arises when the pelvic operator attempts to open the presacral space before the correct plane has been defined by the surgeon from above, since the dissection is then placed too far posteriorly and causes the sacral nerves carrying the nervi erigentes to be damaged. There is also an increased risk of infertility in women the evidence here pointing to blockage of the Fallopian tubes. Whether this is the result of pelvic inflammation due to the disease itself or to the results of surgery it is, at present, impossible to say.

Life with an ileostomy is unimpaired. Of a group of 100 patients (62 women, 38 men) selected only in one respect, to ensure that they had had an ileostomy for not less than 5 years, 95 were fully employed 3 having retired. One patient was a surgical cripple after numerous operations for intestinal obstruction; another regarded herself incapable of work though no physical reason could be found for this. All forms including heavy work were being undertaken; no evidence could be elicited to indicate limitation of prospects of promotion. All women undertaking full housework and bringing up families were considered to be fully employed; 13 of these undertook, in addition, work outside their homes. Recreations included camping, gliding, swimming, gardening and dancing.

The Ileostomy Bag

These results can only be achieved by efficient management of the ileostomy bag, of which numerous varieties are obtainable. Basically these fall into one of two categories: the bag in which flange and its body are united in one piece and the type with separate flange over the rim of which the body of the bag can be fitted. It is wise to select one and start all patients with this in the convalescent period. Most will adapt to this; that other varieties are available will be apparent from contacts with the Ileostomy Association and its literature, so that each individual patient can later select what to him seems more suitable should the original choice made by his surgeon appear in some way inappropriate for his own needs.

The bag is usually cemented to the skin with latex or Karaya gum reinforced with adhesive strapping, but cement is not essential and some patients dispense with this. It is usual to change the bag for cleaning every third day though for some patients the interval is less, for some as long as a week.

An important development has been the establishment of the Ileostomy Association which now covers the British Isles and is ready to be called upon at any time. Amongst its numerous functions it provides a hospital visiting service to clarify problems in the minds of those about to undergo operation, an after-care service for those with problems regarding bag management and makes available films and literature for the instruction of patients and nurses. It also takes part in research without which much of the information in this chapter would not have been obtained.

References

BARON, J. H., CONNELL, A. M., LENNARD-JONES, J. E., AVERY JONES, F. (1962) Sulphasalazine and salicylazo-sulphadimidine in Ulcerative Colitis. *Lancet*, **1**, 1094; (1965) **1**, 185.

BROOKE, B. N. (1961). Malignant Change in Ulcerative Colitis. *Dis. Colon & Rectum*, **4**, 393.

BROOKE, B. N. (1962). Inflammatory Disorders of Colon. *Dis. Colon & Rectum*, **5**, 138.

BROOKE, B. N., SAMPSON, P. A. (1964). An Indication for Surgery in Acute Ulcerative Colitis. *Lancet*, **2**, 1272.

DALY, D. W., BROOKE, B. N. (1967). Ileostomy and Excision of the Large Intestine for Ulcerative Colitis. *Lancet*, **2**, 62.

EDWARDS, F. C., TRUELOVE, S. C. (1963). The Course and Prognosis of Ulcerative Colitis. *Gut*, **4**, 299; (1964) **5**, 1.

SLANEY, G., BROOKE, B. N. (1959). Cancer in Ulcerative Colitis. *Lancet*, **2**, 694.

TRUELOVE, S. C., WITTS, L. J. (1955). Cortisone in Ulcerative Colitis. *Brit. Med. J.*, **2**, 1041.

Chapter 14

HIRSCHSPRUNG'S DISEASE

J. H. Louw

The eponym "Hirschsprung's disease" indicating a specific type of congenital megacolon, is so well known and through common usage so firmly established, that it will probably stay. It is as well to note, however, that credit for the first description of the disease should go to a Dutch anatomist, Frederic Ruysch, who published a detailed report in Latin in the seventeenth century and that at least 20 other reports preceded Hirschsprung's paper of 1888 (Benson *et al.*, 1962). In recent years there has been a tendency to refer to the disease simply as *aganglionosis* or *congenital aganglionic megacolon*, or, more correctly, *congenital intestinal aganglionosis* (Nixon, 1964, 1966).

Aetiology and Pathogenesis

Hirschsprung in 1888 described the characteristic clinical feature of the disease, viz., "sluggishness of the stool in the newborn" but he attributed this to the dilatation and hypertrophy of the proximal colon. In 1946 Ehrenpreis produced evidence that the primary fault was "dysfunction of evacuation" and that the megacolon developed secondarily because of an obstruction which, he suggested, was of neurogenic origin. Swenson, Rheinlander and Diamond (1949) demonstrated that the motility of the distal colon was disturbed in Hirschsprung's disease and in 1948 Swenson and Bill made history by showing that the condition could be cured by resection of the abnormally functioning rectum and sigmoid. Although absence of ganglia from the affected bowel was described by Tittel as long ago as 1901 and confirmed by several others thereafter, it was not until 1949 when Bodian, Stephens and Ward published their classic paper, that the histological features of aganglionosis were fully described and correlated with the clinical findings.

It is now well established that the essential lesion is congenital absence of ganglia in the submucous and intermuscular myenteric plexuses of the distal part of the bowel and that their place is taken by clusters of enlarged unmedullated nerve fibres. Characteristically, the aganglionosis commences at the lower end of the rectum and extends proximally for a variable distance. In about 80 per cent of cases the anomaly does not extend beyond the sigmoid (short segment) while in the remainder it extends proximally to involve variable lengths of the colon and may even involve the terminal ileum (long segment). Rarely the aganglionosis involves the whole of the small as well as the large bowel, but this type differs from the usual in that there are no large nerve fibrils present (Nixon, 1964). Cases with "skip areas" or "segmental aganglionosis" have been described (Keefer and Makrohisky, 1954; Sprinz *et al.*, 1961) but must be very rare because most workers have failed to confirm the existence of such a variation (Swenson, 1957; Wyllie, 1957a; Hiatt, 1958; Nixon, 1964; Kottmeier and Clatworthy, 1965). Roviralta (1962), Bentley (1964) and Pagés and Duhamel (1966) have described hypoganglionosis localized to the distal rectum but most authors are agreed that "diminution in ganglion cells" or "atypical ganglion cells" cannot be regarded as consistent with a diagnosis of Hirschsprung's disease (Kottmeier and Clatworthy, 1965; Nixon, 1966). It should be noted that Smith (1960) has found considerable variation in the histology of ganglion cells in foetal and neonatal life and that this immaturity should not be mistaken for the aganglionosis of Hirschsprung's disease (Kottmeier and Clatworthy, 1965; Ehrenpreis, 1966). It must also be remembered that ganglion cells are normally absent or scanty in the terminal anal canal up to about 2 cm. from the mucocutaneous junction (Bentley, 1964; Kiesewetter *et al.*, 1965; Nixon, 1966); biopsies from this area will, therefore, be misleading.

The early studies of Swenson and his associates (1949) and also those of Hiatt (1951b) showed clearly that the "narrow" aganglionic segment of Hirschsprung's disease is incapable of progressive peristaltic contractions, whereas the dilated proximal colon retains relatively normal functional activity. The aganglionic bowel contracts or relaxes *en masse* and so causes a functional obstruction with secondary hypertrophy and dilatation of the normal bowel proximal to it. The severity of symptoms, however, does not depend entirely on the length of the aganglionic segment. As a rule, short segment cases tend to be mild but some long segment cases may have equally mild symptoms while some short segment cases may have extremely severe symptoms. Hiatt (1958) explains this paradox by suggesting that the hypertrophy of the proximal normal bowel results in increased activity which, in turn, stimulates the aganglionic segment to contract *en masse*. On the other hand, State (1965) claims that X-ray studies in the usual short segment case show the left side of the colon to be markedly dilated with little if any evidence of peristalsis or haustrations. In contrast, the right side of the colon presents good peristaltic activity and haustral markings. He points out that these differences can also be seen at surgery, viz., the wall of the right side of the colon is normal in thickness while the wall of the left side is markedly thickened and hypertrophied. These observations require further investigation by radiographic and intraluminal pressure studies.

Several workers have studied the response to drugs of strips of aganglionic and of ganglion-containing bowel taken from cases of Hirschsprung's disease. The response of the dilated (ganglion-containing) portion to both cholinergic and adrenergic drugs is similar to that of normal colon (Kamijo *et al.*, 1963; Wright and Shepherd, 1965). Muscle from the aganglionic segment is less sensitive to acetylcholine than normal muscle suggesting that a cholinergic system is present (Wright and Shepherd, 1965). Kamijo and others (1953) found an increase of both specific and non-specific cholinesterase activity in the aganglionic bowel and by histochemical studies showed that this finding was closely associated with the abnormal nerve fibres. Ehrenpreis and Pernow (1952) have shown that substance P (a biologically active polypeptide found in nerve tissue) which stimulates smooth muscle activity, is greatly reduced in the aganglionic segment and increased in the hypertrophied proximal colon.

Wright and Shepherd (1965) found that the aganglionic muscle responds normally to adrenaline but, unlike normal muscle, it is contracted by nicotine and dimethylphenylpiperazinium (D.M.P.P.). Therefore, they suggest that an adrenergic inhibitory system is either absent or functionally subnormal. Ehrenpreis (1966) and his associates have pursued this matter further by histochemical studies using a highly specific fluorescence method. They have shown that adrenergic nerve fibres to normal intestines are distributed mainly to the intramural plexuses where they make synaptic contacts with the parasympathetic ganglion cells. In Hirschsprung's disease these adrenergic synapses are lacking in the intramural plexuses of the aganglionic segment but present in the proximal, hypertrophied bowel. Further studies along these lines are clearly indicated and may be rewarding.

The aetiology of the aganglionosis is not yet fully understood. The great rarity of the anomaly in premature infants (Berdon *et al.*, 1964; Hofmann and Rehbein, 1966) suggests that the ganglia might be destroyed late in foetal life. Support for the concept of selective destruction of ganglia is to be found in the similarity between Hirschsprung's disease and Chaga's disease in which the myenteric plexuses are selectively destroyed by the toxins of Trypanosoma cruzi (Ferreira-Santos, 1961). Furthermore, McElhannon (1959) has shown that the myenteric plexus in dogs can be selectively destroyed by injecting the inferior colic artery with Urokon and that the animals develop all the symptoms and signs of Hirschsprung's disease. It is now well known that interruption of the blood supply to a segment of the foetal bowel may result in certain congenital malformations such as atresia and stenosis (Louw, 1959, 1966) and Hukuhara and others (1961) have claimed that selective destruction of ganglia can be produced by temporary ischaemia of the colon. It has, therefore, been suggested that a similar mechanism acting late in foetal life might be responsible for aganglionosis (Ehrenpreis, 1966; Lister, 1966).

Ehrenpreis (1966) records a case of Hirschsprung's disease where complete excision of the aganglionic segment failed to relieve the constipation. Barium studies done 4 years later showed a recurrence of the megacolon with a "narrow segment" extending to the promontory of the sacrum. Examination of the excised "narrow segment" revealed that ganglion cells were sparse with degenerative changes and that the blood vessels had inclusions of hyaline material in their walls. He presumed that these changes were due to temporary impairment of the vascular supply to the distal colon as a result of the previous pull-through procedure and cites the case as evidence in favour of the vascular origin of aganglionosis. Lister (1966) has reported changes in the blood vessels supplying the transitional zone in 3 out of 10 cases of histologically proven Hirschsprung's disease. At operation the vessels were firm and thickened and had the appearance of an inflammatory peri-arteritis but microscopy revealed hamartomatous changes. He suggests that the vascular changes might indicate a poor foetal blood supply with consequent degeneration of the myenteric plexus in utero.

Although the theory of the vascular origin of Hirschsprung's disease may appear attractive, there are certain features of the disease which render the hypothesis unlikely. In the first place, it fails to explain the natural distribution of aganglionosis which always starts most distally and extends proximally. Secondly, it does not account for the extreme rarity of "skip lesions". Thirdly, it cannot be reconciled with the fact that aganglionosis is only rarely associated with lesions known to be due to vascular interference, viz., intestinal atresia and stenosis (Louw, 1959a, 1964, 1966a). In this connection Parkkulainen and others (1959) reported detailed studies of 25 patients with anorectal malformations of whom 15 had absence of ganglia from the terminal gut but these lesions have not been shown to be due to vascular interference and the findings are contrary to the experience of all other writers on the subjects. Indeed, to test the validity of Parkkulainen's observations, Kiesewetter and others (1965) collected data from 32 major paediatric centres in the United States and Canada. Nineteen reported that they had never encountered the association. Thirteen reported on specific histological examinations done in 296 cases with anorectal malformations and of these 10 had associated aganglionosis, i.e. an incidence of 3·4 per cent. It would appear, therefore, that a real association is unlikely.

The evidence in favour of the vascular theory may also be questioned. Ehrenpreis's (1966) solitary case of "secondary aganglionosis" remains unproven because his initial proximal transection might have been through the transitional zone between aganglionic and normal bowel and, moreover, the secondary "narrow segment" was not completely devoid of ganglia. Lister's (1966) observations are inconclusive because in only three of 10 cases were vascular anomalies present and he describes similar vascular changes in a case of apparent Hirschsprung's disease where subsequent examination showed that the myenteric plexus was normal. We have, therefore, investigated the problem along two lines. Firstly, the experiments described by Hukuhara and others (1961) have been repeated in our laboratories in an attempt to produce aganglionosis by temporary ischaemia of a segment of colon. These experiments were carried out on 18 dogs and, although a variety of lesions of the bowel wall were produced, intramural ganglion cells were consistently present in adequate numbers and of normal structure in both the submucosal and myenteric plexuses of all the specimens examined (de Villiers, 1966). Secondly, experiments were performed on foetal puppies whereby the blood supply to the terminal colon was interrupted and although colonic atresia and stenosis were produced, it was impossible to produce aganglionosis (Louw, 1964). Furthermore, re-examination of all our experimental and clinical material on intestinal atresia and stenosis has failed to reveal any abnormality of ganglia in the bowel adjacent to the atretic areas.

Considerable evidence has now accumulated to incriminate genetic factors in the aetiology of Hirschsprung's disease. Dalla Valle in 1924 commented on the familial incidence of the disease and in 1951 Bodian and others reported the first systematic family study. In 1962 Althoff reported a family study based on 68 index cases, in 1963 Bodian and Carter published their findings based on 207 index cases and in 1966 Gordon and others from Cape Town reported a study based on 71 index cases. Several important findings have emerged from these studies, viz.:

1. The overall male to female ratio is approximately 4 to 1 but this decreases with increasing length of the aganglionic segment, being almost equal for long segment cases and 5 to 1 for short segment cases.

2. The proportion of sibs affected is consistently and significantly higher for the long segment than for the short segment cases. Bodian and Carter (1963) estimate that the proportion of affected sibs of short-segment cases is 1 in 20 for brothers and 1 in 100 for sisters while the proportion of affected sibs of long segment cases is 1 in 10 irrespective of sex.

3. There is no evidence for autosomal dominant or sex-linked in-

heritance (Bodian and Carter, 1963), but the occurrence of parental consanguinity and the presence of affected relatives in the pedigrees of some of the studied families are consistent with a recessive type of inheritance (Gordon *et al.*, 1966).

4. There are families containing both long and short segment cases (Gordon *et al.*, 1966) and therefore it is unlikely that the two types are caused by different mutant genes. However, the variation in length may be attributed to modification by environmental factors acting at the genetic level (Bodian and Carter, 1963). This is supported by the tendency of the mothers of index cases to be older than those in the general population (Gordon *et al.*, 1966). Since maternal age also plays a role in the incidence of Down's syndrome (Mongolism) it is of interest that this is the only condition which has a significant association with aganglionosis. From collected figures it would appear that the incidence of Down's syndrome in patients with aganglionosis is about 1 in 60 while in the general population the incidence of the syndrome is 1 in 600 (Gordon *et al.*, 1966).

Further information on the genetic aspects of Hirschsprung's disease has come from animal experimentation. Derrick and St. George-Grambauer (1957) of Brisbane have reported both long and short segment aganglionosis in a colony of mice. In this colony the incidence was about 1 in 200, the sex ratio unity and it was not uncommon to find more than one member of a litter affected. Bielschowsky and Scho-field (1962) have studied the incidence of megacolon in an inbred New Zealand strain of mice and in descendants of this strain outcrossed with two other strains. The results of this study leave no doubt that aganglionosis in mice is due to genetic factors transmitted by both males and females.

The best indication of the way in which the genetic predisposition might act comes from the experimental work of Yntema and Hammond (1954, 1955) on chick embryos. They found that complete extirpation of the cranio-cervical neural crest before the ten somite stage led to aganglionosis from oesophagus to rectum. Incomplete or later extirpation led to aganglionosis in the distal part of the gut only. These experiments suggest that Hirschsprung's disease is due to a disturbance in the migration of cells from the cranio-cervical portion of the embryonic neural tube to the gut (Bodian and Carter, 1963). The increase in sex ratio with decreasing length of aganglionic bowel may be due to sex differences in the rate of development (Bodian and Carter, 1963). The association of anophthalmos with aganglionosis in one of the cases reported by Gordon *et al.* (1966) (Fig. 14.1) may be significant because this anomaly is due to a disturbance in outgrowth and migration of cells from the same region of the neural tube. Furthermore, Bodian and Carter (1963) report associated congenital cataract in one of their cases and occipital encephalocoele in another: these lesions are also associated with disturbances of development affecting the cranio-cervical portion of the neural tube.

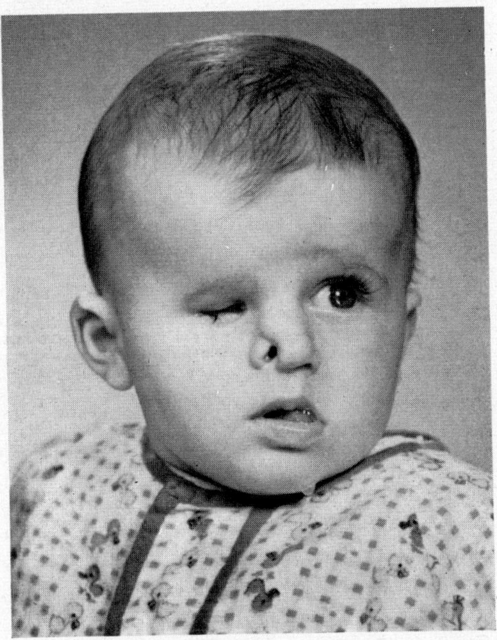

FIG. 14.1. A case of aganglionosis associated with anophthalmos. See text.

Diagnosis

Clinical features: With increasing awareness of the symptomatology of Hirschsprung's disease it is now realized that the child with "classical" abdominal distension, severe constipation, stunted growth and wasted limbs is the survivor of a relatively minor form of the disease (Nixon, 1964; Berdon and Baker, 1965). Often the disease causes more urgent symptoms (obstruction or diarrhoea) in the neonate or during early infancy and if untreated, at least 50 per cent will succumb during the first year of life (Louw, 1959; Nixon, 1964; Hofmann and Rehbein, 1966). The important point is that, whatever the presentation, it is *almost always possible, on careful questioning to elicit a history of bowel trouble since birth.* Often the initial symptoms are so slight or so transitory that hospitalization is not considered necessary, but with a high index of suspicion the diagnosis can be made during the first days or weeks of life long before actual "megacolon" develops. Paediatricians are now aware of this and consequently more patients are being referred for confirmation of the diagnosis during early infancy, e.g. during the past five years over 80 per cent of our new cases of Hirschsprung's disease have been neonates.

It is most important to be familiar with the early symptoms because of the grave risks of acute obstruction and enterocolitis. Usually the infants are well at birth but within a few days they become distended and often vomit bilestained material. A significant feature described by Hirschsprung himself is "sluggishness of the stool", i.e. the passage of meconium is delayed (90 per cent of normal infants pass meconium within 24 hrs.). The obstipation is sometimes relieved spontaneously or more often after digital examination of the rectum. This acute episode which may be mild and transient or severe and life-threatening represents the initial "decompensation period" (Berdon and Baker, 1965) and, although not entirely related to the length of the aganglionic segment, is almost always present. It is this episode which must be recognized so that radiological studies can be undertaken to make the diagnosis promptly and accurately.

Failure to recognize the lesion during the initial period of decompensation may be responsible for a disastrous outcome or prolonged suffering depending upon the subsequent progress which may conform to any of the following patterns (Nixon, 1964):

GROUP I: Acute obstruction persists until death or relieved by colostomy. (Most of these patients have long segments and in those with total colonic aganglionosis ileostomy may be necessary.)

GROUP II: Recurrent obstructive episodes occur which render early colostomy mandatory.

GROUP III: Recurrent obstructive episodes occur but respond well to washouts. Remissions may last for several weeks or months.

GROUP IV: The "compensated" case. Mild obstructive symptoms occur during infancy but tend to settle although constipation is often a problem. Over a period of a year or so the "classical" clinical picture may develop.

GROUP V: Attacks of enterocolitis occur and these are lethal in 25 to 50 per cent of affected infants.

It should be emphasized that infants belonging to Groups II and III may develop enterocolitis at any time during the course of their illness and that even those in Group IV are at risk. Indeed, this dreaded complication of the disease is said to occur in almost 50 per cent of infants suffering from aganglionosis (Berdon and Baker, 1965; Bill and Chapman, 1962; Dorman, 1957; Louw, 1959). The attacks are characterized by severe prostration, massive abdominal distension despite enemas and suppositories, foul, watery diarrhoea and sometimes vomiting. Dehydration develops out of proportion to the external losses probably because of accumulation of massive amounts of fluid in the dilated bowel, and the child may die within 24 hrs. Those who recover from the attack are prone to further attacks and the condition may become chronic with persistent anorexia, failure to gain weight and intermittent attacks of bloody diarrhoea with fever, leucocytosis and "toxic megacolon" resembling ulcerative colitis. The cause of this complication is not clearly understood. Colonic ulceration may be extensive and although pathogenic bacteria cannot be cultured in the early stages, secondary infection does occur and may extend through the bowel wall to give rise to peritonitis and septicaemia (Swenson, 1964). Presumably the condition is related to colonic stasis with an increase in intraluminal pressure and reduction in blood flow (Swenson, 1962 and 1964; Bill and Chapman, 1962), and there is also an apparent defect in water metabolism and electrolyte control (Swenson, 1962). The important point, however, is that the enterocolitis can be avoided by the timely performance of a proximal colostomy (Bill and Chapman, 1962; Dorman, 1957; Swenson, 1962; Berdon and Baker, 1965).

X-Ray Studies:

In the newborn. Plain X-Rays of the abdomen during the first period of clinical decompensation will usually show multiple gas-filled loops with air-fluid levels. Differentiation of large and small bowel is often impossible but lateral films may facilitate recognition of gas in the descending colon. Barium enema examination—which should be routine in all infants with suspected intestinal obstruction—is necessary to differentiate large from small bowel distension and to provide proof of the diagnosis (Fig. 14.2).

Contrast studies must be done with great care using a soft catheter without a balloon taped to the buttocks. Barium is run into the *unprepared* bowel and observed running up the "narrow" terminal bowel until it flows through the cone of transition into the dilated bowel above. At this point the enema is stopped and immediate frontal and lateral films are taken. The dilated bowel should not be filled because large amounts of liquid barium may obscure the essential lesion and carry the risk of water intoxication. No attempt should be made to promote evacuation and delayed films are taken at 24 hrs. and, if necessary, at 48 hrs. (Berdon and Baker, 1965). The most distinctive feature of aganglionosis in the neonate, first emphasized by Ehrenpreis in 1946, is retention of the barium for 24 hrs. and longer and persistence of colonic distension (Berdon and Baker, 1965) (Fig. 14.2(*b*)). In the newborn infant the proximal colon has not yet become permanently

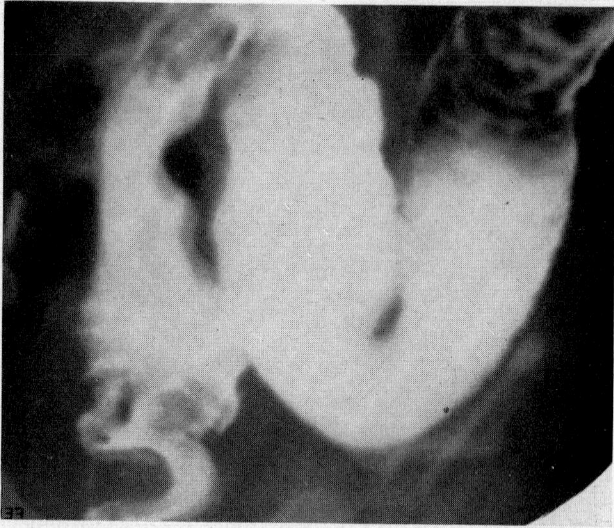

FIG. 14.2(*a*). Barium enema in a neonate suffering from aganglionosis. A "narrow segment" can be recognised but is not well defined.

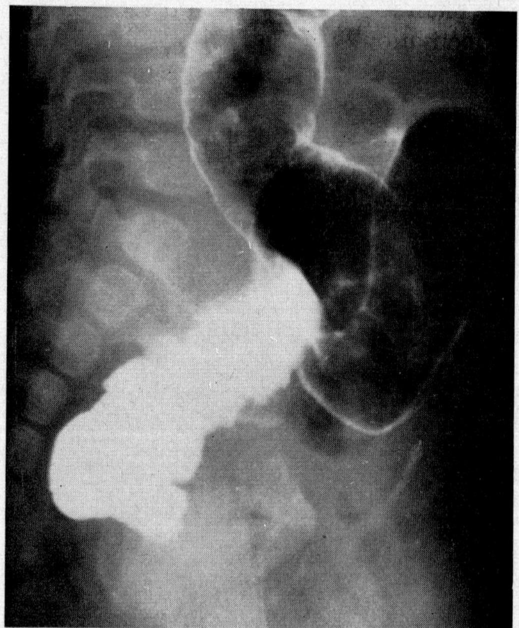

FIG. 14.2(*b*). 24-hour Film in the same patient. Note the retention of barium and persistence of colonic distension.

dilated and therefore a change in calibre between aganglionic and normal bowel is not well defined (Fig. 14.2(*a*)) and may not be seen at all especially when films are taken after deflation (Hofmann and Rehbein, 1966; Berdon and Baker, 1965).

The *meconium plug syndrome* may mimic aganglionosis (Fig. 14.3) but in many cases the barium enema alone produces complete relief of the

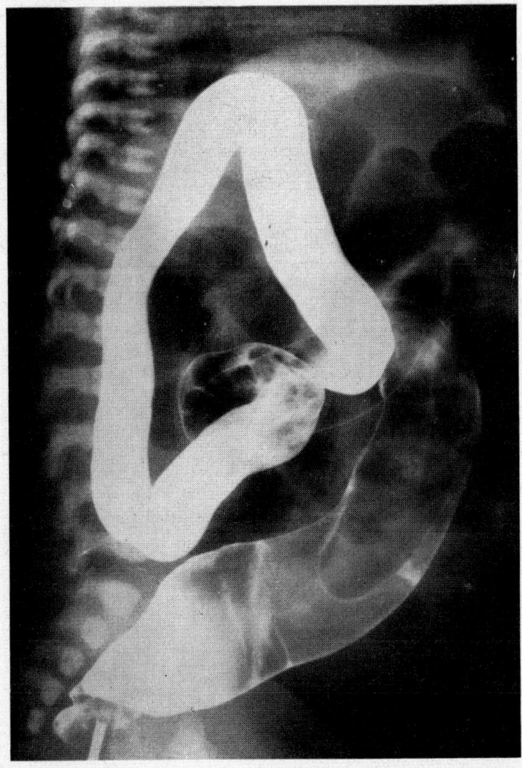

Fig. 14.3. Meconium plug obstructing the distal colon. The clinical picture resembled Hirschsprung's disease but the symptoms were completely relieved after passage of the plug.

obstructive symptoms and the plug may be recovered at the time of evacuation (Hofmann and Rehbein, 1966; Kottmeier and Clatworthy, 1965). The *faecal plug* (Zachary and Emery, 1957) and *inspissated milk* syndromes may also be confusing. In both some meconium is passed before obstruction develops and in both palpable hard concretions block the bowel and may be visualized on the barium enema. Moreover, the inspissated milk syndrome, unlike Hirschsprung's disease, occurs almost exclusively in premature infants. *Immaturity of bowel function* may also account for some cases of distension, vomiting and constipation in premature babies (Nixon, 1966). *Necrotizing enterocolitis* in premature infants not associated with Hirschsprung's disease may occur and may be equally confusing because barium studies may even reveal a transitional zone between "narrow" and "dilated" bowel (Fig. 14.4) (Berdon *et al.*, 1964; Berdon and Baker, 1965).

When there is total colonic aganglionosis the diagnosis is more difficult. Barium enema films reveal massive distension of the small bowel

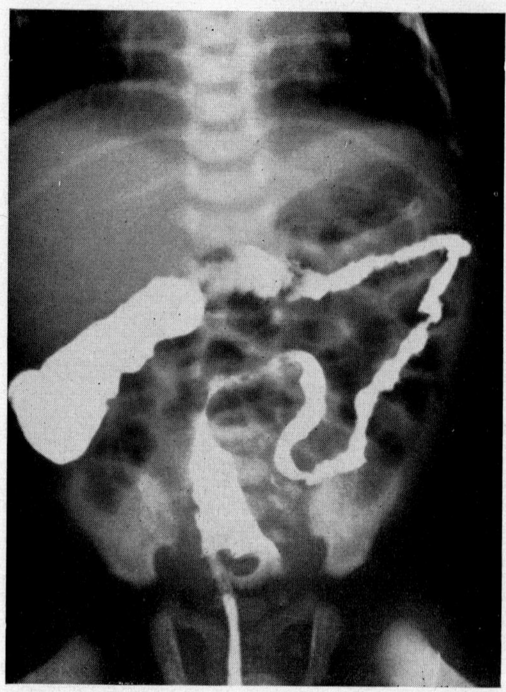

FIG. 14.4. Necrotising enterocolitis in a premature infant resembling Hirschsprung's disease. On rectal biopsy the "narrow segment" contained normal ganglia and nerve fibres and the child recovered completely.

and "microcolon", but these are also features of ileal atresia, malrotation or meconium ileus. The problem usually does not pose a practical difficulty because of the need for urgent laparotomy whatever the cause of the obstruction. However, some of the long-segment cases of Hirschsprung's disease deflate spontaneously and may live for weeks or even months without surgical relief (Dorman, 1957; Louw, 1959). The characteristic features of Hirschsprung's disease, viz., a colon of *normal* calibre but *shortened* length and evidence of stasis on the delayed films should, therefore, be sought for. (Berdon and Baker, 1965).

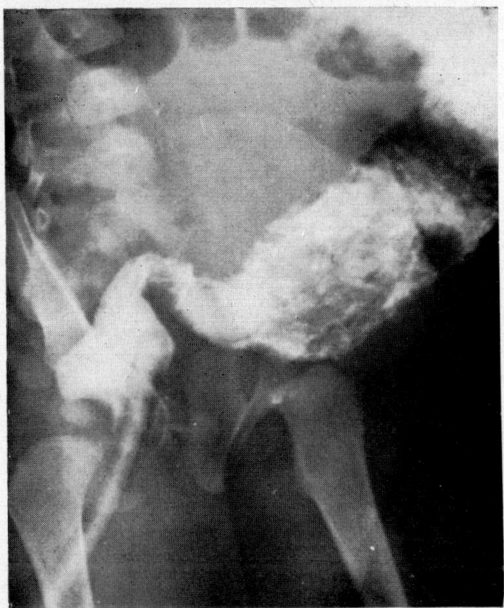

Fig. 14.5. The typical barium enema picture of Hirschsprung's disease in older children. Note the narrow distal segment, the transitional "cone" and the dilated proximal colon.

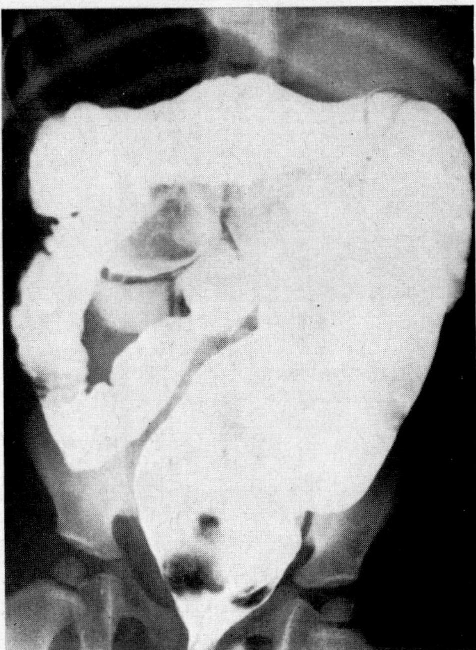

Fig. 14.6. Barium enema in a case of very short segment Hirschsprung's disease. The appearance is similar to that found in idiopathic megacolon with no evidence of the aganglionic segment.

In older infants and children. The characteristic radiological findings are well known (Fig. 14.5), viz., the narrow aganglionic distal colon, the funnel-shaped transition zone and the increasingly dilated proximal colon which, if over-filled, tends to obscure the distal bowel. However, the diagnosis cannot be made on the radiological picture alone. Firstly, variations from the classical pattern are common and have been well-documented (Keefer and Makrohisky, 1954; Louw, 1959). Secondly,

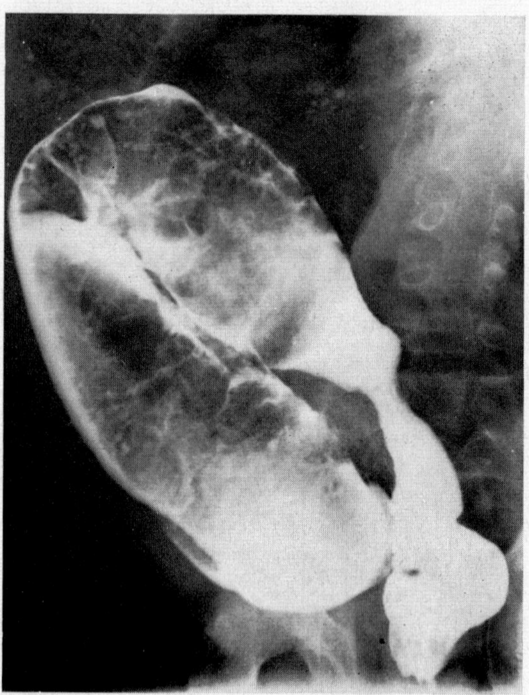

FIG. 14.7. Barium enema in a case of pseudo-Hirschsprung's disease. Rectal biopsy and histological examination of the excised "narrow segment" revealed normal ganglia and nerve fibres.

when the aganglionic segment is very short the picture may resemble that of colonic inertia or idiopathic megacolon (Fig. 14.6). Although there is still no general acceptance of the occurrence of an extremely short aganglionic segment involving little more than the internal sphincter, Pagès and Duhamel (1966), Bentley (1964) and Roviralta (1962) have provided some evidence that such a *forme anale* might exist. Thirdly, the radiological findings in other types of megacolon may simulate those of aganglionosis in every respect (Fig. 14.7). This has been well illustrated in Chaga's disease (Ferreira-Santos, 1961) and

also in other types of so-called pseudo-Hirschsprung's disease (Ehrenpreis, 1965, 1966: Nixon, 1966; Katz, 1966).

Rectal Biopsy:

From above it should be clear that confirmation of the diagnosis by
histological examination of the affected bowel is necessary before
definitive treatment is carried out. This can be established by rectal
biopsy because in Hirschsprung's disease adequate microscopic
sections of the rectal wall will reveal the *characteristic absence of*

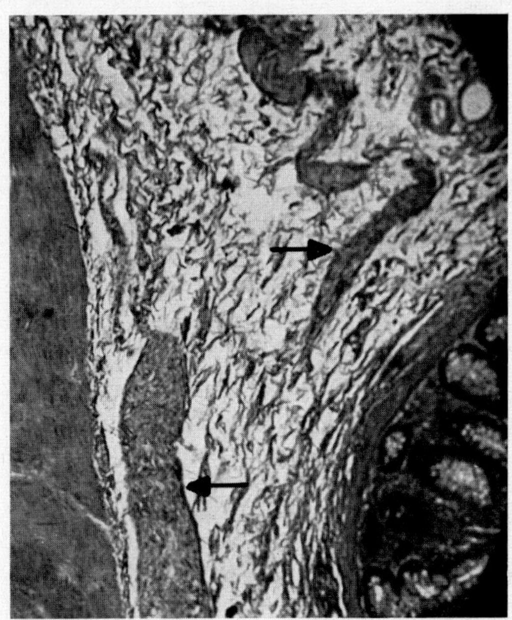

FIG. 14.8. Rectal biopsy in Hirschsprung's disease. No ganglion cells could be
detected but in their place there are large nerve trunks (indicated by arrows).

*ganglion cells in the submucous and intramural myenteric plexuses as
well as the presence of large nerve trunks in the bowel wall in place of
the ganglia* (Fig. 14.8). The demonstration of the typical histological
picture may be facilitated by sections prepared histochemically. It must
be re-emphasized that the histological diagnosis should be based on the
"all or none" characteristic of aganglionosis, (see above) and that the
biopsy specimen must be taken at least 2 cm. from the mucocutaneous
junction because below this point ganglion cells are often scanty or
absent in normal subjects (Bentley, 1964; Kiesewetter *et al.*, 1965).

The biopsy technique described by Swenson, Fisher and MacMahon
in 1955 has been widely adopted. It involves the removal of a 5 mm.

by 10 mm. full-thickness section of the rectal wall at least 2 cm. from the mucocutaneous junction and formal repair of the defects in muscle and mucosa with two layers of interrupted sutures. The procedure is not easy especially in newborn infants, requires general anaesthesia and may interfere with subsequent definitive surgery. Other methods of obtaining the biopsy specimen have, therefore, been devised. In 1958 Hiatt described a biopsy technique which involves an approach to the posterior rectal wall through an incision in the natal cleft midway between anus and coccyx. By this approach the bowel lumen is not entered thus avoiding faecal contamination but it also requires general anaesthesia and is more difficult than the Swenson technique. In 1960 Bodian pointed out that the diagnosis of aganglionosis could be made by examination of a biopsy of a 2 cm. strip of mucosa and submucosa only. This involves examination of the submucous nerve plexuses only and requires general anaesthesia. Nixon (1966) has found the method completely reliable but many pathologists are not prepared to commit themselves on such limited material. In 1961 Shandling described a technique for obtaining biopsy material from Houston's valves. General anaesthesia is not required but, although he found the method simple and reliable, our subsequent experience at the same hospital has shown that the biopsy specimens are often inadequate. *In the author's opinion Swenson's original biopsy procedure remains the method of choice.*

The importance of obtaining histological confirmation of the diagnosis before proceeding with definitive surgery has been emphasized by many authors (Kottmeier and Clatworthy, 1965; Louw, 1959; Nixon, 1964; Shandling, 1961). In a recent publication Kottmeier and Clatworthy (1965) draw attention to 7 of 21 patients who were subsequently proven to have ganglion cells in the rectum but who were unnecessarily subjected to enterostomy, colostomy or even rectosigmoidectomy. In addition, several patients who were subsequently proven to have aganglionic megacolon were treated conservatively for up to 12 years with a mistaken diagnosis of acquired functional megacolon. Such mistakes could have been overcome and years of morbidity avoided by timely rectal biopsy.

The timing of the rectal biopsy is important. In older infants and children it should be done as a routine procedure as soon as the diagnosis is suspected and the bowel has been cleansed. Swenson (1962) has found it possible to perform the definitive resection of the aganglionic segment at any time following the biopsy, usually after 2 to 3 days to allow the pathologist adequate time to prepare the sections. However, although the bowel containing the biopsy site is resected, there is always some surrounding inflammatory reaction and a tendency for the biopsy scar to split during the mobilization of the rectum, and sometimes active infection may interfere with subsequent healing of the anastomosis. It is, therefore, preferable either to obtain a frozen section report at the time of the biopsy and to proceed with the resection immediately or, better still, to postpone resection for several weeks to allow for adequate healing of the biopsy site.

In newborn infants the position is more difficult. Those presenting with acute obstruction which cannot be relieved by washouts, require immediate colostomy. This should be sited proximal to the transition zone between contracted and dilated bowel and in cases with the usual short segment, transverse colostomy is preferred. It is important to obtain a biopsy of the colonic wall at the site of the proposed colostomy and to have it examined by frozen section to ensure that the bowel will be decompressed above the aganglionic segment. At the same time, if the condition of the infant permits, biopsies should be taken of the distal collapsed bowel and of the transition zone to confirm the diagnosis of Hirschsprung's disease and to determine the site of subsequent resection. (The biopsy sites should be marked by sutures.)

In infants who have been (correctly) treated for the obstructive episode by suppositories, enemas and/or colonic irrigation and in whom the diagnosis has been confirmed by radiological studies, it might be tempting to omit or postpone rectal biopsy. Benson and Lloyd (1964) and Hofmann and Rehbein (1966) feel that the biopsy procedure is too difficult and hazardous in infants under 3 months to justify its routine use and they rely on the clinical and radiological findings to make a diagnosis. Nixon (1964) also believes that routine biopsy is not essential but Swenson (1962) favours it and the experiences described above serve to emphasize how important it is to make an accurate diagnosis before embarking on surgical treatment. Infants who develop enterocolitis present the most difficult problem because any type of surgical intervention in these seriously ill patients is associated with a prohibitive mortality. In some of them it may be wiser to defer the rectal biopsy and to proceed to colostomy as soon as the diarrhoea and distension have been controlled. In others it may be possible to obtain a rectal biopsy during a remission.

Methods of Treatment

An important milestone in the progress of paediatric surgery was reached in August, 1948 when Swenson and Bill published a method of curing Hirschsprung's disease by excision of the "narrow" (aganglionic) distal portion of the bowel with preservation of the sphincters. Before this time the disease was treated by a variety of methods including intensive medical measures, forcible dilatation of the anal sphincters, spinal anaesthesia, sympathectomy and partial or total excision of the dilated proximal colon without a significant improvement in the nearly hopeless prognosis. Since that time the outlook for child or infant has become a bright one with the prospect of living an essentially normal lifespan. However, it was not long before various modifications of the Swenson procedure and alternative methods of treatment were introduced and this has resulted in considerable controversy concerning the ideal method of managing the malady. Before discussing the relative merits of the various procedures, however, the place of colostomy in the overall management of the disease should be considered.

Colostomy

As already indicated above, emergency or urgent colostomy may be required to save the life of an infant born with Hirschsprung's disease. The acute episode of obstruction in the neonate is often relieved by digital examination of the rectum which stimulates the passage of meconium and large quantities of flatus. If not, a rectal washout with saline (after a diagnostic barium enema) usually succeeds but if this fails, emergency colostomy (with appropriate colonic biopsies) should be performed. Cases with aganglionosis of the entire colon usually fall into this category (Group I) and in them ileostomy should be performed. In some infants regular daily washouts may keep the baby adequately decompressed (Group III) until definitive surgery can be undertaken at the age of 6 to 12 weeks but this requires prolonged hospitalization because of the risks of recurrent acute obstruction and/or enterocolitis. Not infrequently, however, the washouts fail to provide adequate relief (Group II) and then colostomy becomes mandatory because of the risk of perforation either spontaneously or by the washout. This applies particularly to infants with very long aganglionic segments and in such cases early colostomy or ileostomy should be performed even if washouts achieve adequate decompression. Infants presenting with enterocolitis (Group V) also require urgent colostomy but it is agreed that the colostomy should preferably be done either before this complication develops or during a remission. The attack itself should be treated by energetic fluid replacement and decompression by means of a very large rectal tube which is irrigated frequently to dislodge any particles that might block the lumen. Usually two or three days of treatment are sufficient but if relief is not prompt, urgent colostomy should follow (Bill and Chapman, 1962). There are many who believe that colostomy (or ileostomy) should be performed on all cases of Hirschsprung's disease diagnosed during the neonatal period and early infancy, leaving the definitive procedure until the baby is a year to eighteen months old.

However, colostomy in infants is not without dangers (Louw, 1966) and recently there has been an increasing tendency towards much earlier definitive surgery without preliminary colostomy (Hofmann and Rehbein, 1966). But all who are familiar with the disease and its complications are agreed that when the diagnosis is suspected in infancy it must be confirmed forthwith and that *operation, either colostomy or definitive resection, should be performed before the baby is discharged from hospital.*

In patients who present in later infancy or childhood (Group IV) primary resection without preliminary colostomy is often possible. In such cases the bowel should be thoroughly cleansed with washouts using saline and not plain water to avoid the risk of serious water intoxication. Pre-operative chemotherapy or antibiotics are best omitted because of the risk of super-infection. If there have been attacks of enterocolitis or the proximal colon is grossly enlarged it is wiser to perform colostomy even if cleansing by washouts is apparently satisfactory.

The siting of the colostomy has already been mentioned. It is essential that it should be made well above the aganglionic segment and therefore biopsy with frozen section at the time of surgery is necessary and should be done in all cases except perhaps in very ill newborn infants with acute obstruction (Benson and Lloyd, 1964). The transition zone between narrow and dilated segments is usually clearly recognizable at surgery but in infants who have been well-prepared the colon may appear normal and the same applies to older patients with very short segments. It should also be noted that the radiological and operative transition zones frequently do not correspond (Berdon and Baker, 1965) and that both may differ considerably from the true transition between aganglionic and ganglion-containing bowel (Bodian *et al.*, 1951). This applies particularly to older patients in whom peristalsis and faecal masses can dilate part of the aganglionic bowel.

For the average short-segment case many surgeons prefer a transverse colostomy which leaves a clean operative field for the definitive procedure and which can be closed after the child has completely recovered from the resection. Others (Benson and Lloyd, 1964; Hofmann and Rehbein, 1966; Nixon, 1966; Swenson, 1962) prefer to site the colostomy just above the transition zone and to resect it together with the aganglionic bowel at the time of definitive surgery. The latter method has the advantage of being completed in two stages but at the expense of one of the great benefits of a proximal colostomy, viz., protection of the suture line after resection. In very long-segment cases it is important to site the colostomy close to the transition zone to ensure the maximum amount of available bowel for the definitive procedure. However, when the aganglionosis reaches the ascending colon, ileostomy is probably preferable (Nixon, 1964).

Definitive Surgical Procedures

Of the various surgical procedures that have been introduced since 1948 only those of Swenson and Bill (1948), Duhamel (1956) and Soave (1963) will be discussed (Fig. 14.9), but others will be briefly mentioned.

In 1952 State described an abdominal resection leaving 6 to 10 cm. of the rectum below the peritoneal reflection but extending the proximal transection beyond the dilated colon. The rationale of this operation is to remove the dilated left half of the colon, which State (1965) believes,

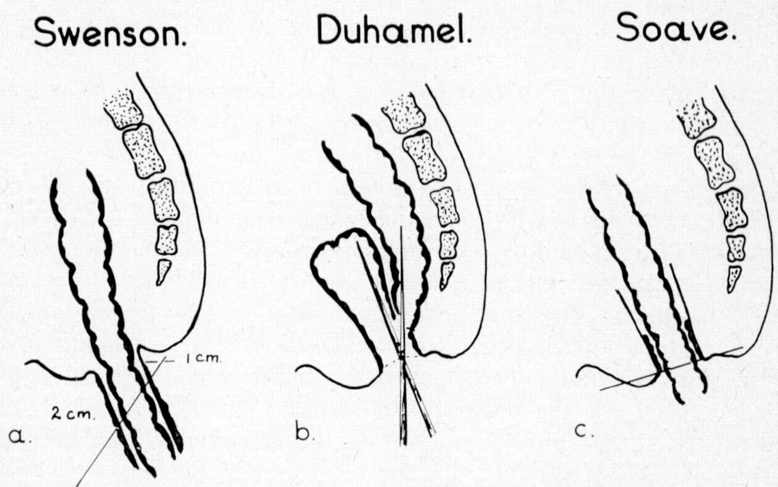

FIG. 14.9. Procedures used in the treatment of Hirschsprung's disease—see text.

does not function normally. In 1963 he reported surprisingly good results considering that the operation leaves most, if not all, the pathological (i.e. aganglionic) bowel *in situ*. In 1964 Rehbein and Nicolai reported their results in treating 110 cases by a modification of States' operation combined with "energetic digital dilatation of the anal canal". The results of this operation leave a good deal to be desired but, as recently stated by Nixon (1964), "perhaps the most surprising thing, considering the pathology of the disease, is that it *ever* succeeds"!

In 1956 Weiss, Hollander and Schwingt described their operation of rectosigmoid myotomy for Hirschsprung's disease. Myotomy has been effective in the treatment of neuromuscular disorders of other parts of the alimentary tract, notably at the cardia and has also been used with some benefit in Chaga's disease (Bentley, 1964) but to date it has received little acceptance as a method of treating aganglionic megacolon.

Recently, Bentley (1964) has revived the concept of an ultra-short aganglionic segment and claims that some of these cases may be cured by "ano-rectal excisional myotomy". The procedure which consists of removing a strip of internal sphincter 5 to 7 mm. wide and up to 10 cm. long, has obvious limitations and further clinical trials are necessary before its value can be assessed.

Swenson procedure: The details of the Swenson operation are well known (Fig. 14.9(*a*)). Suffice it to say that it is a sphincter-saving pull-through procedure in which all the aganglionic bowel is removed down to a point close to the mucocutaneous junction (Swenson, 1962). During the eighteen years that have elapsed since the introduction of the procedure, many surgeons in all parts of the world have used it with satisfactory results in hundreds of cases. Hiatt (1951a) and Browne (1955) introduced modifications to avoid opening the bowel within the abdomen but Swenson and Idriss (1964) object to these "refinements" on the grounds that the resection may be inadequate and that the anal sphincters and mucosa may be damaged. Time has shown that the success of the operation depends mainly on three factors, viz., dissection *on* the muscular wall of the rectum, adequate resection of the aganglionic segment and meticulous technique (Swenson, 1964; Swenson and Idriss, 1964). The purpose of mobilizing the rectum by tedious sharp dissection on the muscular wall instead of by wide blunt dissection is to preserve the pelvic nerves and thereby to avoid interference with bladder and ejaculatory function. To ensure adequate removal of the aganglionic segment the proximal transection must be through normally innervated bowel while the distal transection must be as close as possible to the mucocutaneous junction. The former can be achieved only by taking multiple frozen section biopsies of the colonic wall at the proximal line of section. The latter is achieved by removing as much of the anal canal as is consistent with anal continence. In his original operation Swenson left an anal cuff of 2 to 3 cm. (Swenson, 1962), but since 1961 he has extended the resection to leave (in infants) only 1·5 to 2·0 cm. anteriorly and 1 cm. or less posteriorly (Swenson, 1964). This modification includes a substantial portion of the internal sphincter posteriorly and thereby overcomes post-operative tightness of the sphincter (which is an important cause of post-operative enterocolitis). The necessity for meticulous technique has been repeatedly stressed by Swenson who points out that he is usually "able to accomplish a resection in about four hours with the use of two operative teams" (Swenson, 1964). This technique requires painstaking dissection on the rectal wall, absolute haemostasis and precision anastomosis using two layers of the finest interrupted sutures.

In Swenson's hands the results have been outstandingly good. In a review of his first 200 cases (Swenson, 1957) he reported an early mortality of 3 per cent, a later mortality of 3·5 per cent (mainly due to enterocolitis), a complication rate of 7 per cent and satisfactory long-term results in 97·5 per cent of survivors. In a more recent series of 32 cases treated by his modified technique the mortality and complication rates were zero but 8 of the patients suffered from subsequent entero-colitis requiring hospitalization (Swenson, 1964). Other surgeons have not, as yet, been able to emulate Swenson's success (Wyllie, 1957b) and overall results covering 425 cases treated at other paediatric clinics reflect an early mortality rate of 5 per cent, later mortality rate of 4 per cent, complication rate of 20 per cent and a satisfactory long-term out-come in 70 per cent (Clausen and Davies, 1963). The main problem has been enterocolitis and dilatation of the residual bowel (Clausen and Davies, 1963; Swenson *et al.*, 1960; Swenson, 1964; Nixon, 1964). Swenson (1964, 1965) has found that the cases who develop post-operative enterocolitis have tight anal sphincters and that subsequent sphincterotomy has had a most beneficial effect in a few selected cases. This has led to his recent modification of the operation which has reduced the incidence of enterocolitis without interfering with anal continence. The rarity of incontinence after the Swenson procedure which leaves only 1 to 2·0 cm. of the anal canal has been questioned because Goligher (1961) has shown that at least 5 cm. of anorectal mucosa are required to provide the sensory component needed for adequate control. Goligher's findings, however, apply to adults in whom the total length of rectum and anal canal is about 16·5 cm. In infants up to the age of 18 months the length of the rectum and anal canal is 4 to 6 cm. and, by analogy, the length of mucosa required for continence should be 1·2 to 2 cm. (Louw, 1959).

Whatever the reason might be for the poorer results obtained by others—Nixon (1964) bluntly attributes it to "bad operating"—it has led to a search for a superior operation. In this way certain modifica-tions of the Swenson procedure have evolved and among these the operations of Pellerin (1963) and Grob (1962) should be mentioned. Pellerin leaves the remnant of the anal canal everted over the pulled-through colon with a large indwelling tube in its lumen for 14 days before delayed suture anastomosis. The rationale is to avoid leaks and he has performed over 60 resections with no mortality. Grob (1962) after trying out modifications of the Duhamel operation has now reverted to the Swenson procedure using a modification which ap-proaches that of Swenson himself. He limits the anterior dissection of the rectum but continues the posterior dissection well down to the pelvic floor. A very oblique suture anastomosis is then performed which extends right down to the anal canal posteriorly but much higher up anteriorly. The long-term results of these modifications are not yet known but it should be emphasized that strict attention to every detail of the technique practised by Swenson can, and will, achieve results to equal his.

Duhamel procedure: The retro-rectal transanal pull-through operation described by Duhamel in 1956 (Fig. 14.9(*b*)) has been accepted (with modifications) in many parts of the world (Grob, 1960; Louw, 1961; Eek and Knutrud, 1961; Kostia, 1962; Martin and Altemeier, 1962; Sieber and Kiesewetter, 1963; Forshall, 1964; Beardmore, 1965; Meeker and Kincannon, 1965; Ehrenpreis *et al.*, 1966; Hofmann and Rehbein, 1966). Duhamel's approach to the problem recognizes the principles established by Swenson, viz., resection of the aganglionic bowel, but differs from Swenson's procedure in that only the posterior half of the rectal wall is removed while the anterior part is preserved as a "pouch". The main objects are to limit dissection deep down in the pelvis and to retain the sensory reflexes of the rectum (Duhamel, 1960, 1963).

Duhamel (1964) has claimed results as good as those of Swenson, viz., an early mortality of 2·6 per cent, a complication rate of 10 per cent and satisfactory results in 96 per cent of survivors. More important is the fact that others who have adopted the procedure or one of its modifications have achieved similar successes and consequently many surgeons have adopted it in preference to the Swenson procedure. Enterocolitis is extremely uncommon after the Duhamel procedure but problems with incontinence, faecal impactions in the pouch and anastomotic leaks have occurred. Grob in 1960 reported a modification to decrease incontinence by making the anastomosis above the internal sphincter and some authors now refer to the Duhamel-Grob procedure (Benson and Lloyd, 1964). Martin and Altemeier in 1962 described a modification to overcome faecal impaction by extending the anastomosis to include the entire length of the rectal pouch (Martin, 1965). The author has attempted to overcome impaction by reducing the length of the pouch (Louw, 1961) and further modifications have been described by Grob (1962), by Roviralta (1962), by Duhamel himself (1963) and by Sieber and Kiesewetter (1963). Indeed, the need for continuing modifications has encouraged further exploration for a better surgical approach.

Soave operation: In 1963 Soave described a method whereby the normal colon is pulled through a retained segment of the aganglionic rectum denuded of its mucosa from the abdominal side (Fig. 14.9(*c*)). The objects of the procedure, which is a modification of Ravitch's (1948) anal ileostomy, are to limit pelvic dissection, preserve the rectal sensory receptors and reduce the chances of anastomotic leaks without creating a pouch as in the Duhamel procedure. In 1964 Soave reported his results in 14 patients treated by this method with no mortality, no morbidity and an excellent outcome without enterocolitis or diarrhoea. In 1966 he reported a three year follow up on 34 patients treated by his operation. The mortality was 6 per cent and complication rate 2·9 per cent. The overall results were much better than those obtained in patients operated on by him according to the Swenson and Duhamel methods especially as far as post-operative constipation, diarrhoea and faecal impaction were concerned. Simonson, Habr and Gazal (1960) reported a similar operation for acquired and congenital megacolon. Nixon (1964, 1966) independently, has used the same technique on chosen cases since 1958 with good results but he warns that "simple and safe as is this operation, details of technique and after care are of importance in avoiding complications, and further experience needs to be gained". In 1964, Boley, apparently unaware of what had gone before, described the operation again—perhaps the procedure should be called the Simonson-Habr-Gazal-Soave-Nixon-Boley operation! Whatever it may be called, however, the early results are promising. Since October 1967 we have performed the operation on 9 children, aged 8 months to 3 years, and have not encountered any serious early complications. It is certainly a much simpler procedure than either the Swenson or the Duhamel.

Comparative Results

Carefully controlled clinical trials *by the same team* are clearly required to determine the relative merits of the various procedures. No such study has been published to date and therefore the author's experience is given below.

During the period 1952 to 1965 one hundred consecutive cases of congenital intestinal aganglionosis were dealt with by the author and his team at the Red Cross War Memorial Children's Hospital, Cape Town. On admission to hospital 50 per cent of the patients were newborn and a further 20 per cent were less than 1 year old. Prior to 1960 the only definitive procedure adopted was Swenson's operation (45 consecutive cases). This was changed to the Duhamel procedure for the period 1960 to 1964 (40 consecutive cases). Since the beginning of 1965 both Swenson and Duhamel procedures have been used. To facilitate comparison we have ignored the results of the first five Swenson procedures (when errors in technique due to inexperience were inevitable) and also those of cases operated upon since 1964 (because the follow-up is still too brief). This has left for comparison 40 primary Swenson procedures and the same number of primary Duhamel procedures. The two series are comparable also in other respects, viz.

age of the patients at resection, staging of the operations and lengths of aganglionic segments removed. All the children have been followed up and carefully assessed particularly from the point of view of attacks of diarrhoea (enterocolitis), constipation, rectal incontinence (soiling) and urinary problems.

TABLE I. *Comparative Results*

	Swenson (40)	Duhamel (40)
EARLY:		
Postoperative Deaths ..	2	2
Complications	7	5
Temporary Dysfunction	12	9
LATE:		
Persistent Dysfunction ..	11	3
Secondary Operations ..	5	1
Late Deaths	1	1
GOOD FINAL RESULTS:	31 (78%)	35 (88%)

Table I summarizes the overall results. It shows that as far as early deaths and complications were concerned, there is not much to choose between the two procedures but the late results of the Duhamel operation appear to be more satisfactory than those of the Swenson procedure. It should be noted, however, that in the Swenson series most of the

TABLE II. *Results—Age at Surgery less than 1 Year*

	Swenson (22)	Duhamel (28)
EARLY:		
Postoperative Deaths ..	1	2*
Complications	6	4
Temporary Dysfunction	7	3
LATE:		
Persistent Dysfunction ..	10	1
Secondary Operations ..	4	—
Late Deaths	1	1**
GOOD FINAL RESULTS:	14 (64%)	26 (93%)

* 1 Case had aganglionosis up to the jejunum.
** Death due to endocardial fibroelastosis.

problems (principally enterocolitis) arose in patients operated upon during the first year of life while in the Duhamel series the age factor was of less significance. Table II which reflects the results in patients operated upon before the age of 1 year shows that both the early and the late results of the Duhamel procedure were better than those of the Swenson procedure. This applied particularly to cases with very long aganglionic segments. On the other hand, Table III, which reflects the results in patients operated upon after the age of 1 year shows a somewhat better outcome with the Swenson than with the Duhamel procedure mainly because of the frequency of faecal impactions when the latter was used.

TABLE III. *Results—Age at Surgery more than 1 Year*

	Swenson (18)	Duhamel (12)
EARLY:		
Postoperative Deaths ..	1*	—
Complications	1	1
Temporary Dysfunction	5	6
LATE:		
Persistent Dysfunction ..	1	2
Secondary Operations ..	1	1
Late Deaths	—	—
GOOD FINAL RESULTS:	17 (94%)	10 (83%)

* Probably a case of pseudo-Hirschsprung's disease.

Three further points require elaboration. Firstly, in regard to the Duhamel procedure—since we have taken care to divide the whole septum between rectal pouch and pull-through colon (by re-application of clamps if necessary) problems with faecal impaction have been practically eliminated. Secondly, in regard to the Swenson procedure—since we started using Swenson's modified technique about two years ago, the results in 16 consecutive cases have been excellent regardless of age and to date not a single case has developed enterocolitis. Thirdly, in regard to secondary operations after an inadequate Swenson procedure—the Duhamel procedure has been far more satisfactory than a secondary Swenson. In performing the secondary Duhamel procedure injury to the vessels supplying the terminal colon must be carefully avoided by drawing the bowel down to one side of the midline. We have had to do this in 5 cases and the results in all have been good.

In view of above, we feel that at the present time the following conclusions are justified:

1. Swenson's procedure, meticulously performed, is more suitable for older children. The results are excellent if the posterior rectal wall is excised down to 1 cm. of the mucocutaneous junction but there may still be a small risk of post-operative enterocolitis.

2. Duhamel's procedure has distinct advantages in infants under 1 year of age especially when the aganglionic segment is very long and it is the operation of choice after a failed Swenson procedure.

3. Neither the Swenson nor the Duhamel procedure will satisfy every-

body and the continuing appearance of alternative procedures shows that there is room for further improvement. Whether the Soave operation will stand the test of time and prove to have any advantage over the others still remains to be seen.

The final chapter on this perlexing disease has not yet been written. Further investigations into the aetiology and patho-physiology are clearly required while the results of the various methods of treatment need to be carefully assessed and, who knows, with advances in our knowledge of neuro-chemistry and smooth muscle activity the ultimate management of Hirschsprung's disease may yet prove to be non-surgical?

References

ALTHOFF, W. (1962). Zur Genetik der Hirschsprungschen Krankheit, Z. Menschl. Vererb. Konstitutionsl., **36,** 314.

BEARDMORE, H. E. (1965). Newer Surgical Approaches to Megacolon. Problems in Neonatal Surgery, Report of 49th Ross Conference on Pediatric Research, 62.

BENSON, C. D. and LLOYD, J. R. (1964). An Evaluation of the Surgical Treatment of Hirschsprung's Disease. *S. Clin. N. Amer.*, **44,** 1495.

BENTLEY, J. F. R. (1964). Some new Observations on Megacolon in Infancy and Childhood with Special Reference to the Management of Megasigmoid and Megarectum. *Dis. Colon and Rectum*, **7,** 462.

BERDON, W. E., GROSSMAN, H., BAKER, D. H., MIZRAHI, A., BARLOW, O. and BLANC, W. A. (1964). Necrotizing Enterocolitis in the Premature Infant. *Radiology*, **83,** 879.

BERDON, W. E. and BAKER, D. H. (1965). The Roentgenographic Diagnosis of Hirschsprung's Disease in Infancy. *Amer. J. Roentgenol., Radium Therapy and Nuclear Med.*, **93,** 432.

BIELSCHOWSKY, M. and SCHOFIELD, G. C. (1962). Studies on Megacolon in Piebald Mice. *Aust. J. Exp. Biol. and Med. Sci.*, **40,** 395.

BILL, A. H. and CHAPMAN, N. D. (1962). The Enterocolitis of Hirschsprung's Disease. *Amer. J. Surg.*, **103,** 70.

BODIAN, M. (1960). Pathological Aids in the Diagnosis and Management of Hirschsprung's Disease. In: "Recent Advances in Clinical Pathology", Series 3, edited by S. C. Dyke, J. and A. Churchill Ltd., London.

BODIAN, M., STEPHENS, F. D. and WARD, B. C. H. (1949). Hirschsprung's Disease and Idiopathic Megacolon, *Lancet, i*, 6.

BODIAN, M., CARTER, C. O. and WARD, B. C. H. (1951). Hirschsprung's Disease, *Lancet, i*, 302.

BODIAN, M. and CARTER, C. O. (1963). A Family Study of Hirschsprung's Disease. *Ann. Hum. Genet., Lond.*, **26,** 261.

BOLEY, S. J. (1964). New Modification of the Surgical Treatment of Hirschsprung's Disease. *Surgery*, **56,** 1015.

BROWNE, D. (1955). Megacolon: Hirschsprung's Disease. In: "Abdominal Operations", 3rd Edition, edited by R. Maingot, Lewis, London.

CLAUSEN, E. G. and DAVIES, O. G. (1963). Early and late Complications of the Swenson Pull-through Operation for Hirschsprung's Disease. *Amer. J. Surg.*, **106,** 372.

DALLA VALLE, A. (1924). Familial Megacolon. *Pediatra*, **32,** 569.

DERRICK, E. H. and St. GEORGE-GRAMBAUER, B. M. (1957). Megacolon in Mice. *J. Path. Bact.*, **73,** 569.

DE VILLIERS, D. R. (1966). Ischaemia of the Colon: An Experimental Study. *Brit. J. Surg.*, **53,** 497.

DORMAN, G. W. (1957). Hirschsprung's Disease: Lethal Problem in Early Infancy. *A.M.A. Arch. Surg.*, **75,** 906.

DUHAMEL, B. (1956). Une Nouvelle Opération pour le Megacôlon Congénital. *Presse méd.*, **64,** 2249.

idem (1960). A new Operation for the Treatment of Hirschsprung's Disease. *Arch. Dis., Childh.*, **35,** 38.

idem (1963). Technique et Indications de l'abaissement Retrorectal et Transanal en Chirurgie Colique. *Gaz. méd. Fr.*, **70,** 599.

idem (1964). Retrorectal and Transanal Pull-through Procedure for the Treatment of Hirschsprung's Disease. *Dis. Colon and Rectum,* **7,** 455.

EEK, S. and KNUTRUD, O. (1961). Megacolon congenitum Hirschsprung. *J. Oslo City Hosp.*, **12,** 245.

EHRENPREIS, T. (1945). Megacolon in the Newborn: A Clinical and Roentgenological Study with Special Regard to the Pathogenesis. *Acta. Chir. Scand.*, **94,** Suppl. 112.

idem (1965). Pseudo-Hirschsprung's Disease. *Arch. Dis. Childh.*, **40,** 177.

idem (1966). Some Newer Aspects on Hirschsprung's Disease and Allied Disorders. *J. Pediat. Surg.*, **1,** 329.

EHRENPREIS, T. and PERNOW, B. (1952). On the occurrence of Substance P in the Recto-sigmoid in Hirschsprung's Disease, *Acta. Physiol. Scand.*, **27,** 380.

EHRENPREIS, T., LIVADITIS, A. and OKMIAN, L. (1966). Results of Duhamel's Operation for Hirschsprung's Disease. *J. Paed. Surg.*, **1,** 40.

FERREIRA-SANTOS, R. (1961). Megacolon and Megarectum in Chaga's Disease. *Proc. Roy. Soc. Med.*, **54,** 1047.

FORSHALL, I. (1964). Hirschsprung's Disease. *J. Roy. Coll. Surg.*, **10,** 31.

GOLIGHER, J. C. (1961). "Surgery of the Anus, Rectum and Colon". Cassell & Col, Limited, London.

GORDON, H., TORRINGTON, M., LOUW, J. H. and CYWES, S. (1966). A genetical Study of Hirschsprung's Disease. *S. Afr. Med. J.*, **40,** 720.

GROB, M. (1960). Intestinal Obstruction in the Newborn Infant. *Arch. Dis. Childh.*, **35,** 40.

idem (1962). "Quoted in Recent Advances in Paediatric Surgery". Edited by A. W. Wilkinson, Churchill, London. 159 and 160.

HIATT, R. B. (1951a). The Surgical Treatment of Congenital Megacolon. *Ann. Surg.*, **133,** 321.

idem (1951b). The Pathological Physiology of Congenital Megacolon. *Ann. Surg.*, **133,** 313.

idem (1958). The Physiological Basis for Surgery in Congenital Megacolon. *S. Clin. N. Amer.*, **38,** 561.

Hirschsprung, H. (1888). Stuhlträgheit neugeborener infolge von Dilatation und Hyper-trophie de Colons, Jb. Kinderheilk., **27,** 1.

HOFMANN, VON S. and REHBEIN, F. (1966). Hirschsprungsche Krankheit im Neugeborenealter, Z. Kinderchi., **3,** 182.

HUKAHARA, T., KOTANI, S. and SATO, G. (1961). Effects of Destruction of Intramural Ganglion Cells on Colon Motility: Possible Genesis of Congenital Megacolon. *Jap. J. Physiol.*, **11,** 635.

KAMIJO, K., HIATT, R. B. and KOELLE, G. B. (1953). Congenital Megacolon. A Comparison of the Spastic and Hypertrophied segments with respect to Cholinesterase Activities and Sensitivities to Acetyl-choline, D.F.P. and the Barium Ion. *Gastroenterology*, **24,** 173.

KATZ, A. (1966). Pseudo-Hirschsprung's Disease in Bantu Children. *Arch. Dis. Childh.*, **41,** 152.

KEEFER, G. P. and MAKROHISKY, J. F. (1954). Congenital Megacolon (Hirschsprung's Disease). *Radiology*, **63,** 157.

KIESEWETTER, W., SUKAROCHANA, K. and SIEBER, W. K. (1965). The Frequency of Agang-lionosis Associated with Imperforate Anus. *Surgery*, **58,** 877.

KOSTIA, J. (1962). Results of Surgical Treatment in Hirschsprung's Disease. *Arch. Dis. Childh.*, **37,** 167.

KOTTMEIER, P. K. and CLATWORTHY, W. (1965). Aganglionic and Functional Megacolon—a Diagnostic Dilemma. *Pediatrics*, **36,** 572.

LISTER, J. (1966). Abnormal Arteries in Hirschsprung's Disease. *Arch. Dis. Childh.*, **41,** 149.

Louw, J. H. (1959a). Some aspects of Hirschsprung's Disease with Special Reference to Hirschsprung's Disease in the Newborn. *Med. Proc.*, **5**, 208.

idem (1959b). Congenital Intestinal Atresia and Stenosis in the Newborn. Observations on its Pathogenesis and Treatment. *Ann. Royl. Coll. Surg. Eng.*, **25**, 209.

idem (1961). The Duhamel Operation for Hirschsprung's Disease. *S. Afr. Med. J.*, **35**, 1033.

idem (1964). Investigations into the Etiology of Congenital Atresia of the Colon. *Dis. Colon and Rectum*, **7**, 471.

idem (1966a). Jejunoileal Atresia and Stenosis. *J. of Ped. Surg.*, **1**, 8.

idem (1966b). Colostomy in Infants. *S. Afr. J. Surg.*, **4**, 39.

McElhannon, F. M. (1959). Experimental Production of Megacolon Resembling Hirschsprung's Disease. *Surg. Forum.*, **10**, 218.

Martin, L. W. and Altemeier, W. A. (1962). Clinical Experience with a new Operation (Modified Duhamel Procedure) for Hirschsprung's Disease. *Amer. Surg.*, **156**, 678.

Martin, L. W. (1965). Preservation of the Rectum (Modified Duhamel operation) in Hirschsprung's Disease. In: "Current Surgical Management III". Edited by E. H. Ellison, S. R. Friesen and J. H. Mulholland. W. B. Saunders Co., Philadelphia.

Meeker, I. A. and Kincannon, W. N. (1965). The Duhamel Approach for Surgical Correction of Congenital Megacolon (Hirschsprung's Disease). Narration from the motion picture produced by Wexler Films, Los Angeles, California.

Nixon, H. H. (1964). Hirschsprung's Disease. *Arch. Dis. Childh.*, **39**, 109.

idem (1966). Progress in Hirschsprung's Disease. In: "Modern Trends in Surgery 2". Edited by W. T. Irvine, Butterworths.

Pagés, R. and Duhamel, B. (1966). Intrinsic Non-propulsive Colon. *Arch. Dis. Childh.*, **41**, 15.

Parkkulainen, K. V., Hjelt, L. and Sulama, M. (1959). Anal Atresia Combines with Aganglionic Megacolon. *Acta. Chir. Scand.*, **118**, 252.

Pellerin, D. (1963). Rectosigmoidectomie pour megacolon congenital. In: "Extrait du Fascicule XXI de la Nouvelle Pratique Chirurgical Illustre. Paris, Doên.

Pilling, G. P. IV and Cresson, S. L. (1962). "Pediatric Surgery". Edited by C. D. Benson, W. T. Mustard, M. M. Ravitch, W. H. Snyder and K. J. Welch. Year Book Medical Publishers, Inc., Chicago, 802.

Ravitch, M. M. (1948). Anal Ileostomy with Sphincter Preservation in Patients Requiring Total Colectomy for Benign Conditions. *Surgery*, **24**, 170.

Rehbein, F. and Nicolai, I. (1964). Operative Treatment of Hirschsprung's Disease. *German Med. Monthly*, **9**, 51.

Roviralta, E. (1962). Nouvelle Orientations Chirurgicales dans le Traitement du mégacôlon congénital. *Ann. Chir. Infant.*, **3**, 155.

Shandling, B. (1961). A New Technique in the Diagnosis of Hirschsprung's Disease. *Canadian J. Surg.*, **4**, 298.

Sieber, W. K. and Kiesewetter, W. B. (1963). Duhamel's Operation for Hirschsprung's Disease. *A.M.A. Arch. Surg.*, **87**, 111.

Simonson, O., Habr, A. and Gazal, P. (1960). Rectosigmoidectomia endo anal com resseccas de mucosa rectal. *Rev. Paul. Med.*, **57**, 116.

Smith, B. (1960). Pre- and Post-natal development of the Plexuses of Meissner and Auerbach. Thesis presented in partial fulfillment of the requirements for the Degree of Master of Medical Science, Ohio State University.

Soave, F. (1963). Le Colon-ano-stomia senza sutura dopo mobilizzazione ed abbassamento extramuscoso del rettosigma. *Osped. Ital.-Chir.*, **8**, 285.

idem (1964). A New Surgical Technique for Treatment of Hirschsprung's Disease. *Surgery*, **56**, 1007.

idem (1966). Hirschsprung's Disease—Technique and results of Soave's Operation. *B. J. Surg.*, **53**, 1023.

Sprinz, H., Cohen, A. and Heaton, L. D. (1961). Hirschsprung's Disease with Skip Area. *Ann. Surg.*, **153**, 143.

State, D. (1952). Surgical Treatment for Idiopathic Megacolon (Hirschsprung's Disease). *Surg. Gynec. Obstet.*, **95**, 201.

STATE, D. (1963). Segmental Colon Resection in the Treatment of Congenital Megacolon (Hirschsprung's Disease). *Amer. J. Surg.*, **105**, 93.

idem (1965). Rationale for Segmental Colon Resection in the Treatment of Congenital Megacolon (Hirschsprung's Disease). In: "Current Surgical Management III". Edited by E. H. Ellison, S. R. Friesen and J. H. Mulholland. W. B. Saunders Co., Philadelphia.

SWENSON, O. (1957). Follow-up on 200 patients treated for Hirschsprung's Disease during a 10 year period. *Ann. Surg.*, **146**, 706.

idem (1962). "Pediatric Surgery 2nd Edition". Appleton-Century Crofts Inc., New York.

idem (1964). Partial Internal Sphincterectomy in the Treatment of Hirschsprung's Disease. *Ann. Surg.*, **160**, 540.

idem (1965). Prevention of Enterocolitis following segmental resection of congenital megacolon. In: "Current Surgical Management III". Edited by E. H. Ellison, S. R. Friesen and J. H. Mulholland. W. B. Saunders Co., Philadelphia.

SWENSON, O. and BILL, A. (1948). Resection of rectum and rectosigmoid with preservation of sphincter for benign spastic lesions producing megacolon: An experimental study. *Surgery*, **24**, 212.

SWENSON, O., RHEINLANDER, H. F. and DIAMOND, I. (1949). Hirschsprung's Disease: A new concept of the etiology. *New. Eng. J. Med.*, **241**, 551.

SWENSON, O., FISHER, J. H. and SCOTT, J. E. S. (1960). Diarrhoea following Rectosigmoidectomy for Hirschsprung's Disease. *Surgery*, **48**, 419.

SWENSON, O., FISHER, J. H. and MACMAHON, H. E. (1955). Rectal Biopsy as an aid in the diagnosis of Hirschsprung's Disease. *New Eng. J. Med.*, **253**, 632.

SWENSON, O. and IDRISS, F. (1964). Surgical Treatment of Hirschsprung's Disease: Technical Details Essential to Good Results. *Dis. Colon and Rectum*, **7**, 451.

TITTEL, K. (1901). Uber eine angeborene Missbilding des Dikdarmes, Wein. *Klin. Wschr.*, **14**, 903.

WEISS, A. G., HOLLANDER, L. and SCHWINGT, E. (1956). La Recto-sigmoidomyotomie, Nouvelle Thérapeutique Chirurgicale du Mégacôlon Congénital. *Strasbourg méd.*, **7**, 171.

WRIGHT, P. G. and SHEPHERD, J. J. (1965). Response to Drugs of Isolated Human Colonic Muscle. *Lancet, ii*, 1161.

WYLLIE, G. G. (1957a). Course and Management of Hirschsprung's Disease. *Lancet, i*, 847.

idem (1957b). Treatment of Hirschsprung's Disease by Swenson's operation. *Lancet, i*, 850.

YNTEMA, C. L. and HAMMOND, W. S. (1954). The Origin of Intrinsic Ganglia of Trunk Viscera from Vagal Neural Crest in the Chick Embryo. *J. Comp. Neurol.*, **101**, 515.

YNTEMA, C. L. and HAMMOND, W. S. (1955). Experiments on the Origin and Development of the Sacral Autonomic Nerves in the Chick Embryo. *J. Exp. Zool.*, **129**, 375.

ZACHARY, R. B. and EMERY, J. (1957). Meconium and Faecal Plugs in the Newborn. *Arch. Dis. Childh.*, **32**, 22.

Chapter 15

HAEMORRHOIDS

Alan Parks

It might be thought that a condition known and described since the origin of writing itself would at least have a universally agreed description, yet this is not the case. It is usually stated that haemorrhoids are varicosities of the terminal part of the superior haemorrhoidal plexus, situated in the upper half of the anal canal. This is true, but it is also true that many patients diagnosed as having haemorrhoids do not have this condition. They have all the symptoms of haemorrhoids, they may have prolapsing mucosa on stress or straining but no varicosities are present in the submucosal veins. For a variety of reasons, which will be discussed, they have prolapsing mucosa but not varicose haemorrhoids (Graham Stewart, 1963).

Anatomy

There are some anatomical points of importance relating to haemorrhoids (Fig. 15.1). At the mid-point of the anal canal the mucosa changes; the lower half is stratified squamous, the upper half columnar as in the remainder of the large bowel. The lower mucosa is dry, not mucus producing; but for this, mucus soiling of the perineal skin would be constantly causing irritation and soreness. It is also a very sensitive mucosa playing an important part in the mechanism of anal continence. It is richly supplied with sensory nerve endings (Duthie and Gairns, 1960). Where the mucosa changes there is an attachment to the underlying muscle (Parks, 1956). The mucosa of the large bowel itself is very mobile on the muscle coat and this is true of the upper anal canal. Were this state of affairs to continue to the anal margin, mucosa would prolapse all the time; the muscle attachment peculiar to the region prevents this.

In many patients with haemorrhoids the mucosal attachment is attenuated and the muco-cutaneous junction is permanently at a lower level than normal. An essential part of any operation for cure of haemorrhoids with restoration of normal anal function is to restore the muco-cutaneous junction to its original level in the anal canal.

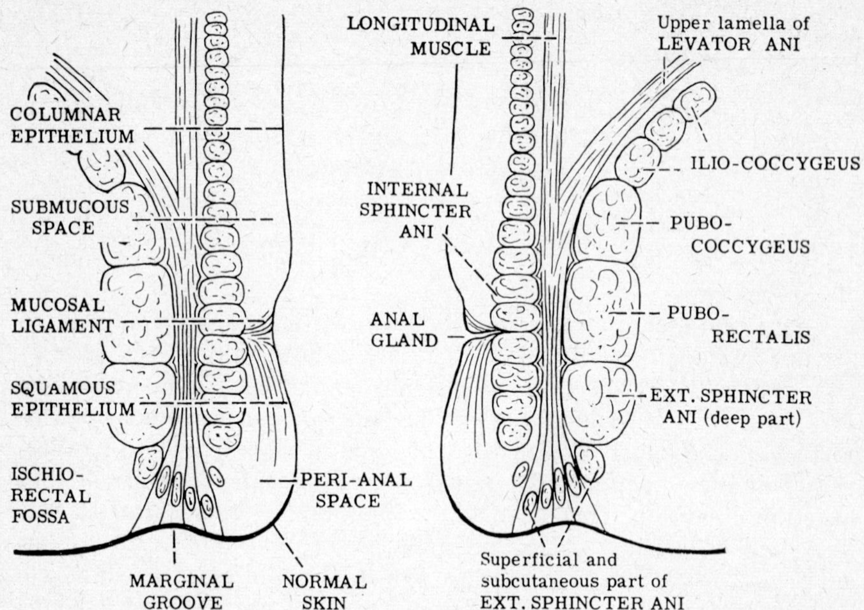

FIG. 15.1. Diagramatic section through the anorectal junction. A number of changes take place at the mid point of the anal canal; mucosa changes from columnar to squamous, the innervation from autonomic to somatic, and the mucosa is adherent to the underlying internal sphincter.

(Parks, A. G., 1958, *Postgrad. Med. J.*, **34,** 360).

Physiology

The physiology of the ano-rectal mechanism is important in the formation of haemorrhoids and the production of symptoms. The pelvic floor muscles, by their tonic contraction, maintain the support for the abdominal viscera and also (through the contraction of the external sphincter muscles) close the anal canal. If the pelvic floor muscles lose their tone, the perineum drops and the anal canal loses length. This situation arises due to age, excessive defaecation straining, or rarely due to neuro-muscular disease. Prolapse of upper anal mucosa occurs even in the absence of true haemorrhoids; if they exist as well then prolapse is even more marked. As the pelvic floor descends under stress so will prolapse occur at this time and what is often called third degree haemorrhoids will be found. This syndrome of perineal descent is an interesting one and may well be an important factor in the pathogenesis of haemorrhoids; it is certainly the most significant factor in recurrence following operation. (Parks, Porter and Hardcastle, 1966.) It follows that an attempt should be made to correct the abnormal physiology of the pelvic floor in all cases who have symptoms and in all who have had an operation for third degree haemorrhoids.

The symptoms of haemorrhoids are too well known to be reiterated in an article of this nature. When the syndrome of perineal descent is present as well several new symptoms occur; these are anal aching, a sense of obstructive constipation and repetitive call to stool. These may be partially relieved by treatment of any haemorrhoids present but will certainly recur if no attempt is made to deal with the lax perineal musculature.

Investigation

Although the investigations required in a patient who has haemorrhoidal symptoms need no emphasis here, mistakes still commonly occur due to omission of one or other of them. Sigmoidoscopy is an essential part of management and anyone not prepared to do it should not treat the condition. If there is any suspicion that the bleeding is of colonic origin (clotted blood, mixed with the stool) then a barium enema must be performed. The counsel of perfection would be for all patients with bleeding to have a barium enema but it is doubtful whether this is justifiable. The incidence of colonic cancer begins to rise at about the age of 45 and it is desirable to include a barium enema as part of routine investigation in those with rectal bleeding above this age. It is often said that if this counsel were given effect (i.e. to sigmoidoscope and X-ray the colon) the demand for investigation would far exceed the facilities available. If this is true, facilities must be provided.

Most conditions considered in the differential diagnosis of haemorrhoids are well known. One relatively uncommon one which is frequently misdiagnosed is a small villous papilloma of the upper anal canal. When it prolapses it looks like a haemorrhoid; if missed at routine examination it is usually recognized at operation and removed. The condition most frequently misdiagnosed as haemorrhoids is the mucosal prolapse associated with the syndrome of perineal descent. These patients often have a long history of straining during defaecation. Straining inhibits the postural tone of the pelvic floor so that the muscles become flaccid. In this state they are liable to be stretched by the straining force. Over the years they are lengthened and the pelvic floor drops; during straining mucosal prolapse occurs. It also happens under stress, such as coughing and sneezing as the stretched pelvic floor is no longer capable of reacting to rapid rises in intra-abdominal pressure. The diagnosis is readily made as the pelvic floor drops four to five centimetres when the patient strains. On proctoscopy no haemorrhoids may be seen, but when the patient strains mucosa flows into the end of the instrument. As mentioned previously both conditions can co-exist.

Conservative Treatment

Too many patients found to have haemorrhoids are subjected to operation. It is true that symptoms may recur with conservative management but this may not happen for many years and further therapy may give another long period of relief. Certain principles may be established as a guide to the suitability of the two main methods of treatment.

Generally speaking it is not justified to operate on patients with haemorrhoids unless they are in distress due to soreness, intractable pruritis, pain or soiling. Prolapse is no reason to operate unless it is causing discomfort; neither is bleeding by itself an indication for surgery. Occasionally bleeding cannot be stopped by conservative means; in this event the patient fears the presence of a malignancy every time blood appears; operative treatment may then be justified. Rarely bleeding is so severe as to cause profound anaemia; conservative measures are not recommended in this case, except in the elderly.

Submucosal injection is, of course, the principal weapon of conservative treatment. Whatever the substance used the chief effect is to cause adherence of the upper anal mucosa to the underlying muscle. There is no thrombosis of veins and the size of any vascular haemorrhoids remains unchanged; the pile no longer prolapses however and symptoms cease.

A vegetable oil (almond or arachis) is the most frequent substance used in this country, to which is added 5 per cent phenol as an anti-bacterial agent; phenol itself in this concentration is probably without effect. The oil induces a foreign body reaction and fibrous tissue is deposited in the submucosa. The site of injection is important, initially the oil should be placed as high in the anal canal as possible. Successive injections may need to be placed somewhat lower. It is important not to inject the lower anal submucosa, under the squamous epithelium, as this is richly innervated and great pain may ensue. Also important is the depth of the injection; it must be placed in the submucosa only. If placed a fraction too deeply it may pass through the muscle and give rise to severe perianal or peri-rectal inflammation.

Complications from this treatment are rare provided the injection is correctly placed. A florid reaction due to hypersensitivity may cause pain, partial narrowing of the upper anal canal or superficial ulceration but these are very rare.

Recently another form of conservative management has been described (Barron, 1963). A rubber ring is slipped over the supra-pectinate portion of the haemorrhoid; the tissue gripped by the ring necroses and sloughs off. By this means a portion of the upper part of the haemorrhoid is removed and the scarring causes adhesion of the mucosa to the underlying muscle; prolapse is thereby prevented. Encouraging results have been reported from the use of this method but it is too early to comment on the long term position. It should be remembered that the short term results of injection therapy are good. A 2 per cent secondary haemorrhage rate has been reported using the rubber band. An intrinsic defect in the method is that it cannot deal with infra-pectinate changes such as tags etc. If long term results are good it may come to occupy a mid position between injection therapy and operation.

Many anal symptoms are relieved by simple hygienic measures and the plethora of preparations in the form of ointments and suppositories afford varying degrees of relief. There is no doubt that relief of constipation is important and the regular use of a bland laxative is not to be too readily discouraged. More important than the constipation itself is the straining efforts it engenders and every attempt should be made to encourage the patient to avoid them. Straining weakens the pelvic floor and encourages the development of increasing prolapse. Sphincter exercises, if practised conscientiously, can restore, to a degree, the tone of the pelvic floor and prevent the development of prolapse.

Principles of Operative Treatment

There are three abnormalities in patients with advanced haemorrhoids, (*a*) varicose change in the submucous veins, (*b*) permanent downward displacement of the muco-cutaneous junction, (*c*) skin tag formation. It is desirable to remedy all these conditions. The downward displacement of the muco-cutaneous junction results in more of the anal canal than usual being lined with mucous secreting epithelium; it also leads to redundant skin and squamous mucosa at the anal margin. One objection to the usual operative methods is that they involve extensive removal of the apparently redundant anal margin mucosa. It is this mucosa, which had dropped from the anal canal, that is supplied with a highly sensitive innervation. If it is removed the anal canal will be mostly lined in its upper two-thirds by insensitive columnar, mucus-secreting epithelium and in its lower part by squamous epithelium which has grown over the wounds from the cut skin edges. Though in practice this leads to much less trouble than might be imagined it is desirable on theoretical grounds to try to restore the anal canal to its normal anatomy. To do this it is necessary to replace and fix in the anal canal the mucosa that has dropped.

Three steps then are essential in the operation of haemorrhoidectomy, (*a*) excision of the submucosal vascular tissue, (*b*) advancement of prolapsed squamous mucosa into the anal canal to reline it with appropriate epithelium, (*c*) excision of excess anal margin skin to prevent tags forming. (*a*) and (*c*) can be satisfactorily achieved, as in classical operations, by extensive removal of squamous and mucous epithelium with the underlying haemorrhoids, but this leaves large areas to heal by epithelialization. These areas do not appear to be considerable when the anal canal is closed by tonic muscle activity; at this stage, with a diameter of say only 1 cm. the circumference of the anal wall (i.e. the mucosal lining) would only need to be 3 cm. During defaecation however, when a diameter of 4–5 cm. is necessary the circumference would be more than 15 cm. It is desirable that the latter figure be the one occupied by a normal mucosa—not the former. It is well known that patients who have untoward long term symptoms after haemorrhoidectomy, have them during defaecation. It is for reasons such as this that the author considers the standard operative procedures not to be ideal as the greater proportion of the anal mucosa may be removed in their performance. Even though stenosis is rare these days the mucosal lining is secondary in origin. The type of operation which meets these objections is that originally described by J. L. Petit in 1774. He dissected the venous plexus from the submucosa leaving most of the mucosa intact. His method was not generally adopted at that time as contemporary surgeons found it difficult, understandably so in view of the absence of anaesthesia. The principle has been revived from time to time but has met with little acceptance. Using modern anaesthetic and operative techniques, however, the method is now practicable.

Most techniques of haemorrhoidectomy depend on traction to bring the tissues to the anal verge so that excision can be performed. This distorts anatomy and exaggerates the downward displacement which has already taken place. The only way in which the natural state of affairs can be seen is when the anal canal is opened up by appropriate retractors—in this manner the canal is inspected as it exists when naturally dilated during defaecation. Most of the mucosa can be seen at the same time so that any tendency to remove excess can be avoided. Most haemorrhoids are seen to be broad based when thus inspected (Fig. 15.2), the pedicle so often described being an artefactual appearance due to traction; however, occasionally one is found with a narrow base. The intra-anal method of operating also makes easy the replacement of the mucosa at the correct level.

Watts *et al.* (1964) have shown that, when the standard haemorrhoidectomy is performed, the attempt to cover the bare area of the anal canal by suturing the pedicle ligature low down to the internal sphincter usually fails. At some stage post-operatively, probably when the first bowel action occurs, the suture pulls out and the ligature returns to the upper part of the anal canal. The wound then heals by secondary epithelialization.

It is a principle of plastic surgery that skin cannot be sutured away from its original site until its underlying connections have been severed; it cannot be sutured under tension or the stitches will tear out and the skin resume its original position. The same principle applies in the anal canal. Epithelium is attached to the underlying internal sphincter, more firmly in the lower half than the upper half. Unless the connective tissue binding the mucosa to the muscle is undermined, any attempt to transpose mucosal flaps will be defeated. In the Petit type of operation the flaps are undermined and tendency to retract is minimal. By avoiding the unnecessary removal of mucosa, and by the

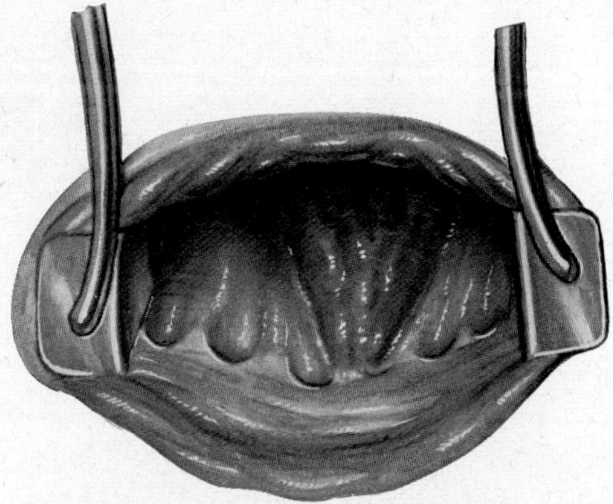

Fig. 15.2. The haemorrhoid is seen lying between the blades of the retractors and has a broad base.

replacement of the mucosal landmarks in their natural site without tension the principles of plastic surgery are adhered to. It is not proposed to describe the various types of conventional haemorrhoidectomy— they are well documented in standard manuals—the majority of them having the advantage that they are simple and rapid. The results are generally satisfactory. Nor is it suggested that the operative technique which follows is the only one conforming to the principles previously enunciated; it is a specific example of a type.

Operative Technique

The operation can be performed in any of the usual positions, the lithotomy or the jack knife are equally suitable. Whatever the method of anaesthetic used it is important that the pelvic floor muscles be relaxed so that the anal retractor can be inserted without stress. The

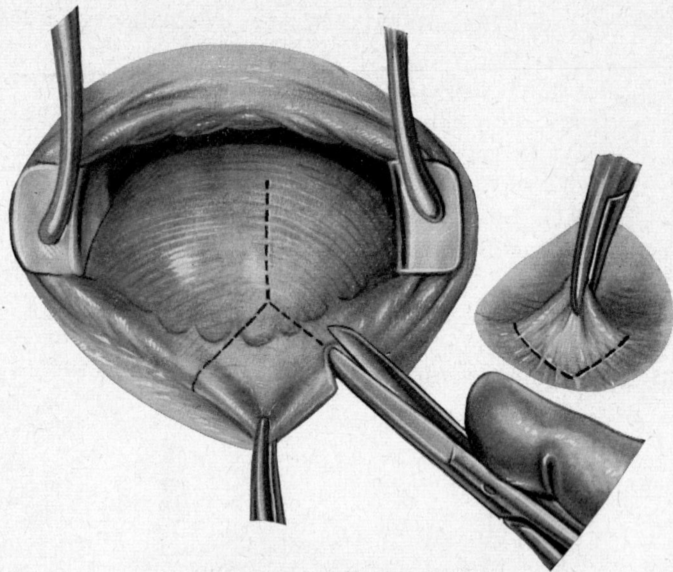

Fig. 15.3. A racquet incision is made in such a way that an adequate amount of anal margin skin is removed; the limb of the racquet passes up over the haemorrhoid for about an inch and a half.

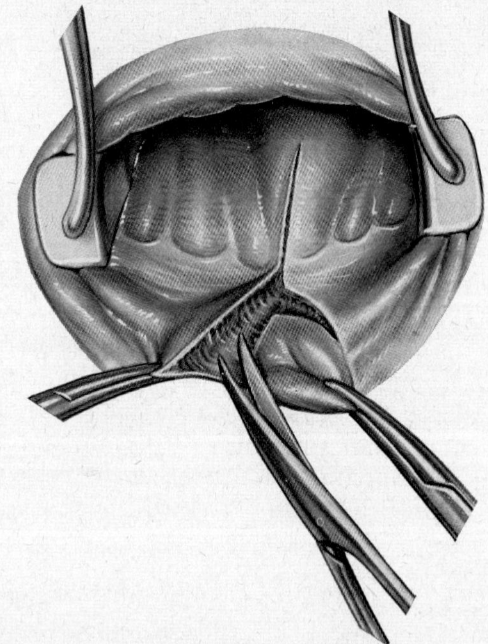

Fig. 15.4. The squamous mucosa of the lower anal canal is dissected off the veins of the perianal space. The fibrous tissue attaching the mucosa to the underlying internal sphincter is then divided.

instrument is inserted opposite each haemorrhoidal area in turn
(Fig. 15.2). The tissues are adjusted so that the muco-cutaneous junction
is situated at its normal level, that is about $\frac{1}{2}$ in. within the anal canal.
The veins constituting a vascular haemorrhoid are found in a thin layer
of connective tissue between the mucosa and the internal sphincter.
This layer is distended with saline containing 1:300,000 parts of epine-
phrine (Adrenaline) to create a larger plane for dissection. An incision
is made into the skin of the anal margin in the form of a raquet; only
a small amount of anal margin skin is taken in the first instance, any

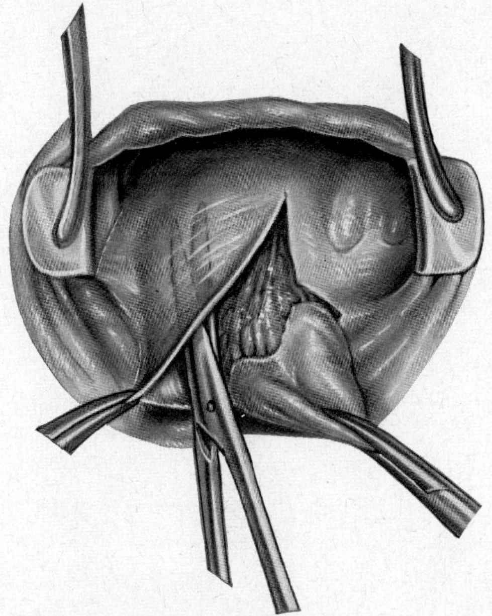

Fig. 15.5. The upper anal mucosa is lifted off the haemorrhoidal veins. In this
way two mucosal flaps are created.

excess to prevent tag formation is removed at the end of the operation.
The incision is then continued up over the surface of the haemorrhoid
for about $1\frac{1}{2}$ in. (Fig. 15.3). The skin on either side of the lower part of
the incision is undermined, and lifted off the veins lying in the submucosa of the lower anal canal. The muco-cutaneous junction itself
is lifted off the underlying tissue; an essential step here is to divide the
fibres in the submucosa which bind the junction to the internal sphincter
(Fig. 15.4). This is the most important part of the mucosa to conserve
and also the most difficult to dissect. Above this level the colonic type
mucosa is extensively undermined so that all the abnormal haemorrhoidal plexus is uncovered (Fig. 15.5).

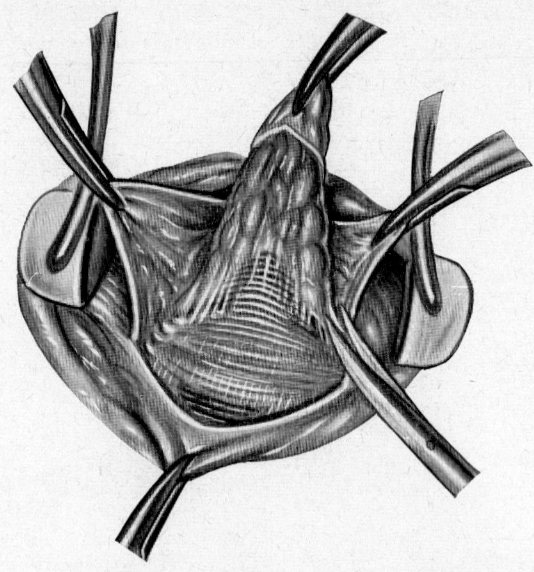

FIG. 15.6. The vascular tissue of the haemorrhoid is now dissected off the internal sphincter.

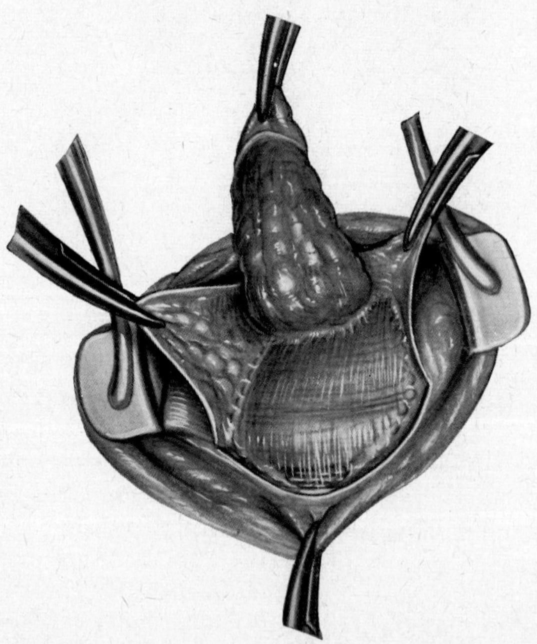

FIG. 15.7. The dissection is completed and the haemorrhoid is now only attached at its uppermost margin. The internal sphincter and both flaps are clearly seen.

At the end of this stage the submucosa is seen denuded of its epithelial covering. In the next step the submucosal tissues themselves are carefully dissected off the internal sphincter commencing at the lowest point (Fig. 15.6). At the mid point of the canal the internal sphincter is more closely adherent to the submucosal tissues and must be carefully freed from them. A point is then reached when the mucosa and submucosa are no longer densely adherent and the dissection is complete. By this means an isolated wedge of submucosa is created containing

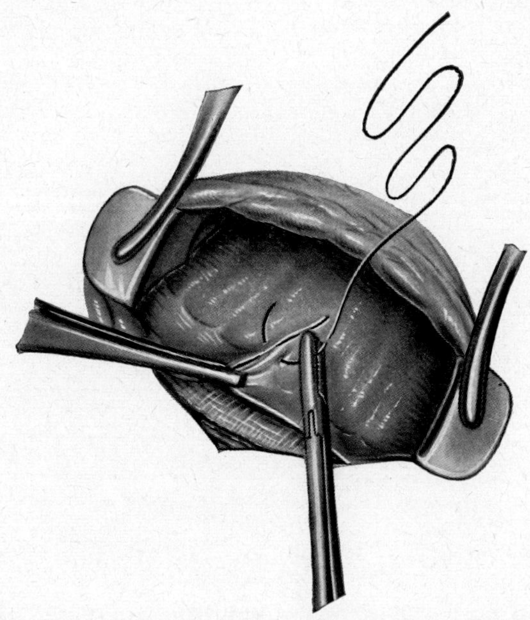

FIG. 15.8. With one or two stitches the two edges of the mucocutaneous junction are opposed. The stitch includes a bite of the underlying internal sphincter to fix the mucosa in the anal canal at the correct level.

mostly blood vessels attached at its upper border. (Fig. 15.7). The base of the wedge, sometimes called the pedicle is then ligated and excess tissue removed. There remains the denuded internal sphincter constituting the floor of the wound, and two mucosal flaps one on either side.

During the dissection of the submucosa from the internal sphincter, small arteries are encountered which enter the submucosal tissue having passed through the internal sphincter. They are best coagulated; occasionally these vessels are so numerous and large as to prolong the length of time taken quite considerably.

When the excision of all three areas has been completed, each wound is inspected for bleeding. The mucosal flaps on either side of each

wound are then brought together to cover the exposed internal sphincter. The muco-cutaneous junction on each side is picked up with a fine
catgut stitch (Fig. 15.8). A bite of internal sphincter about half an
inch above the anal verge is taken in the stitch so that the muco-cutaneous junction is firmly fixed at the correct level. If necessary similar
stitches can be placed at a higher level.

The anal margin is then inspected and any excess skin, which might
form a tag post-operatively, is removed. The skin edges are then
sutured with fine catgut to ensure rapid healing and also to prevent
unnecessary tags. No intra-anal packs or drains are used.

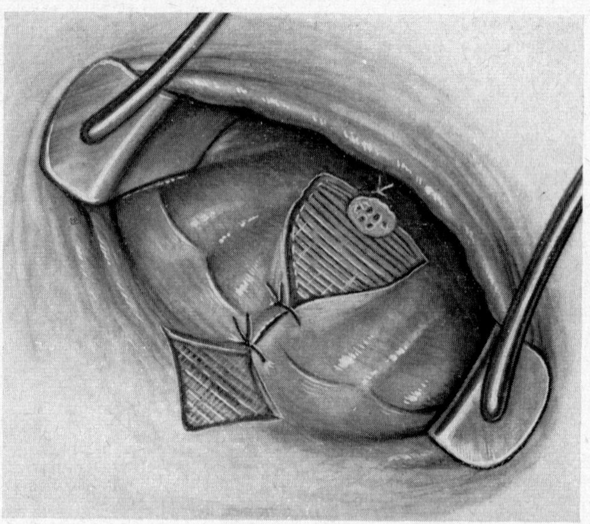

Fig. 15.9. In cases where the pelvic floor muscles are lax and there is a good deal
of mucosal prolapse present, a wedge of upper anal mucosa is removed.

A modification of this technique is required if the patient has lax
perineal muscles with mucosal prolapse. In this case mucosa of the
upper anal canal and lower rectum is removed in each haemorrhoidal
area (Fig. 15.9). In this way excess mucosa is removed, and the fibrosis
which results from the healing wound anchors mucosa in place so that
the tendency to future prolapse is greatly reduced.

Post-operative Care

In the post-operative period the wounds are interfered with as little
as possible. One or more baths a day greatly increase the comfort of
the patient and after each a simple external dressing only is applied.
Early bowel action is encouraged as in this way the anal canal is
dilated at an early stage by a soft stool; paraffin emulsion is usually

sufficient, given both pre-operatively and post-operatively. Codeine and morphine are avoided because of their constipating tendencies; pethidine suffices for severe pain, aspirin or paracetamol for mild symptoms. Rectal examination is performed on the fourth or fifth post operative day to detect spasm, though this is usually obvious if present, because of the symptoms it gives rise to. Secondary haemorrhage rarely occurs, as after other haemorrhoidal operations, but for this reason the patient is usually kept in hospital for ten days.

Assessment of pain and discomfort after operation is difficult as so much depends upon the personality of the patient. Pain seems to be less following this technique than after ligature and excision. Silen and Brown (1960) described a control trial of 96 patients using the two methods; pain was less following the Petit type procedure. Watts *et al.* (1964) also reported less pain with this operation but ascribed it to the sphincter stretching effect of the anal retractors.

Long term results are good provided the patient has a tonic pelvic floor. Recurrent symptoms are liable to occur after any type of haemorrhoidectomy in those patients who have lax perineal muscles; they do not get actual haemorrhoids as a rule but mucosal prolapse which gives similar symptoms. With care the patient can minimize the chances of getting recurrent trouble. He is encouraged to practise sphincter exercises regularly and indefinitely; further weakening of the pelvic floor by straining at stool can be prevented by the usual simple measures.

Acknowledgement

The author and publishers are pleased to acknowledge the co-operation of Butterworth & Co. for allowing reproduction of Figs 15.2–15.8 from 'Operative Surgery' edited by C. G. Rob and Rodney Smith

References

BARRON, J. (1963). *Amer. J. Surg.*, **105**, 563–570.
DUTHIE, H. L. and GAIRNS, F. W. (1960). *Brit. J. Surg.*, **47**, 585–595.
GRAHAM-STEWART, C. W. (1963). *Dis. Colon and Rectum*, **6**, 5.
PARKS, A. G. (1956). *Brit. J. Surg.*, **43**, 337–351.
PARKS, A. G., PORTER, N. H. and HARDCASTLE, J. (1966). *Proc. R. Soc. Med.*, **59**, 477–482.
PETIT, J. L. "Traite des maladies chirurgicales et des operations". Vol. 2. Paris, Didot, 1774, pp. 137–142.
SILEN, W. and BROWN, W. B. (1950). *Am. Surgeon*, **26**, 3.
WATTS, J. McK., BENNETT, R. C., DUTHIE, H. L. and GOLIGHER, J. C. (1964). *Brit. J. Surg.*, **51**, 808.

CHAPTER 16

CARCINOID TUMOURS AND THE CARCINOID SYNDROME

E. D. WILLIAMS and R. B. WELBOURN

The term "carcinoid" was used first by Oberndorfer in 1907 to describe an intestinal tumour which, while resembling a carcinoma histologically, did not behave in a malignant fashion clinically. For many years these tumours were regarded as pathological curiosities and of little clinical importance. In 1954, however, Waldenstrom and his colleagues (Thorson, Björck, Bjorkman and Waldenstrom, 1954) drew attention to the fact that patients with widespread metastatic carcinoids often showed a specific syndrome. At about the same time Lembeck, (1953) discovered that carcinoids contained 5-hydroxytryptamine (5-HT) and Page *et al.* (1955) found that patients with the carcinoid syndrome excreted large amounts of 5-hydroxyindoleacetic acid (5-HIAA) in the urine. These observations led to a great burst of interest in all aspects of carcinoid tumours. We shall summarize the basic knowledge of carcinoid tumours, paying particular attention to recent advances and discussing briefly some special features of the surgical treatment of these tumours.

Cell of Origin

The typical carcinoid tumour is found in the small intestine, and its cell of origin is known as the basigranular, enterochromaffin or Kulchitsky cell. These cells are present in intestinal mucosa from the stomach to the anus and in smaller numbers in other sites, including the pancreas, biliary tract and prostate. In the intestine they usually occur singly at the bases of the crypts of Lieberkühn. Each cell is triangular in shape, with its apex towards the lumen and its base lying against the basement membrane. It contains eosinophilic cytoplasmic granules which lie mainly at the base of the cell, their orientation suggesting that the cellular secretions have a local action. The granules give a number of histochemical reactions which suggest the presence of a high concentration of a substance with a phenolic group. The techniques used most commonly are the argentaffin reaction and the alkaline diazonium reaction. After formalin fixation the granules show a yellow-green fluorescence in ultraviolet light, suggesting that they contain 5-hydroxytryptamine (5-HT, serotonin, enteramine).

Microscopical Appearance

Most small intestinal carcinoids contain large numbers of cells with cytoplasmic granules giving the same histochemical reactions as those

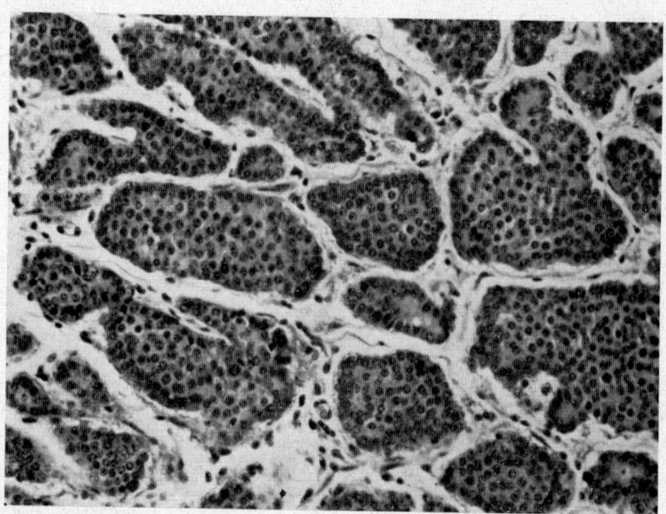

FIG. 16.1. The typical histological appearance of an ileal carcinoid tumour, with islands of uniform cells separated by connective tissue. (H & E ×230).

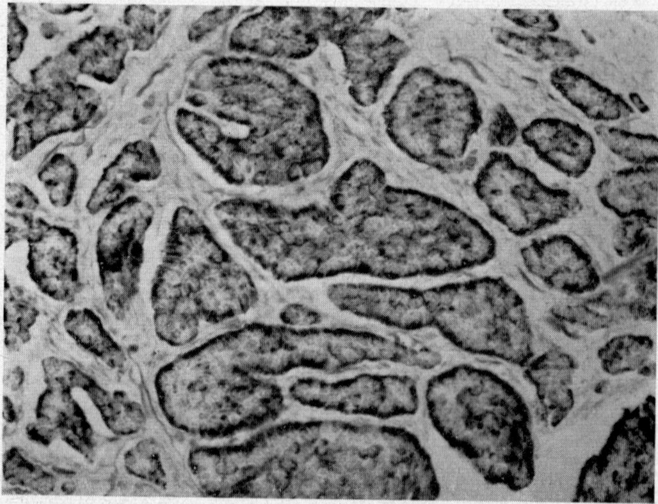

FIG. 16.2. The argentaffin reaction in an ileal carcinoid tumour. The 5-HT rich cells show a black cytoplasmic granularity. (Masson-Fontana ×230).

of the Kulchitsky cell. In the tumours the cells tend to form solid islands or trabeculae, separated by a connective tissue stroma which is often made up of dense fibrous tissue (Figs. 16.1 and 16.2). The tumours are not encapsulated, and groups of cells invade the muscle coat of the bowel. Perineural invasion is not infrequent. Despite the local invasion the cells tend to be regular, with abundant granular cytoplasm and few mitoses, and to show little of the anaplasia usually associated with malignancy.

Macroscopical Appearance

The local invasion of muscle produces a puckering or kinking of the bowel wall which is often the only external abnormality in the intestine. In the small bowel the tumour is commonest in the lower ileum, and may be multiple. From within the lumen the tumour is seen as a small nodule, which rarely shows central ulceration. On section the cut surface is yellow and raises the mucosa. In some cases there is massive local extension. The metastases are frequently much larger than the primary tumour and occasionally the hepatic lesions are enormous in size, but few in number. While all carcinoids show malignancy in pathological terms, only about 30 per cent of small intestinal carcinoids give rise to metastases. The sharp angulation of the bowel at the primary site not uncommonly causes subacute intestinal obstruction, and this is frequently the presenting feature.

Carcinoid Syndrome

The carcinoid syndrome may occur many years after resection of the primary tumour, or it may be the cause of the initial complaint. In some patients the syndrome is absent despite widespread metastases and in the Mayo Clinic series only 40 per cent of patients with small intestinal carcinoids and liver metastases suffered from it (Fontana, Tyce, Flock and Dockerty, 1963). The main features of the carcinoid syndrome are:

1. **Episodic flushing.** The skin of the head and neck, and often of the upper trunk, shows a brick red or cyanotic appearance, sometimes with conjunctival suffusion. The flush in many patients is precipitated by food, alcohol or emotion, and lasts for a few minutes. In patients who have had the syndrome for many years the face may show a permanent dusky red colour, often with prominent telangiectasia.

2. **Diarrhoea.** The motions are usually profuse and watery, with little mucus and without blood. Diarrhoea may be accompanied by colic and sometimes follows the flushing attacks.

3. **Asthma.** A minority of patients complain of intense wheezing during the flushing attacks.

4. Cardiac lesions. The most dangerous feature of the carcinoid syndrome is valvular and endocardial fibrosis, which usually occurs in patients who have had the syndrome for many years. It affects the tricuspid and pulmonary valves (Fig. 16.3) most frequently, the right atrium and right ventricle occasionally, and the aortic and mitral valves rarely. Macroscopically the valves show diffuse fibrous thickening, with contraction and fusion of the cusps, and tricuspid incompetence and pulmonary stenosis are common. Microscopically the lesions consist of

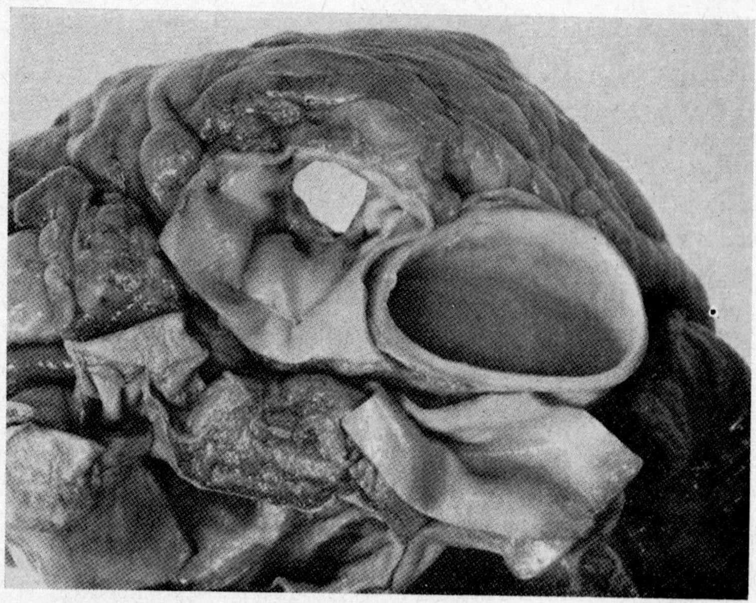

FIG. 16.3. Argentaffinomatosis—stenosed pulmonary valve and normal aorta, viewed from above.
(Montgomery, D. A. D. and Welbourn, R. B. 1963. "Clinical Endocrinology for Surgeons"; London, Edw. Arnold.)

fibrous tissue superimposed on the normal valvular structure. In rare cases, with a patent foramen ovale or with the main mass of functioning tumour in the lungs, left sided lesions may be severe.

5. Other features. Oedema, peptic ulcer, arthralgia and mental abnormalities have all been recorded as part of the carcinoid syndrome in some patients, but they are not constant. Lesions resembling scleroderma may be seen in the skin of the legs, and pellagra may occur as a secondary phenomenon.

Biochemical findings. Initially the carcinoid syndrome was attributed to the secretion by the tumour of 5-HT, but evidence against this view has accumulated gradually. The syndrome may occur with only minimal elevation of urinary 5-HIAA, and the blood level of 5-HT does not rise at the initiation of a flush (Robertson, Peart and Andrews, 1962). Sjoerdsma's group at the National Institutes of Health have now found, in a number of patients with the carcinoid syndrome, high levels of circulating bradykinin, a small polypeptide with the property of causing marked contraction of smooth muscle (Oates *et al.*, 1964, Oates, Pettinger and Doctor, 1966). Moreover, the tumours tested contained the enzyme kallikrein which, when released into the circulation, liberates kinins from the precursor kininogen, an α-2 globulin. The biochemical pathways at present known to be of importance in the carcinoid syndrome can be tabulated as follows:

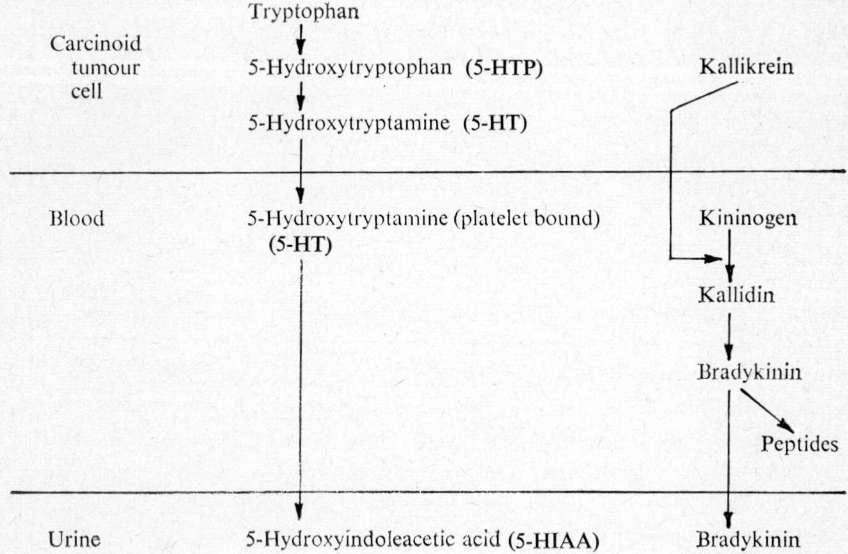

The relative importance of 5-HT and kinins in the genesis of the carcinoid syndrome is not yet clear, but it seems likely that kinins play the major role.

5-HT is metabolized to 5-HIAA, under the influence of the enzyme monoamine oxidase, mainly in the liver and in the lungs. It was assumed formerly that this fact accounted for the development of the carcinoid syndrome only when large metastases in the liver secreted 5-HT directly into the systemic circulation. It was also held to account for endocardial fibrosis in the right side of the heart predominantly. The sites of metabolic breakdown of kinin are not known precisely, but there is evidence that its concentration in the blood falls greatly during passage from the hepatic vein to a peripheral artery (Oates *et al.*, 1964).

Estimations of kinin levels in blood and in urine are difficult, partly because the kinins are released spontaneously from their precursors. Estimation of 5-HIAA in the urine is relatively simple and it remains the most useful routine biochemical test. Excretion is raised markedly in the great majority of patients with the carcinoid syndrome and false positive results are rare.

Carcinoid Tumours in Sites other than the Small Intestine

While the small intestine is the most common site for tumours giving rise to the carcinoid syndrome, carcinoid tumours do occur in other sites. Figures for the incidence of tumours of different organs are influenced by the specialized interests of the collecting centres. In the following list the sites are mentioned in approximate order of frequency, based mainly on the papers by Sanders and Axtell (1964), Fontana *et al.* (1963) and Linell and Mansson (1966).

Appendix (36 per cent). The appendiceal carcinoid is usually discovered at the tip of an appendicectomy specimen as a small yellow nodule. Histologically it shows the typical carcinoid histology and is usually considered to be benign. However, metastases have been reported in 2·5 per cent of cases (Sanders and Axtell, 1964). The age incidence of these tumours is well below the average reported for carcinoids in other sites, partly because appendices resected surgically appear to be examined more carefully than those found at autopsy. The carcinoid syndrome with widespread metastatic tumour from an appendiceal primary has been recorded in a very few cases (Markgraf and Dunn, 1964).

Jejunum and ileum (30 per cent). The typical jejuno-ileal tumour has been described already. Metastasis occurs in about one third of these cases. The carcinoid syndrome develops in about 7 per cent and in about 40 per cent of those with hepatic metastases (Fontana *et al.*, 1963). Multiple primary tumours are found in approximately 30 per cent of cases.

Bronchus (10 per cent). Most bronchial "adenomas" are in reality carcinoids, and in Pershall's series of 125 tumours (Fontana *et al.*, 1963), 12 per cent metastasized, 4 per cent metastasized to the liver, and 2 per cent produced the carcinoid syndrome. Histologically these tumours resemble ileal carcinoids, but show a trabecular pattern (Fig. 16.4) more often. Positive argentaffin and diazo reactions are found much less frequently and the content of 5-HT is correspondingly low (Even *et al.*, 1965; Fontana *et al.*, 1963). The tumours, although often largely endobronchial, invade the bronchial wall. Metastases usually involve the local lymph nodes first and distant organs, particularly the liver, later. Skeletal and cutaneous deposits are more frequent with bronchial than with ileal carcinoids. The bony secondaries are often osteoblastic (Toomey and Felson, 1960). More than 50 cases of the carcinoid syndrome have been reported with primary bronchial tumours, the majority being bronchial carcinoids and a minority oat cell carcinomas. The clinical picture in some cases differs from that seen in the carcinoid syndrome with an ileal primary, in that the flush may be of a brighter red, may last longer and may affect geographic areas of the trunk, sharply separated from the unaffected areas. Biochemical studies show that in a proportion of cases the tumour produces 5-hydroxytryptophan (5-HTP) rather than 5-HT The 5-HTP

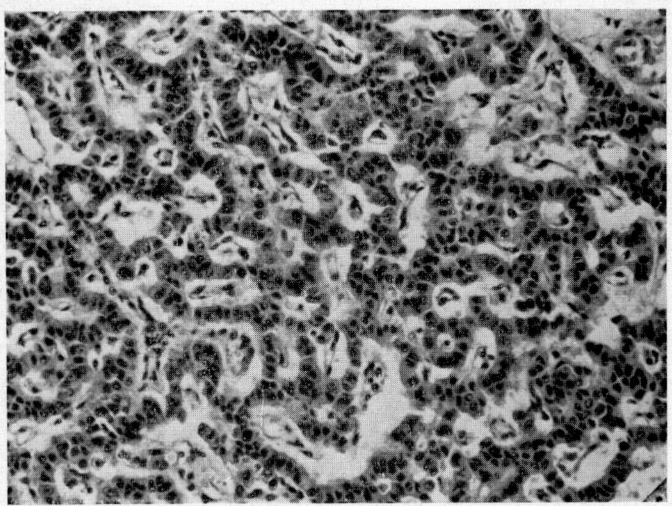

FIG. 16.4. The ribbon like cellular pattern commonly seen in bronchial carcinoids. (H & E × 230).

is decarboxylated in peripheral tissues and 5-HIAA is still the main urinary metabolite.

Rectum (10 per cent). Most rectal carcinoids are small mucosal and submucosal nodules, similar macroscopically to the ileal tumours. They differ histologically in that they are often composed exclusively of cells arranged in a ribbon pattern, and rarely show marked argentaffin reactions. The 5-HT content was elevated slightly in two out of three tumours studied by Fontana *et al.* (1963), but no well documented case of rectal carcinoid with the carcinoid syndrome has yet been published. In a large series of tumours collected by Bates (1966) 14 per cent had metastasized, most commonly to the lymph nodes and liver, although spread to other sites, including skin and bone, has been recorded (Roth, 1961; Krikler, Lackner and Sealy, 1958). Most tumours larger than 2 cm. in diameter metastasize, while most of those smaller than 1 cm. do not do so (Bates, 1966).

Stomach (3 per cent). Carcinoids of the stomach are usually polypoid tumours and may be multiple. They are frequently non-argentaffin and in 4 cases, where the 5-HT content of the tumour was estimated, it was normal in 2 and slightly raised in the other 2 (Fontana *et al.*, 1963). Metastasis occurs in about 16 per cent of cases, the commonest sites being the local lymph nodes and the liver. Osteoblastic bone secondaries have been recorded (Pochaczevsky and Sherman, 1959). The carcinoid syndrome has been described in a number of patients and, as in the bronchial carcinoids, the tumour may secrete 5-HTP and the syndrome may be atypical. One added peculiarity of gastric carcinoids is that in a few cases with the carcinoid syndrome a raised urinary level of histamine has been found (Waldenstrom, Pernow and Silwer, 1956; Campbell *et al.*, 1963).

Duodenum (2·5 per cent). Duodenal carcinoids have been reviewed by Warren, McDonald and Logan (1964). They are found particularly in the first part of the duodenum or at the ampulla of Vater. Metastasis occurred in 4 of 9 cases and one showed the carcinoid syndrome (Warren *et al.*).

Ovary (2 per cent). Primary carcinoids of the ovary are usually found in ovarian teratomas, and may occur in association with either intestinal or respiratory epithelium. Metastasis is rare, and ovarian carcinoids are the best examples of primary lesions causing the syndrome in the absence of metastases (Thorson *et al.*, 1958; Sauer *et al.*, 1958). Histologically they are usually typical and give positive histochemical reactions. It should be remembered that metastatic carcinoid in the ovary has been recorded on several occasions (Quinn, 1965; Roberts and Sjoerdsma, 1964).

Meckel's diverticulum, Caecum, Ascending colon (1–2 per cent each). Carcinoids of these sites are infrequent, but tend to behave like typical ileal primaries. The number of reported caecal primaries is low, partly because tumours in the region of the ileocaecal valve have been classed as ileal in origin. The very rare carcinoids of the descending and sigmoid colon may resemble the rectal more than the ileal tumours. The incidence of metastasis in caecal and colonic carcinoids is said to be high (Sanders and Axtell, 1964).

Pancreas, Biliary tree. (0·2–1 per cent each). These are extremely rare primary sites for carcinoids, but tumours in both have been recorded with the carcinoid syndrome (Oates and Sjoerdsma, 1962, Peart *et al.*, 1963). Only 7 examples of gallbladder carcinoids were traced by Shiffman and Juler, (1964). Carcinoids of the pancreas raise an interesting problem in pathological semantics. It is now accepted that many carcinoids give negative argentaffin and diazo reactions and that the diagnosis rests on the basic histological pattern and on the ability of some examples of the tumour group to cause the carcinoid syndrome together with an elevated excretion of 5-HIAA. Separation of carcinoids from islet cell tumours in the pancreas may be impossible on histological grounds and the same problem is found with ectopic islet cell tumours in the duodenum. It might be thought that the biochemical separation would be clear cut, but cases have been recorded where pancreatic tumours have produced both 5-HT and insulin (Van der Sluys Veer *et al.*, 1964). It is probable that the cells of origin of carcinoids and of islet tumours are closely related and that the two groups of tumours merge into one another.

Other sites. Carcinoids have been recorded on extremely few occasions in other sites, including the testis (Berkheiser, 1959) and parotid (Nicod, 1958).

Classification of Carcinoid Tumours

The features of many of these tumours can be grouped together in a broad classification based on the embryological origin of the primary tumour (Williams and Sandler, 1963). While this inevitably involves some over-simplification, it forms a useful basic classification, and is repeated here in a modified form.

	Foregut	Mid gut	Hind gut
Histology	Trabecular	Typical	Trabecular
Argentaffin and Diazo reaction	Usually negative	Positive	Usually negative
Carcinoid syndrome	Frequent*	Frequent*	Not recorded
Tumour 5-HT	Low-medium	High	Low
Urinary 5-HIAA	Medium-High*	High*	Normal
5-HTP excretion	Frequent	Rare	Not recorded
Bone and skin metastasis	Common	Unusual	Recorded

* when metastases are extensive.

Treatment

The treatment of primary carcinoid tumours is well established (Montgomery and Welbourn, 1963), and needs no detailed description. The treatment of patients with metastatic carcinoid, particularly if they show the carcinoid syndrome, raises certain interesting problems. No method is curative but, since patients may survive for years with metastases, every effort should be made to alleviate symptoms. The severity of the syndrome depends on the amount of functioning tumour and therefore, even in a case which is "inoperable" in that a radical excision of all tumour is not possible, the removal of a considerable mass of tumour may bring relief. Indeed considerable temporary improvement in symptoms followed massive resections of liver on two occasions in one patient (Wilson, Storer and Star, 1963). The cytotoxic drug 5-fluorouracil has been claimed to be of value in some cases (Rochlin, Smart and Silva, 1965) and the same drug has been given in hepatic artery perfusion with initial improvement (Reed *et al.*, 1963). Radiotherapy in general is of little value in the treatment of carcinoid tumours, and the lack of response to most drugs designed to prevent the synthesis of 5-HT or to block its action is explicable now that it is realized that 5-HT is not the sole chemical cause of the syndrome. Finally, surgical treatment may be of value in patients with carcinoid heart disease. Successful repair of the valvular lesions has been carried out, under cardiopulmonary bypass, with commisurotomy of the pulmonary valve and prosthetic replacement of the tricuspid valve (Aroesty *et al.*, 1966).

Conclusions

Carcinoid tumours are malignant tumours in pathological terms, but are frequently benign in clinical behaviour. Those that do metastasize usually grow slowly, and about half the patients with a considerable mass of tumour tissue show the carcinoid syndrome. The earlier view that the features of the syndrome could be attributed entirely to the secretion of 5-HT by the tumour is no longer tenable, and it has been demonstrated that the tumours also produce kallikrein, a kinin-releasing enzyme. The differences in clinical, pathological, and biochemical features of carcinoid tumours occurring in different sites is noteworthy. In the treatment of these tumours the value of resection of large amounts of tumours, even without the possibility of radical cure, is stressed and the treatment of carcinoid heart disease by cardiac surgery is noted.

Acknowledgements

We wish to thank the Department of Medical Illustration, Royal Postgraduate Medical School, for the preparation of the figures and Mrs. E. Clark for secretarial assistance.

References

AROESTY, J. M., DE WEESE, J. A., HOFFMAN, M. J. and YU, P. N. (1966). Carcinoid heart disease: successful repair of the valvular lesions under cardiopulmonary bypass. *Circulation*, **34**, 105.

BATES, H. R. (1966). Carcinoid tumours of the rectum, a statistical review. *Dis. Colon Rectum*, **9**, 90.

BERKHEISER, S. W. (1959). Carcinoid tumour of the testis occuring in a cystic teratoma of the testis. *J. Urol.*, **82**, 352.

CAMPBELL, A. C. P., GOWENLOCK, A. H., PLATT, D. S. and SNOW, P. J. D. (1963). A 5-hydroxytryptophan secreting carcinoid tumour. *Gut*, **4**, 61.

EVEN, P., GOBERT, J. G., LIOT, F., SAVEL, J., CHRETIEN, J. and BROUET, G. (1965). Dosage des 5-hydroxy-indoles dans les tumeurs carcinoides des bronches. Etude de 10 cas et revue critique de la literature. *Rev. Franc. Et. clin. biol.*, **10**, 935.

FONTANA, R. S., TYCE, G. M., FLOCK, E. V. and DOCKERTY, M. B. (1963). Serotonin and the carcinoid syndrome in patients with bronchial tumours. *Ann. Otol. Rhinol. Laryngol.*, **72**, 1024.

KRIKLER, D. M., LACKNER, H. and SEALY, R. (1958). Malignant argentaffinoma and the carcinoid syndrome. *S. Afr. med. J.*, **32**, 514.

LEMBECK, F. (1953). 5-hydroxytryptamine in a carcinoid tumour. *Nature (Lond.)*, **172**, 910.

LINELL, F. and MANSSON, K. (1966). On the prevalence and incidence of carcinoid in Malmo. *Acta. med. scand.*, **179**, Suppl. 445, p. 377.

MARKGRAF, W. H. and DUNN, T. M. (1964). Appendiceal carcinoid with carcinoid syndrome. *Amer. J. Surg.*, **107**, 730.

MONTGOMERY, D. A. D. and WELBOURN, R. B. (1963). Clinical Endocrinology for Surgeons. Arnold, London.

NICOD, J.-L. (1958). Carcinoide de la parotide. *Bull. Ass. Et. Cancer*, **45**, 214.

OATES, J. A. and SJOERDSMA, A. (1962). A unique syndrome associated with secretion of 5-hydroxytryptophan by metastatic gastric carcinoids. *Amer. J. Med.*, **32**, 333.

OATES, J. A., MELMON, K., SJOERDSMA, A., GILLESPIE, L. and MASON, D. T. (1964). Release of a kinin peptide in the carcinoid syndrome. *Lancet*, i, 514.

OATES, J. A., PETTINGER, W. A. and DOCTOR, R. B. (1966). Evidence for the release of bradykinin in carcinoid syndrome. *J. clin. Invest.*, **45**, 173.

OBERNDORFER, S. (1907). Karzinoide tumoren des Dunndarms. *Frankfurt Ztschr. Path.*, **1**, 426.

PAGE, I. H., CORCORAN, A. C., UDENFRIEND, S., SZOERDSMA, A. and WEISSBACH, H. (1955). Argentaffinoma as Endocrine Tumour. *Lancet*, i, 198.

PEART, W. S., PORTER, K. A., ROBERTSON, J. I. S., SANDLER, M. and BALDOCK, E. (1963). Carcinoid Syndrome due to pancreatic-duct neoplasm secreting 5-hydroxytryptophan and 5-hydroxytryptamine. *Lancet*, i, 239.

POCHACZEVSKY, R. and SHERMAN, R. S. (1959). Roentgen appearance of gastric argentaffinoma. *Radiology*, **72**, 330.

QUINN, B. F. (1965). Argentaffin carcinoma in the ovary. *Med. J. Aust.*, **2**, 120.

REED, M. L., KUIPERS, F. M., VAITKEVICIUS, V. K., CLARK, M. D., DRAKE, E. H. and EYLER, W. R. (1963). Treatment of disseminated carcinoid tumours including hepatic artery catheterization. *New Engl. J. Med.*, **269**, 1005.

ROBERTS, W. C. and SJOERDSMA, A. (1964). The cardiac disease associated with the carcinoid syndrome (Carcinoid heart disease). *Amer. J. Med.*, **36**, 5.

ROBERTSON, J. I. S., PEART, W. S. and ANDREWS, T. M. (1962). The mechanism of facial flushes in the carcinoid syndrome. *Quart. J. Med.*, **31**, 103.

ROCHLIN, D. B., SMART, C. R. and SILVA, A. (1965). Chemotherapy of malignancies of the gastrointestinal tract. *Amer. J. Surg.*, **109**, 43.

ROTH, M., (1961). Carcinoid of the rectum. A case report with observations on radiosensitivity of nodular metastases to the skin. *Amer. J. Roentgenol.*, **86**, 97.

SANDERS, R. J. and AXTELL, H. K. (1964). Carcinoids of the gastrointestinal tract. *Surg. Gynec. Obstet.*, **119**, 369.

SAUER, W. G., DEARING, W. H., FLOCK, E. V., WAUGH, J. M., DOCKERTY, M. B. and ROTH, G. M. (1958). Functioning carcinoid tumours. *Gastroenterology*, **34**, 216.

SHIFFMAN, M. A. and JULER, G. (1964). Carcinoid of the biliary tract. *Arch. Surg.*, **89**, 1113.

THORSON, A., BJÖRCK, G., BJORKMAN, G. and WALDENSTROM, J. (1954). Malignant carcinoid of the small intestine, with metastases to the liver, valvular disease of the right side of the heart, peripheral vasomotor symptoms, bronchoconstriction and an unusual type of cyanosis. *Amer. Heart. J.*, **47**, 795.

THORSON, A., HANSON, A., PERNOW, B., SODERSTROM, N., WALDENSTROM, J., WINBLAD, S. and WULFF, H. B. (1958). Carcinoid tumour within an ovarian teratoma in a patient with the carcinoid syndrome. *Acta. med. scand.*, **161**, 495.

TOOMEY, F. B. and FELSON, B. (1960). Osteoblastic bone metastasis in gastrointestinal and bronchial carcinoids. *Amer. J. Roentgenol.*, **83**, 709.

VAN DER SLUYS VEER, J., CHOUFOER, J. C., QUERIDO, A., VAN DER HEUL, R. O., HOLLANDER, C. F. and VAN RYSSEL, T. G. (1964). Metastasizing islet-cell tumour of the pancreas associated with hypoglycaemia and carcinoid syndrome. *Lancet*, i, 1416.

WALDENSTROM, J., PERNOW, B. and SILWER, H. (1956). Case of metastasizing carcinoma (argentaffinoma?) of unknown origin showing peculiar red flushing and increased amounts of histamine and 5-hydroxy-tryptamine in blood and urine. *Acta. med. scand.*, **156**, 73.

WARREN, K. W., MCDONALD, W. M. and HUME LOGAN, C. J. (1964). Periampullary and duo denal carcinoid tumours. *Gut*, **5**, 448.

WILLIAMS, E. D. and SANDLER, M. (1963). The classification of carcinoid tumours. *Lancet*, i, 238.

WILSON, H., STORER, E. H. and STAR, F. J. (1963). Carcinoid tumours, a study of 78 cases. *Amer. J. Surg.*, **105**, 35.

CHAPTER 17

THE KIEL BONE GRAFT

D. CHURCHILL-DAVIDSON

The earliest recorded heterogenous bone graft was performed in the middle of the seventeenth century by a Russian doctor and reported by Meekeren. A cranial defect of a nobleman who had been wounded in a sabre duel was repaired with a piece of dog's skull. Apparently the graft was a great success, the delighted patient exhibiting himself to his friends and anybody he could persuade to take an interest. The authorities of the Church soon heard of the operation and he was forced to have it removed under threat of excommunication.

Bone grafting did not progress significantly till the advent of anti-septic surgery. Contributions were then made by MacEwen (1881), Albee (1911), Phemister (1931) and later by Groves, all of whom helped to establish grafting of autogenous bone as a safe method of treatment. There are disadvantages, however, in using autogenous bone since the donor area, be it iliac crest or shaft of tibia, often remains painful and swollen and large quantities of bone may be needed. In addition it may not be possible to get the correct shape of the graft and the tibial shaft may have to be protected against fracture. Furthermore, the operation is prolonged and a second site is necessary. For these reasons, the search for a satisfactory heterogenous material has continued. The first attempts were made in 1867. Although these were unsuccessful it was suggested that bone for grafting could be stored frozen. This idea lay dormant till 1945, since when deep-freeze banks of homogenous bone have become commonplace. In 1948, supplies of homogenous bone on the Continent began to fall behind demand. A fresh search was made for a satisfactory material for heterografting and deep-frozen calf bone was introduced. This material was widely used but it gradually became apparent that it stimulated an immune response from the host with a resultant high rejection rate of the graft. Experimental work was then directed towards removing the antigens from the graft without changing its other properties. This problem would now appear to have been solved and non-antigenic calf bone is being used in increasing quantities throughout the world, although its acceptance in this Country has been slow.

Development of the Kiel Graft

In 1951, Maatz, working in Kiel, noted that even in implanted autografts, every bone cell dies, the dead material having to be replaced by the host; he called this process "creeping substitution". This observation suggested that a dead, cleaned bone would be a satisfactory scaffold for a graft. As a means of comparing materials for grafting, he introduced the "Spongiosa Test". Briefly, this consists of making boreholes of a predetermined size in the spongy bone near a joint, usually the knee. Into these holes were placed equal sized cores of the graft material under test. At intervals samples were taken and examined microscopically for the amount of substitution with living bone that had occurred.

Working with Bauermeister, Maatz then developed a method of preparing calf bone in which the antigenic properties had been removed but, at the same time, largely preserving its mineral and protein structure. The new graft was then subjected to the spongiosa test; there was a hundred per cent reproduction in the Kiel Grafts and autografts but relatively poor substitution of other available materials such as deep-frozen heterografts and grafts treated with formamide. Maatz and Bauermeister called this new heterograft "the Kiel Graft".

Manufacture of the Graft

Young calves are the donor source, a young animal is said to be better because it has larger intertrabecular spaces in the marrow cavity which makes for easier substitution. The adherent soft tissue is removed and blood is washed from the bone with water. The washed bone is treated with 30 per cent hydrogen peroxide (weight/volume) at room temperature for up to 2 days, the temperature never exceeding 35°C. It is washed again with water to remove the hydrogen peroxide, then with acetone, air dried and finally sterilized with ethylene oxide, a gas with a small molecular weight allowing complete penetration into the porous cavities of the bone. The final graft material consists only of fibrils and crystallites with a residue of 31 per cent protein; at present the exact pattern of its distribution is not known. This protein residue is of great importance since it is recognized that new bone formation decreases as the protein content of a graft decreases. Although the catalyst for osteoblastic activity remains unknown, it has been suggested by some workers that a chemical is responsible and that this chemical may be a glycoprotein. Burwell has recently suggested, however, that the fresh red marrow from an autogenous graft plays an important part in stimulating osteogenesis. It is important to realize that Kiel bone is not anorganic in composition, but that it has nearly the same protein content as an autograft.

Kiel bone is now available in sterile packs in many shapes and sizes with varying amounts of cancellous or cortical bone. The simple cancellous blocks (Fig. 17.1) which are used for filling cavities are callus promoting but are non-load bearing. The mainly cortical grafts are load-bearing but slower in substitution and can be used for keeping open an oesteotomy wedge.

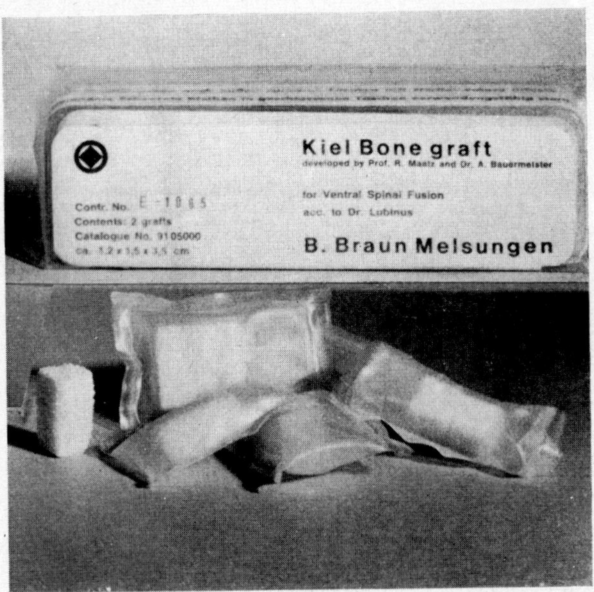

FIG. 17.1. The Kiel Bone Pack.

Experimental Work

Maatz and Bauermeister have shown with the spongiosa test that the Kiel graft is substituted as rapidly as an autograft. According to these workers it may even be faster since the soft tissue has already been removed from the heterograft making for quicker substitution. They call this phenomenon "callus promoting".

Kienholz and Kemkes experimented with the graft and found it to be antigen free. Fuchs, Stegeman and Eger confirmed that the graft was substituted as quickly as an autograft.

Koch and Dahman have investigated this new material by means of animal experiments and by conducting a large clinical trial. Comparative x-ray and histological examinations were carried out on Kiel grafts and on freeze-dried grafts. Implants of pure spongiosa and pure cortex grafts were placed in the quadriceps femoris of rabbits. The calcium uptake of the implants was measured after intravenous injection of the calcium replacement thorium X and compared with the activity of samples taken from the spongiosa and cortex of the host's tibia. The Kiel graft showed a considerable increase in the uptake over the freeze-dried graft. In addition this uptake started much sooner and was very similar to that of the host bone. They also showed histologically that the absence of fat and tissue from the marrow spaces of the Kiel graft produced a quicker vascularization of the graft by the host.

Clinical Use

At the University Hospital in Kiel where Maatz worked until 1957, the graft was used in 350 cases. In his own hospital in Berlin, he had operated on 351 cases up to the end of 1963. From his experience of these cases, he made certain recommendations concerning the use of

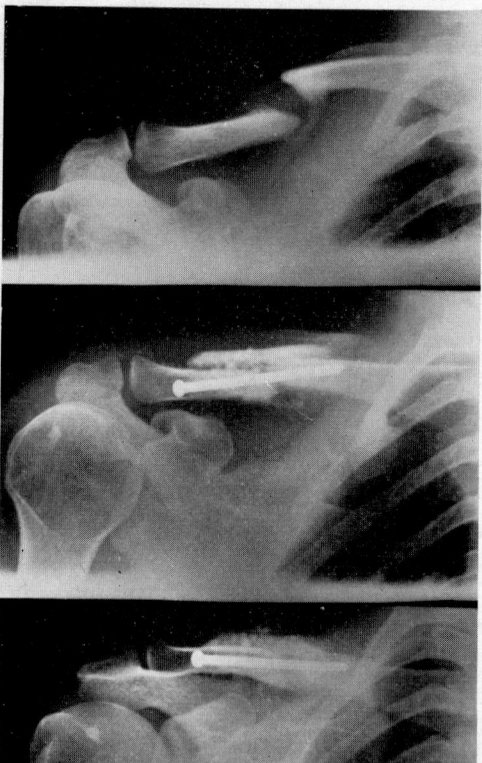

Fig. 17.2. Ununited Fracture of Clavicle. 18 months old.

Fig. 17.3. Ununited clavicle three months after grafting with Kiel bone and internal fixation.

Fig. 17.4. Ununited clavicle showing union six months after grafting.

the graft, stressing the importance of preparing an adequate bed. Since the graft is replaced by substitution, it cannot be expected to bridge a gap and in such cases an autograft is preferable. The framework of the graft must not be destroyed by hammering because this closes the intertrabecular spaces making substitution difficult or impossible. Maatz found the graft highly satisfactory in all situations when correctly used.

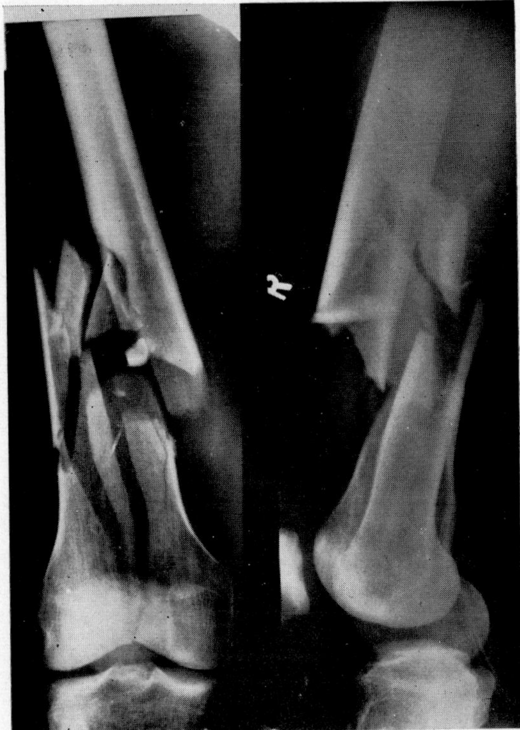
Fig. 17.5. Comminuted fracture lower end of femur.

Koch and Dahman reported a clinical trial of the graft in 1962. They had used it in 208 cases, including 11 grafting operations in osteomyelitis and 16 cases of bone and joint tuberculosis. Out of this trial of 208 cases, there were 136 successful grafts. Of the failures, 63 were caused by the graft and 9 by incorrect technique, early mobilisation and the continued growth of a tumour or cyst. These workers pointed out, however, that in line with their accumulated experience in the use of the graft, their present-day results would be appreciably different. Out of the 133 grafts which were correctly used, 112 were successful and only 14 failures could be attributable to the graft material.

10*

In 1964 Williams reviewed 14 cases of delayed union of fracture of the tibia in which the Kiel bone graft had been used. All the fractures united but in one case the graft refractured and was treated by a sliding tibial graft.

In 1967 Churchill-Davidson, Bendall and Dunkerley reported their initial impressions of the use of the Kiel bone graft. 82 grafts were reviewed, 64 were successful and 18 were failures. These cases were

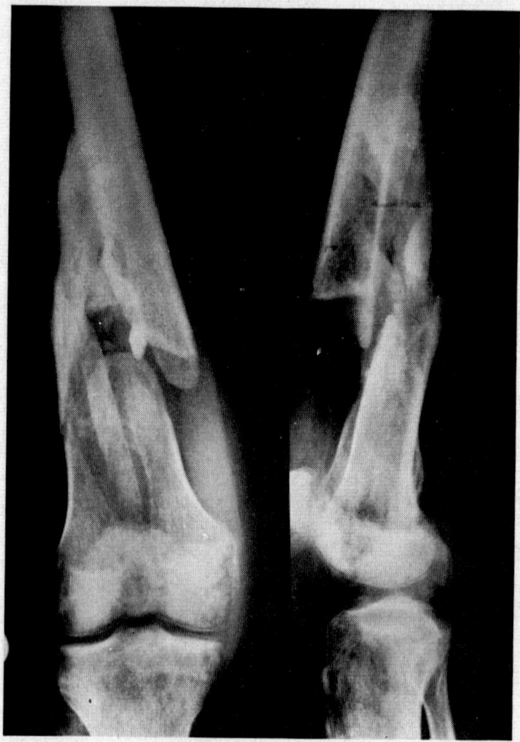

FIG. 17.6. Fractured femur 5 months after treatment on traction and in a hip spica. Fracture ununited.

widely representative of grafting operations and it was found that the cancellous grafts were successful when used as inlays, but, when used as onlays, the failure rate was high, probably because the graft bed was inadequate. The grafts containing a high proportion of cortical bone were slowly substituted and were not so successful. The failures were due to a recurrence of tumour (1 case); avascular necrosis of femoral head after a shelf operation for congenital dislocation of the hip (1 case); graft correctly used but failed to take (6 cases); wrong use of the graft or badly planned operation, e.g. cancellous bone as onlays, or

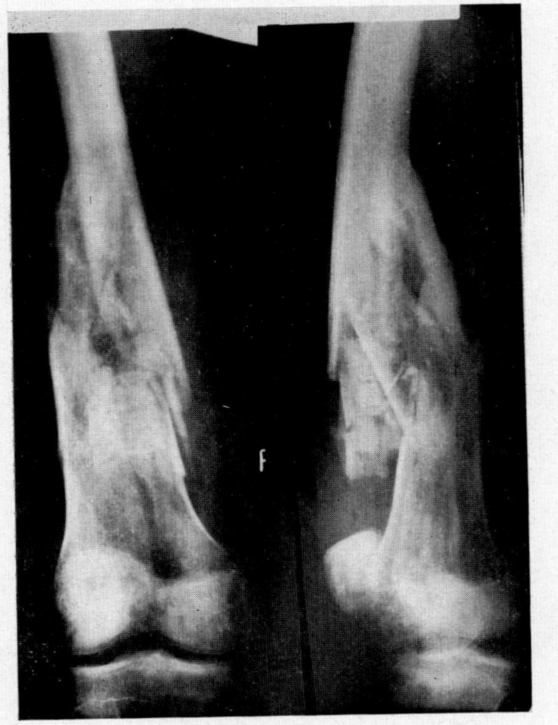

FIG. 17.7. Fractured femur. Post-operative picture after grafting with Kiel bone.

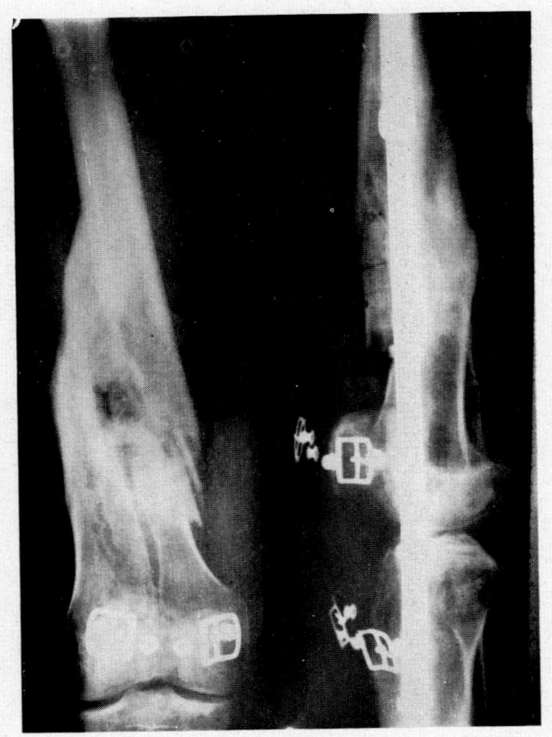

FIG. 17.8. Fractured femur. Two and a half months after the graft. Walking in a weight relieving caliper. Union commencing.

hammering the material (10 cases). Successful use of the graft can be demonstrated by two of their cases. The first is that of a 27 year old male with an ununited fracture of the clavicle of eighteen months duration (Fig. 17.2) which was treated by freshening the fracture site, onlay of cortical and cancellous Kiel bone, followed by internal fixation with a screw. Figure 17.3 shows the fracture at three months and Fig. 17.4 at six months. The second is that of a comminuted fracture of the lower

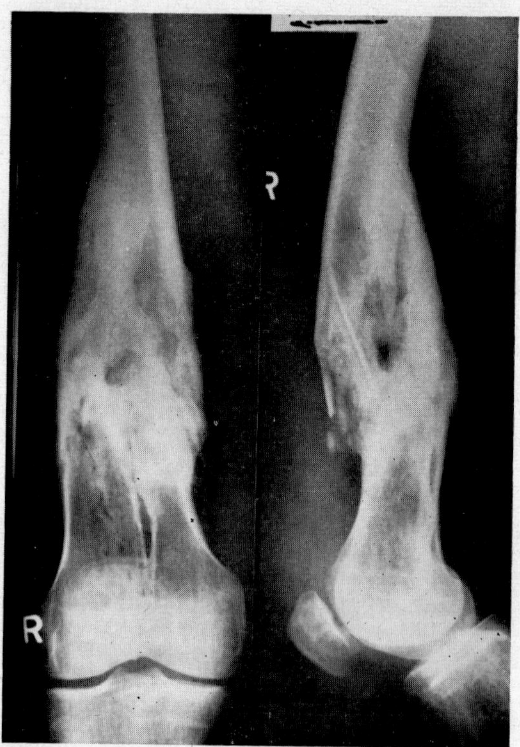

FIG. 17.9. Fractured femur six and a half months after grafting. Union has been achieved and replacement of the graft is apparent.

end of the femur in a 31 year old male (Fig. 17.5). Initially treatment was by traction and then a hip spica, but at 5 months (Fig. 17.6) the fracture was ununited. At operation, the non-union was confirmed, the interposed soft tissue was removed and the gap filled with cancellous Kiel Graft (Fig. 17.7). Two and a half months later the patient was in a caliper (Fig. 17.8) and union was progressing; 6 months later union had been achieved (Fig. 17.9) and modelling of the graft was apparent.

Summary

The Kiel graft is now in wide use on the Continent and in some centres in this country. The cancellous blocks are satisfactory for filling cavities, providing they are correctly packed; crushing is to be avoided. The cortical and cancellous graft placed sub-periosteally is successful for grafting ununited fractures and in short spinal fusions, when close apposition of the grafts to the bed and themselves is carefully achieved. It is most important not to leave a gap requiring bridging; this may account for the high failure rate in long fusions for scoliosis. The mainly cortical graft, which is often placed in situations where weight will be transmitted, is slowly substituted and is of less certain value.

The heterogenous graft has been shown to be incorporated by a process of removal of the dead implant and substitution with living bone. The autogenous graft may, however, contribute a chemical factor which results, not only in replacement of the dead implant, but also a more extensive area of ossification; this factor has been termed "the inductive potential" for producing osteogenesis.

References

ALBEE, F. H. (1911). Transplantation of a portion of the tibia into the spine for Pott's disease. A preliminary report. *J. Amer. med. Ass.*, **57**, 885–6.

BURWELL, R. G. (1966). Studies in the transplantation of bone. VIII. Treated composite homograft-autografts of cancellous bone: an analysis of inductive mechanisms in bone transplantation. *J. Bone Jt. Surg.*, **48b**, 532–566.

CHURCHILL-DAVIDSON, D., BENDALL, R. and DUNKERLEY, D. (1967). Initial impressions of the Kiel Bone Graft. *Proc. roy. Soc. Med.*, **60**, 11, 1077–79.

FUCHS, G., STEGEMAN, H. and EGER, W. (1963). Der transplantierte Knochenspan und seine Qualität nach partieller und vollständiger Enteiweissung bei erhaltener anovganischer Substanz. *Langenbeck Arch. Klin. Chir.*, **303**, 240–60.

GROVES, E. W. H. (1939). New bones for old. *Lancet*, **1**, 69–72.

KIENHOLZ, M. and KEMKES, B. (1956). Untersuchungen über den immunobiologischen Wert heteroplastischer konservierter knochenspäne. *Arch. orthop. Unfallchir.* **48.**, 623–32.

KOCH, W. and DAHMEN, G. (1962). Experimental and clinical experiences with heterologous bone bank graft. *Z. Orthop.*, **96**, 348–78.

MAATZ, R. (1966). In Symposium on Bone grafting materials. Armour Pharmaceutical Co. and B. Braun, Melsungen, p. 22–48.

MAATZ, R. and BAUERMEISTER, A. (1957). A method of bone maceration. Results in animal experiments. *J. Bone Jt. Surg.*, **39A**, 153–166.

MAATZ, R. and BAUERMEISTER, A. (1961). Clinical experience with the Kiel graft. *Langenbeck Arch. Klin. Chir.*, **298**, 239–44.

MACEWEN, W. (1881). Observations concerning transplantation of bones, illustrated by a case of inter-human osseous transplantation, whereby over two thirds of the shaft of the humerus was restored. *Proc. Roy. Soc.*, **32**, 232–47.

MACEWEN, W. (1909). Intra-human bone grafting and re-implantation of bone. *Ann. Surg.*, **50**, 959–968.

MEEKEREN, J. J. V. (1668). Heel-en geneeskonstige aanmerkingen. Amsterdam C. Commelijn.

PHEMISTER, D. B. (1931). Splint grafts in treatment of delayed and non-union of fractures. *Surg. Gynee. Obstet.*, **52**, 376–381.
WILLIAMS, J. J. (1966). In Symposium on bone grafting materials. Armour Pharmaceutical Co. and B. Braun, Melsungen, p. 58–75.

CHAPTER 18

CARCINOMA OF THE BREAST

JOHN HAYWARD

Introduction

Our knowledge of breast cancer has proceeded apace during the last two decades, probably more so than at any other time in history, but differences in the surgical treatment of the early lesion have played little part in this progress. The old topics are still being debated. Is radical mastectomy the most efficient way of treating the early disease? Does a simpler procedure give as good results but with less morbidity and less mutilation? Is the radical operation not radical enough and are better results obtained when it is extended? All methods have their advocates, all views are sincerely held and all protagonists can provide convincing reasons why their method is to be preferred.

Luckily it is now realized that no finite answer will result simply from public or private debate. The concept of the clinical trial has been introduced and accepted as the only logical way of resolving these differences. The results of those trials currently underway are eagerly awaited, and in the interim it may be preferable to turn our interests to those aspects of breast cancer which previously have been neglected. Epidemiology, the problems of detection, the hormonal environment and the use of hormones for treatment, have all been extensively studied and it is here that advances have been made. These in their turn may pose new problems but the appreciation of each is a step forward and must lead to a greater understanding of the disease.

Epidemiology

In England and Wales breast cancer is the commonest cancer in women, and one in every 25 female children born will develop it. But it is not solely a Western disease, nor does its incidence differ greatly between white and coloured races living in the same environment. For instance, in the United States the death rate per 100,000 women is very similar in Negroes and whites. It does, however, have a strong predeliction for certain races and also there are races in which the disease is relatively rare (Fig. 18.1). In Japan the incidence is only about one eighth of that seen in most European and North American countries, with the unaccountable exception of Finland where the condition is also seldom seen.

In recent years these differences in incidence have been investigated more fully and one report has shown (Wynder *et al.*, 1963) that not only is the incidence in Japan much less than in the United States but also that a higher proportion of Japanese patients present with the disease at

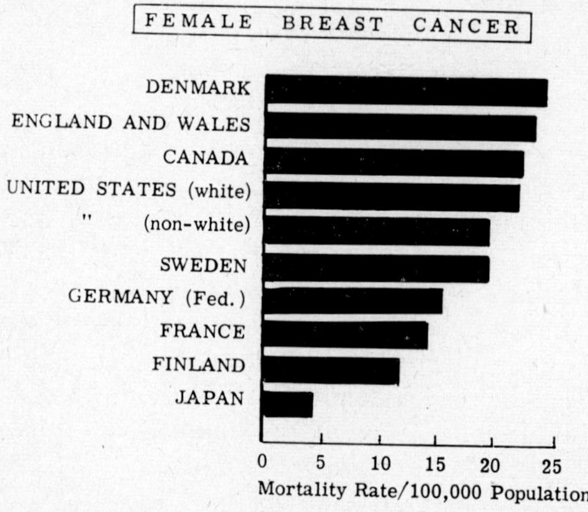

Fig. 18.1. The incidence of breast cancer in various countries as measured by the mortality rate per 100,000 Population. (From Segi, 1957).

an earlier stage. Furthermore, when patients are subjected to radical surgery, a higher percentage of the Japanese in all stages survive to 5 years. (Table I.) It has been suggested that these observations may reflect differences in the internal hormonal environment between the two races and limited studies so far carried out tend to support this supposition. Bulbrook, Thomas and Utsunomiya (1964) have shown significant

Table I. *Breast cancer patients in New York and Japan compared by survival and incidence of lymph node metastases.* (Wynder *et al.* 1963).

	NEW YORK Memorial Hospital 1953–1955	JAPAN Cancer Institute 1946–1955
	581 Cases	401 Cases
5-year survival of all primary operable breast cancer	60%	74%
Stage 1	79%	88%
Stage 2	46%	59%
Percentage with lymph node metastases at time of mastectomy	51%	43%

differences, which could have a bearing on the development of breast cancer, in the androgen excretion of British and Japanese women. Hormone assays have also been carried out on an immigrant Japanese population to see if these differences in androgen excretion may be related to diet and become less marked when the diet becomes Western-ized (Bulbrook *et al.*, 1966). Although no significant data are yet available it seems likely that immigrant Japanese populations may eventually have a cancer incidence similar to that of their country of adoption (Buell and Dunn, 1965).

Aetiology

Almost as little is known of the aetiology of breast cancer as is known of the aetiology of most other cancers; but it is encouraging that sufficient data are available for the subject to be discussed at all.

Antecedent Factors

Some factors that influence the development of breast cancer have been known for many years but may be summarized with advantage.

Heredity plays only a small part, but retrospective studies have shown that in families of patients suffering from breast cancer there is approximately a two-fold increase of the disease in mothers and sisters (Lilienfeld, 1963). From available data there does not appear to be a similar relationship with other close relatives such as aunts or grandmothers (Wynder *et al.*, 1960).

Since Bittner (1937) described a virus-like particle which he believed to be responsible for the transmission of susceptibility to breast cancer in mice, much work has been done to detect similar particles in human milk. Certain particles have been demonstrated but it seems unlikely that their presence is related to the subsequent development of breast cancer (Passey *et al.*, 1951; Gross *et al.*, 1952). A forward study was started by Atkins in 1949 in which the incidence of breast cancer in women, known never to have received mothers milk, will be compared with the incidence in controls (Atkins, 1958).

Breast cancer is less frequent in married than in single women (Wainwright, 1931; Lewison and Allen, 1953; Wynder *et al.*, 1960), and in parous women than in nulliparous (Lane-Claypon, 1926). Indeed it has been stated that the incidence of breast cancer is inversely proportional to the number of children born (Peller, 1940), but there are many factors that may influence this. The time of the menopause, the age a woman has her children, and lactation, all probably play a part.

There is a positive relationship between cancer of the breast and cancer of the uterine body (Wynder *et al.*, 1960; Bailar, 1963) but a negative relationship with cancer of the uterine cervix (Wynder *et al.*, 1960). Also a woman who has had cancer of one breast is 5 to 10 times more likely to get a second primary in the other breast. (Robbins and Berg, 1964.)

Lastly and perhaps the most vexing question is whether there is an association between breast cancer and previous fibrocystic disease of the breast. Most workers report an increased incidence of carcinoma in these patients, but until a stricter definition is obtained of fibrocystic disease and its many vagaries, nothing will be certain. No treatment policy can be based on the present evidence and we are unlikely to know more of this for a long while yet.

Hormone Factors

Of far greater importance is the search for specific host factors which, by their action, may precipitate breast neoplasia. None has yet been found, but current investigations may provide a clue. Bulbrook, Hayward, Spicer and Thomas (1962a) reported that about 50 per cent of their patients who were operated on for early breast cancer had an abnormal hormone excretion. In particular the levels of aetiocholanolone (an androgen metabolite) were lower than normal and those of the 17-Hydroxycorticosteroids (17-OHCS) were higher than normal. Also the clinical behaviour of the tumour seemed different in patients with an abnormal steroid output, and the question arose whether these abnormalities could have been present, and have been an important developmental factor, before the tumour became clinically apparent.

To test this, a large scale field trial was started in 1961 on the island of Guernsey when 5,000 normal women between the ages of 35 and 55 were asked to provide 24-hr. urine specimens (Hayward, 1964). These specimens were partly processed and the extracts stored at $-20°C$. In such a population an incidence of breast cancer of about 1 per 800 women per year could be expected, and when a case occurred the urinary hormones could be compared with those from controls matched for age, weight, parity, etc. In this way hormone abnormalities could be detected before a woman presented with her breast cancer.

Bulbrook and Hayward (1967) have now reported on the preliminary results of this trial. During the first $5\frac{1}{2}$ years, urine specimens were collected from 4,850 volunteers and 19 of the volunteers subsequently developed breast cancer. Comparison of the hormone excretion of the breast cancer patients with that of matched controls showed that many of the breast cancer patients were excreting abnormal amounts of aetiocholanolone and the 17-OHCS. This abnormality was multidirectional, in that very high and very low values were recorded, and was detectable up to 6 years before the cancer became clinically apparent. Bulbrook and Hayward suggested that measurement of these hormones in the general female population might enable women to be identified who had 3–4 times the normal chance of developing breast cancer. Regular surveillance of these women, possibly by clinical examination and mammography, should enable developing tumours to be detected in their very earliest stages.

Detection

The Palpable Lump

The clinical rule remains unchanged that no woman shall be left with an undiagnosed lump in the breast, and biopsy of the whole or part of the lump must still be the policy in all cases. But there are now aids to diagnosis which may help in the management of many of these patients.

1. The frozen section is now a standard procedure in most hospitals. When interpreted by a pathologist who is experienced in the technique, a diagnosis can be provided within 10 mins. and the elective operation performed. A definite diagnosis can be made in 90–95 per cent of cases and those in which the appearances are equivocal can be referred for a rapid paraffin section, which can be done in about 48 hrs. Delay between biopsy and mastectomy does not appear to influence prognosis although most surgeons would prefer the delay to be no longer than four days. It is probably preferable that the entire lump be excised at the original biopsy although there is no evidence that the removal of part of the lump causes a greater hazard to the patient.

2. Drill biopsy is now generally accepted to carry little risk and is particularly valuable to Out Patients. It has the advantage of providing a diagnosis before admission to hospital and hence treatment can be planned in advance. There are, however, disadvantages, and in particular many pathologists are unwilling to give a diagnosis on the small cylinder of tissue that is obtained. Also there is a possibility that the biopsy will miss that part of the lump which shows malignant changes and hence the condition may be considered benign and treatment delayed until further manifestations of malignancy appear.

3. When the lump can confidently be diagnosed as a cyst, it can be treated by aspiration without risk to the patient. Patey and Nurick (1953) described three conditions under which the cyst should be excised.

   (i) if the aspirate was blood-stained
   (ii) if a lump was still palpable after aspiration
   (iii) if the cyst recurred.

4. The management of the patient, with or without a lump, who complains of a discharge from the nipple now seems to have been clarified, and Atkins and Wolff (1964) have proposed a sensible, workable scheme (Fig. 18.2).

Many of their recommendations depend on the presence or absence of blood in the discharge and the use of the Occultest tablet provides an answer to this at the bed-side. Only one drop of the discharge is needed and if haemoglobin is present a colour change occurs within one minute.

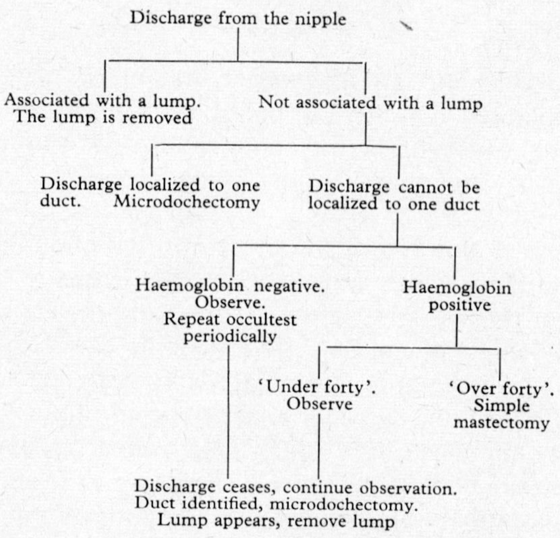

Fig. 18.2. Treatment plan for patients complaining of a discharge from the nipple (Atkins and Wolff, 1964, reproduced by permission of the British Journal of Surgery.)

The Impalpable Lesion

Much attention has been paid recently to the detection of the impalpable lesion, and methods have been proposed for scanning the clinically normal breast. Most of these are still experimental but the concept of pre-symptomatic detection is important and it is to be hoped that a regime similar to the cervical smear for uterine cancer may one day be available for breast disease.

Mammography. This probably has been the method most investigated and offers the greatest hope of detecting impalpable tumours in the breast. Carcinomas can be demonstrated by soft tissue X-rays and are frequently revealed by the presence of local calcification (Fig. 18.3). At the present it is particularly valuable in the routine scanning of the opposite breast in women who have had one breast removed for carcinoma, and also possibly to reinforce clinical opinion when dealing

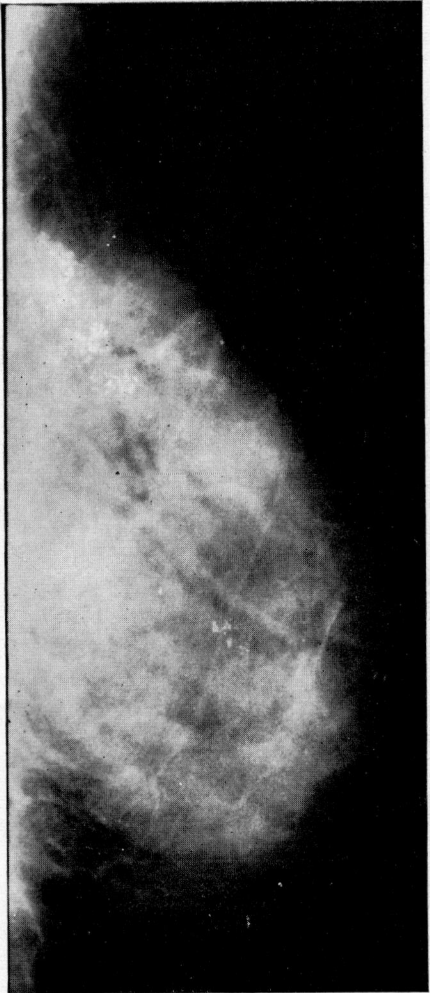

FIG. 18.3. Mammogram showing a carcinoma in a patient clinically free from disease. The calcification shown in the upper part of the picture indicates a duct and its branches involved with carcinoma. (Photograph by courtesy of Dr H. T. Apsimon and the Dept. of Radiotherapy, Cardiff Royal Infirmary; reproduced by permission of the *Proc. roy Soc. Med.*)

with women with fibroadenosis in whom the degree of nodularity makes palpation difficult. Lesions may also be detected in the breasts of obese women in whom again the clinical examination is unreliable. It should be emphasized, however, that mammography is no replacement for biopsy, and that if a lump is palpable, it must be histologically examined even if the mammogram is normal.

A further use of mammography may be in the routine scanning of normal breasts and, when combined with clinical examination, aids in the detection of lesions before they have become apparent to the patient (Stevens and Weigen, 1966). The time involved, the cost, and the frequency of examination would seem at the moment to make this impractical for use as a population study although pilot trials are now being carried out (Shapiro *et al.*, 1966).

Thermography. Malignant lesions are hotter than both normal breast tissue and benign lesions, and this appears to be due both to an in-

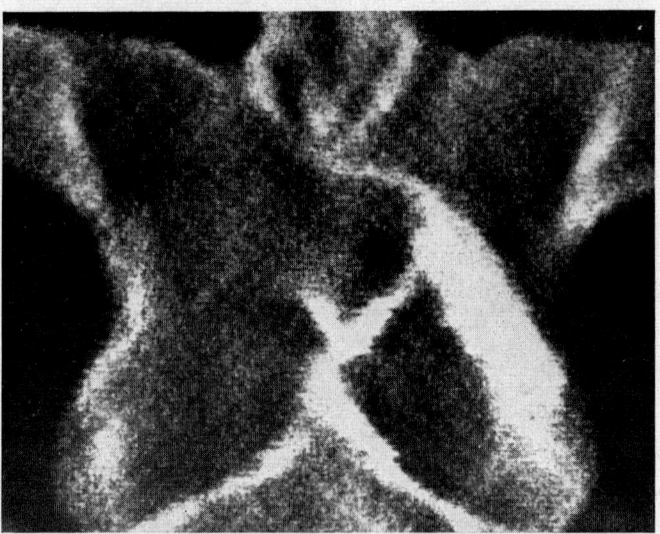

Fig. 18.4. A carcinoma of the left breast as shown by thermography. The white area in the upper half of the breast is at the site of the tumour. (Photograph by courtesy of Mr. W. P. Greening of the Royal Marsden Hospital, London; reproduced by permission of the *Proc. roy. Soc. Med.*)

creased blood supply and increased metabolism. Thermography uses this property by scanning the breast with an infra-red camera and transducing the heat energy to a light pattern which can be recorded by a polaroid camera (Fig. 18.4). The present methods can detect large lesions but further developments in technique are needed for it to be of use clinically.

Xero-radiography. This is another experimental technique depending on the use of a charged metal plate coated with selenium. X-rays cause a loss of charge from this plate and, when it is subsequently dusted with calcium carbonate, provides an image similar, but with greater detail, to that of the standard X-ray (Fig. 18.5). The method holds great promise but there is as yet insufficient experience of its use in distinguishing between benign and malignant breast lesions.

Urinary steroids. As mentioned on p. 306 abnormal steroid patterns have been detected in patients with early breast cancer and also in women who subsequently develop the disease. These abnormalities may enable a group of women to be identified who have a high chance of

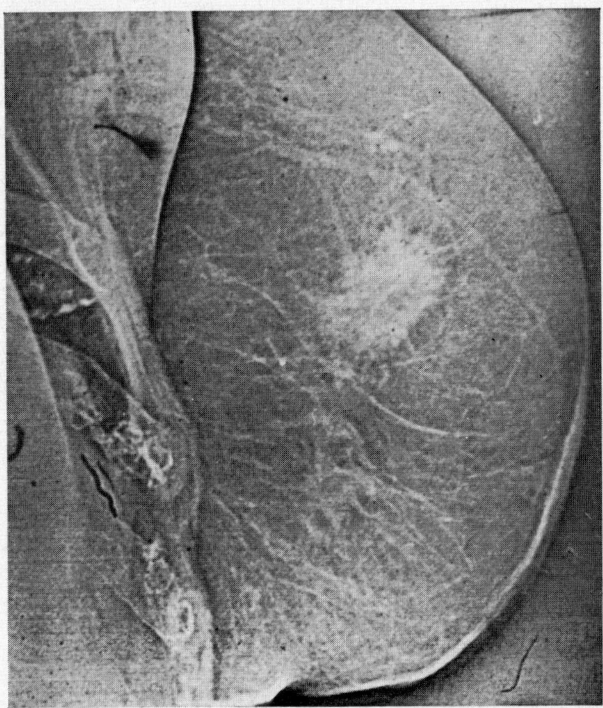

FIG. 18.5. Xeroradiogram showing a carcinoma of the breast. (By courtesy of Dr. F. F. Ruzicka Jr. of the Dept. of Radiology St. Vincent's Hospital and Medical Center, City of New York; reproduced by permission of the *Proc. Roy. Soc. Med.*)

developing subsequent breast cancer. This "high risk group" could then be examined frequently—possibly by a combination of mammography and clinical examination—and treatment instituted when the disease was in its very early stages.

Treatment

Early Breast Cancer

As stated previously, the surgical treatment of early breast cancer has changed little since the beginning of the century. But many surgeons now suspect that the fate of the patient may be decided before treatment is instituted. Either the tumour has metastasized sufficiently widely for a curative operation to be impossible, or it is still localized, and hence a minor operative procedure will suffice. It is certainly obvious that major differences in surgical methods produce only marginal, if any, changes in survival rates. So marginal are these changes that, in a trial comparing similar methods of treatment, the number of cases required for statistically significant differences to be shown might be so great that the results in practical terms would be meaningless. If differences in survival cannot dictate policy then the choice of operation has to be made on other grounds. It is certainly the duty of the many groups now carrying out clinical trials assessing different surgical methods—radical mastectomy compared with simple mastectomy, radical mastectomy compared with excision, radical mastectomy compared with extended radical mastectomy—to ensure that as many factors as possible are taken into account. Morbidity, recurrence rate, recurrence time, and quality of survival (Eisenberg and Goldenberg 1966) can all be measured, and may well prove decisive. Surgical treatment has for too long been influenced by the "5-year survival rate" which, when used to compare the results of two centres, is usually misleading, and even when measured in a properly controlled clinical trial has yet to justify its value.

In the meanwhile, it would be wrong to pre-judge the issue and carry out what may prove to be an inadequate operation because it is expeditious. These problems must be in the hands of those with proper facilities for their solution and in the interim the least hazard will accrue from following traditional therapeutic policies.

Adjunctive Therapy

Whilst the situation regarding surgical treatment remains in a state of flux, new therapies which are adjunctive to surgery have been introduced and evaluated.

Radiotherapy. The techniques of radiotherapy have greatly improved and the indications for both pre- and post-operative irradiation have been fully discussed previously (Riddell, 1954). Recently, however, doubt has been cast on the value of the therapy except as a method of treating recurrences. A clinical trial was carried out by Paterson and Russell at the Christie Hospital in Manchester to compare the survival and recurrence rates of patients with and without post-operative treatment; the choice was made by random sample. Two techniques were used in the treated groups but no significant difference was noticed in the incidence of distant metastases or in the survival rate when these were compared with the controls. Many cases had been followed up for over 7 years and it was concluded that there was no advantage in prophylactic post-operative X-ray therapy provided the patient could be carefully followed up and treated, if and when metastases appeared. (Cole, 1964.)

The trial has been criticized because some radiotherapists feel that the techniques employed did not deliver a high enough dose and that the distribution of the dose was not ideal. Be this as it may, and given that some improvement might be obtained by altering the dosage schedule, it is obvious that post-operative radiotherapy does not alter the survival and recurrence rate to the extent that was previously believed. This does not mean that the treatment should be discarded, but rather that the surgeon and radiotherapist should be aware of its considerable limitations and take into account its many unpleasant side effects. Further enquiry is needed to detect those patients to whom it may give real and lasting benefit but there seems little justification for its use as routine treatment after radical mastectomy. Most surgeons will reserve it for those cases in which the axillary glands are known to be involved or when the growth is situated medially when the mediastinal glands will be principally affected.

Ovarian ablation. The value of ovarian ablation as a prophylactic measure has still not been determined. Neither, is it certain whether destruction of the ovaries by radiotherapy is equivalent to their surgical removal.

To consider the second problem first, it is likely that attempts—particularly in young women—to abolish all ovarian function by radiotherapy frequently fails. Much larger doses are needed than was first apparent and the fact that the periods cease does not necessarily mean that all ovarian secretion has stopped. A dose of at least 2,000 rads is probably needed and, in the very young, even this may be insufficient. There seems a good case for surgical oophorectomy to be the method of choice; it is a simple operation, more certain in its effect, and probably less upsetting to the patient.

Of much greater doubt is the effectiveness of the manoeuvre to postpone recurrence and possibly improve the survival rate. Some protagonists believe it to be a major step in the treatment of breast cancer in young patients. Nissen-Meyer (1966) also recommends ovarian ablation for post-menopausal women and encourages the additional use of oral prednisone. A clinical trial carried out by Paterson and Russell in premenopausal women, compared a group receiving ovarian irradiation with a control group. They showed that the treatment resulted in a decreased incidence of distant metastases at 7 years and an increased survival rate at 10 years after treatment. (Cole, 1964.) The problem with this therapy is that probably a great number of women have to be treated so that few will benefit. Most surgeons and radiotherapists now tend to judge each case on its own merits, taking into account such factors as age, emotional response, degree of malignancy of the tumour etc. What is required is a method of pre-selecting patients who will benefit, and investigations are now proceeding—particularly on the endocrine status of the patient—which may resolve this problem.

Androgens. Evidence accumulated over the past few years has suggested that small doses of androgen following mastectomy may also be effective in postponing recurrences. Bulbrook, Hayward and Thomas (1964) described how the fate of patients could largely be predicted by the post-operative urinary excretion of aetiocholanolone and the 17-OHCS combined in a discriminant function. When the levels of aetiocholanolone (an androgen metabolite) were low and the discriminant was negative (see p. 321) the disease tended to recur early and nearly 50 per cent of these patients succumbed within 3 years. Trials are now going on to test the effect of prescribing small doses of androgens to patients after mastectomy and comparing the recurrence and survival rate with that of a control group.

A similar claim for the prophylactic use of testosterone has previously been made by Prudente (1945) but this was not a controlled trial and the doses of testosterone used were very high.

Cytotoxins. The fact that circulating cancer cells can usually be found in the blood of patients during operations for cancer has prompted the use of cytotoxins synoperatively in an attempt to protect the patient from developing metastases. These circulating malignant cells are difficult to recognize under the microscope, and are frequently confused with blast cells and megalocaryocytes. The prognostic significance of their appearance has variously been claimed and denied.

Several trials are being carried out to determine the use of cytotoxins under these conditions and preliminary results have indicated that in pre-menopausal patients the recurrence rate may be affected favourably by their administration (Chemotherapy Statistical Unit; Surgical Adjuvant Breast Study, 1964).

ThioTEPA is the drug most commonly used and a suitable dose regime would be 2 mg. per stone body weight given intramuscularly with the premedication followed by 1·5 mg. per stone body weight on the 2nd post-operative day and 1 mg. per stone body weight on the 4th post-operative day. The white blood count is seldom lowered by this dosage but should always be measured pre-operatively, and on the 10th post-operative day.

There is no confirmation at the moment whether cytotoxins given at the time of operation play a substantial or indeed any part in the management of the disease, but their use seems logical and is unlikely to cause harm.

Advanced breast cancer

It is in the treatment of the advanced disease that most progress has been made. Starting with a suggestion by Schinzinger (1889) that oophorectomy might benefit these patients, the surgeon now has at his disposal so many medical and surgical measures for palliation as to make the therapy of breast tumours unique in the treatment of cancer. But, though over 70 years have elapsed since Schinzinger's original suggestion, most of these measures are entirely empirical. Little more is known now of their mode of action than was known originally. This state of affairs should not continue much longer and seems principally to be the result of a lack of methods for the precise measurement of small quantities of hormones either in the blood or urine. These methods now exist and in skilled hands should soon place treatment on a more rational basis.

It would seem appropriate at this juncture to outline the treatments available, and to evaluate the part that each may play.

Local surgery. Local surgery still plays a major part in the management of the advanced disease. Many years relief can be obtained by the excision of isolated recurrences; those in the skin are particularly suitable but even solitary deposits in the brain may be removed and no further evidence of disease appear for many years. Particularly, the surgical removal of local offensive lesions—even when the cancer is disseminated—can give relief in the terminal stages. When skeletal deposits are predominant, the prophylactic pinning of a bone rendered weak from a metastasis can prevent a pathological fracture. If such a fracture does occur then it should be treated in the same fashion as a similar fracture in a normal bone—even if this means the use of a nail or plate. Ordinary surgical principles should not be neglected in the treatment of advanced cancer.

Radiotherapy. The use of radiotherapy in the treatment of established lesions far outweighs its value as a prophylactic measure following radical mastectomy. In the treatment of the locally inoperable primary lesion it can give many years of symptom-free life and not infrequently enables the surgeon to carry out a palliative mastectomy. However, it is in the disseminated disease that it has more to offer. Both cutaneous and certain visceral metastases can be treated with advantage and, although the patients continue to deteriorate the symptomatic relief may be considerable. Most of all it should be prescribed to relieve local pain, particularly when caused by skeletal lesions. Pain resulting from vertebral disease can nearly always be alleviated even when accompanied by gross pathological changes, such as the collapse of one or more vertebrae. Such treatment can be prescribed with benefit to those with grossly disseminated disease and, providing this is tempered so that the patient suffers minimally from the treatment itself, can always provide that essential element of hope that something further can still be done.

Ovarian ablation. First described and carried out successfully by Beatson in 1896 this therapy has been practised for nearly three-quarters of a century. It is probably the simplest treatment for the advanced disease and, whilst having few side effects, can produce a remission in a large proportion of cases. The exact remission rate has been variously reported and largely depends on the criteria of success used by each surgeon. When carried out in pre-menopausal women, probably about 40 per cent will obtain some degree of benefit and in about half of these the remission will be really worth while. Surgical removal is probably preferable to irradiation as it ensures a complete cessation of ovarian function. Many clinicians believe that the response to ovarian ablation gives a good indication to the subsequent response to adrenalectomy or hypophysectomy and will not perform these latter procedures following a negative response to removal of the ovaries. Its disadvantages are minimal, but it often cannot be carried out because the ovaries have been removed as a prophylactic measure following mastectomy. Also the operation may be difficult if multiple peritoneal deposits are present in the pelvis.

Androgens. First described by Uhlrich in 1938 this type of therapy now holds a firm place in the treatment of the advanced disease. Its use should probably be restricted to the premenopausal patient or to the patient who is within 5 years of the menopause. It may be exhibited as a supplement to ovarian ablation, or as a substitute; in the latter case the ovaries can be left intact when they have not already been removed as a prophylactic measure.

The great disadvantage of the treatment is its side effects and many surgeons consider these too great a penalty to pay. Virilization with the growth of facial and body hair, deepening of the voice, acne, and increased libido may prohibit its use, particularly in the younger patient. These were certainly major disadvantages when drugs such as methyl testosterone were the only ones available, but now new synthetic androgens with a marked anabolic effect have reduced the in-incidence of masculinization. Nandrolone phenyl-propionate, (Durabolin) 25 mg. twice weekly by intramuscular injection has an equivalent remission rate to testosterone but the side effects are severe only in about 10 per cent of the cases. Longer acting agents are also now available and drugs such as 19-nor-androstanolone decanoate (Deca-durabolin) need only be administered once every three weeks. Much work has been done, particularly in the U.S.A. to produce an androgen with a higher response rate than testosterone. But no significant advance has been reported in spite of the many compounds studied.

Oestrogens. Whatever disadvantages there may be with androgens, the same cannot be said of oestrogen therapy in the post-menopausal woman. The only side effects of consequence are nausea and vomiting which, if one perseveres with the treatment, shortly disappear and are only pronounced in about 10 per cent of cases. Stilboestrol is the drug of choice and should be administered orally in a dose of at least 25 to 50 mg. a day. Usually this dose is easily tolerated but if gastric symptoms are very disturbing ethinyl oestradiol 1 mg. a day by mouth can be substituted. It is important not to give too small a dose of oestrogen as this may actually stimulate the tumour.

Perhaps the most remarkable feature of this treatment is that the remission improves in direct relationship to the age of the patient and, in women over 70, more than 60 per cent obtain a worthwhile response (Hayward, 1957). Twenty per cent of post-menopausal women in their fifties will enjoy a remission but, if the drug is used in pre-menopausal patients, oestrogens may again provoke the tumour to grow faster.

Adrenalectomy. In 1952 Huggins and Bergenstal described the effect of bilateral adrenalectomy on patients with advanced breast cancer. Although the operation had been attempted previously (Atkins, 1966) it had not been performed successfully until the advent of cortisone made adequate replacement therapy possible.

The operation can be carried out in one or two stages but in either case the ovaries must also be removed if this has not been done previously. The one stage procedure is done through an abdominal incision and although the approach may be difficult with an enlarged liver, its advocates claim that it carries no greater risk and has the advantage that only one anaesthetic is needed. When performed in two stages, the right adrenal and both ovaries are removed at the first operation—the former usually approached through the bed of the 11th or 12th rib—and the left adrenal some 10 to 14 days later. The approach is technically easier and, although carrying the disadvantage of two anaesthetics on an ill patient, it does not disturb the patient so severely as the one stage procedure. Cortisone administration must be started before the first operation in case this should prove to be the only viable adrenal (see Table II).

Bilateral adrenalectomy has now stood the test of time and can be expected to result in a response rate of from 30 to 40 per cent. Some of these responses are prolonged and cases have been reported of patients enjoying a complete remission for about ten years. The operation has the great advantage that it can be carried out with little mortality by any competent general surgeon, but the disadvantage that at least 60 per cent of the operations performed will have no effect. Many methods have been advocated for selecting in advance those patients likely to benefit and these will be discussed subsequently.

Hypophysectomy. Like adrenalectomy this operation has only been performed successfully since cortisone has been available for replacement therapy and the first series was reported by Luft and Olivecrona in 1953. They approached the gland by the trans-frontal route and probably this has been the most popular method of removal. Carried out by a neuro-surgeon familiar with the technique, it has few disadvantages other than those associated with any major intracranial operation. But because it demands specific neurosurgical expertise it is beyond the scope of many Units dealing with breast cancer and, therefore, other approaches have been devised. The implantation of Yttrium[90] as described by Forrest and Peebles Brown (1955) seemed for a long time to be the answer. It could be performed by a general surgeon, resulted in very little upset to the patient, and, once the initial snags had been overcome, carried very little morbidity. The unanswered question was whether ablation by this means resulted in as high a remission rate as could be obtained by extirpation via the transfrontal route. Recently its originator has made known his belief that this is probably not so (Forrest and Stewart, 1967), and Forrest now feels that a greater degree of benefit can be obtained from bilateral adrenalectomy.

The transphenoidal operation is now widely practised, and seems to have the advantages of both methods (Westover, Rand and Greenfield, 1960). Here there is dual approach to the gland both through the nose and through a small incision near the inner canthus of the eye. It is usually performed by an E.N.T. surgeon, who, when familiar with the technique, can remove the gland in under one hour. There has not as yet been time to evaluate the degree of remission following removal by this route, but there is very little upset to the patient and usually the gland is removed *in toto*.

Compared with adrenalectomy, hypophysectomy seems the method of choice; in skilful hands both the life expectancy and degree of remission are better (Atkins, *et al.*, 1960), and the operative mortality even on very ill patients is negligible. It is important to emphasize however, that adrenalectomy can be carried out as an occasional operation by any general surgeon and for this reason alone is to be preferred when facilities for hypophysectomy are not available.

Replacement Therapy. Perhaps the most important factor in the successful accomplishment of either adrenalectomy or hypophysectomy is adequate maintenance therapy. Cortisone must be administered to all patients

TABLE II. *Steroid regime showing replacement therapy during adrenal-ectomy or hypophysectomy. In cases of adrenalectomy the same technique applies to both the first and second stages.*

Day	I. M. Cortisone	Oral Cortisone
Op. − 2	100 mg. nocte	NIL (1st stage) 25 mg. b.d. (2nd stage)
Op. − 1	100 mg. b.d.	50 mg. mane 75 mg. at 6 p.m. 75 mg. at midnight (morning op) 50 mg. at midnight (afternoon op)
Op.	MORNING OPERATION	
	100 mg. b.d.	100 mg. at 6 a.m. @ 75 mg. as soon as possible after operation* 75 mg. at 6 p.m.** 50 mg. at midnight.
AFTERNOON OPERATION		
	100 mg. b.d.	75 mg. at 6 a.m. 100 mg. at 11 a.m. 75 mg. as soon as possible after operation * 75 mg. at midnight. **
Op. + 1	100 mg. b.d.	50 mg. 6 a.m., noon, 6 p.m. and midnight.
Op. + 2	100 mg. mane only	50 mg. 6 a.m., 2 p.m. and 10 p.m.
Op. + 3	Nil	50 mg. 6 a.m., 2 p.m. and 10 p.m.
Op. + 4	Nil	50 mg. 6 a.m. 25 mg. noon, 6 p.m., midnight.
Op. + 5	Nil	25 mg. 6 hourly.
Op. + 6	Nil	25 mg. t.d.s. (8 hourly)
Op. + 7 and subsequently	Nil	25 mg. b.d.

* If this dose is vomited it must be repeated.
** Not to be given until 4 hours after the previous dose.
@ This dose should be given approximately 3 hours before the patient goes to the theatre. If the case is to be done late on the morning or afternoon list, it should be administered rather late.

In emergency collapse 100 mg. of hydrocortisone hemisuccinate should be given intravenously (or intramuscularly when its action starts in about 30 min.). This dose must be repeated 8 hourly until the patient's condition is satisfactory in addition to the therapy outlined above.

Occasionally patients need the maintenance dose of oral cortisone to be increased to 25 mg. t.d.s. If this fails to keep the blood pressure at a normal level, it probably means they are short of mineralo-corticoids and 9-alpha-fluoro-hydrocortisone (fludrone) should be given orally in a dose of 0·1 mg. from once to four times daily, in addition to routine cortisone. This hormone may cause water retention.

Any complication post-operatively such as an infection will necessitate a great increase in the cortisone dosage to anything between 100 and 300 mg. daily according to the circumstances.

D.O.C.A. is not as a rule necessary.
Salt may be taken as the patient wishes.

before operation and continued for the rest of their lives. For patients to be subjected to adrenalectomy in two stages, it is important that the drug should be given before the first stage, in case the second adrenal is non-functional. Table II shows a workable scheme for the replacement therapy of patients to be subjected to hypophysectomy and it can easily be modified for adrenalectomy patients. If possible the advice of a physician should be obtained on replacement therapy and ideally each patient should be seen by both a surgeon and a physician at each subsequent visit to Out Patients.

Theoretically, patients who have had an adrenalectomy are slightly more at risk since all sources of glucocorticoids and mineralo-corticoids have been removed. In practice, however, there is little difference in the management following either operation.

The patient should be warned that serious consequences may result from failure to take their cortisone and it is wise for them to carry a card indicating their dependence on the drug and instructions for increasing the dose in case of accident.

Almost all patients after hypophysectomy develop a degree of diabetes insipidus, which passes off after about six months. In the interim it can be alleviated by giving pitressin tannate in oil by intra-muscular injection, or pituitary snuff. They also tend to become hypo-thyroid and usually require about 1 grain of thyroid extract daily to maintain them in good health.

Corticoids and Ovarian Ablation

After adrenalectomy and hypophysectomy had proved successful measures in treating the advanced disease, some physicians felt that a similar result might be obtained by the sole administration of cortisone (this acting as a medical adrenalectomy) and destruction of the ovaries. Nissen-Meyer (1955) was the first to describe a series of patients treated in this manner and there is no doubt that the therapy is effective in some patients. But the results were disappointing when compared with those from surgical removal of the adrenal or pituitary. When prescribed, prednisone or prednisolone are the drugs of choice and should be given in doses of about 5 mg. t.d.s. If not carried out previously, all premenopausal women should also have their ovaries irradiated or removed.

Cytotoxins

Because their side effects are severe, and the response only occasional and unpredictable, cytotoxins have had little place in the treatment of advanced breast cancer. Sometimes, however, a remission can be obtained lasting a year or more, and their use may be considered when all other treatments have failed for patients suffering from multiple offensive cutaneous lesions. Under such circumstances the superficial lesions may heal and symptomatic relief continue until the patient dies from other deep-seated metastases. Cyclophosphamide 100–150 mg. daily is an efficient drug and can be administered orally to patients without the necessity of admitting them to hospital. As with other cytotoxins a careful watch must be kept on the blood picture and the patient warned of the symptoms of leucopenia; total alopecia may occur in a small percentage of patients and this side effect should be explained before treatment starts.

Tests of Prediction

Whilst welcoming the degree of benefit that can be given to patients by adrenalectomy or hypophysectomy, it must be remembered that only about 30 per cent of those submitted to either procedure have a worthwhile response. Much effort has been directed towards finding an accurate pre-operative test which might indicate to the surgeon those patients likely to benefit.

The histology and particularly the degree of differentiation of the tumour does not correlate with the results, nor does the response to previous hormone therapy (Atkins *et al.*, 1966). Certain clinical features give some indication of response and these will be mentioned subsequently; but the most accurate guide to results appears to be obtained from an analysis of urinary hormones. In 1960, Bulbrook, Greenwood and Hayward showed that the response to adrenalectomy or hypophysectomy varied with the urinary levels of aetiocholanolone and the 17-OHCS. The response to ablative surgery was good when the levels of aetiocholanolone were high and those of the 17-OHCS were low, and bad when the converse occurred. To obtain the most accurate prediction a discriminant function was formed to include the pre-operative levels of the hormones:

80–80 (17-OHCS (mg. per 24 hrs.)) $+$ aetiocholanolone μ gm. per 24 hrs. If for any patient the result of this formula is a positive number, this is termed a positive discriminant, and the treatment is likely to succeed. If a negative number results, it is termed a negative discriminant and the treatment is likely to fail. These findings have been confirmed by subsequent work (Hayward and Bulbrook, 1965) and by other workers (Juret, Hayem and Fleisler, 1964; Kumaoka *et al.*, 1966).

The following factors may be taken into account in deciding whether to recommend adrenalectomy or hypophysectomy.

(i) The response to previous oophorectomy. If this has been performed to treat established secondaries and produced a remission, this may be an indication that subsequent adrenalectomy or hypophysectomy will also be successful.

(ii) The age of the patient. It is seldom wise to operate on patients aged over 70.

(iii) The patient's clinical condition. This is difficult to define but for instance it would probably be unjustifiable to operate on a patient who was bedridden due to an irreversible hemiplegia.

(iv) The condition of a patient as an anaesthetic risk. This should be liberally interpreted but there are some in whom an anaesthetic would inevitably be fatal.

(v) The length of the free period. This is the length of time between mastectomy and the first recurrence and, if less than two years, heralds a poor response to subsequent ablation.

(vi) The time since the menopause. If the patient presents within six years of the menopause she is unlikely to respond.

By using the discriminant, the free period, and the time since the menopause, Hayward and Bulbrook (1968) have been able to identify a group of patients in whom the remission rate is only 5 per cent (Table III). They have ceased recommending ablative procedures, for these patients who represent nearly one third of all those presenting with advanced breast cancer.

TABLE III. *A comparison of response to adrenalectomy or hypophysectomy in discriminant positive and discriminant negative patients when the free period and menopausal status are taken into account (Hayward and Bulbrook, 1968).*

	Discriminant Positive		Discriminant Negative	
	Success	Response Rate	Success	Response Rate
Either < 2 yrs. free period or < 6 yrs. potsmenopausal or both	22/55	40%	3/61	5%
> 2 yrs. free period > 6 yrs. postmenopausal or premenopausal	18/50	36%	9/42	21%

Prognosis

Some indication of prognosis can be determined from features noted at the time the patient first presents with operable breast cancer. This not only enables an assessment to be made of the patient's chances of survival and cure, but can also affect the choice of treatment.

Staging

It is unfortunate that there is still no agreement on methods of staging. In Great Britain the Manchester staging (Paterson, 1948) is almost certainly the best known and with variations is used by most surgeons. In the U.S.A. Haagensen (1949) has proposed a staging system based on pre-operative clinical assessment and on the presence or absence of "five grave signs". In Europe the U.I.C.C. have advocated the T.N.M. system first proposed by Denoix (1944). In this system, T. stands for tumour, N. for nodes and M. for metastases; various numbers placed after these letters indicate size or degree of involvement. This method is relatively precise but somewhat complicated and has not yet been universally accepted.

Lastly the American Joint Committee on Cancer Staging and End Result Reporting (1962) have advocated a system similar to the T.N.M. but emphasizing different features of the primary growth.

All these methods give a degree of prediction which can be of value to the surgeon in planning treatment. All have features in their favour and it can only be hoped that in the next few years agreement can be reached on a system which all workers will accept.

Grade

Throughout this century attempts have been made to use the microscopic appearance of a breast tumour as an indication of malignancy and hence prognosis. Many methods were advocated but eventually Bloom (1950) combined the best features of other methods to produce a Grading system which was workable. Briefly this depends on tubule formation, regularity of nuclei and the number of mitoses; from these factors the tumour is graded from I to III, with III being the most malignant. The system seems to work and has since been confirmed independently (Wolff, 1966). It gives as accurate an indication of prognosis as Staging, and a combination of the two methods provides a fair assessment of a patients chances of recurrence and survival.

Immune Response

This is difficult to define, but, when measured, attempts to provide an indication of the host's response to the tumour. It has probably been most successfully demonstrated by Cutler, Black and Goldenberg's (1963) use of sinus histiocytosis in the lymph nodes draining the breast. They showed that sinus histiocytosis was clearly associated with patient survival, and the greater degree of histiocytosis the longer was the survival, irrespective of whether the nodes were involved with secondary carcinoma. They combined this finding with Grade and Stage and were able to provide a valuable prognostic index.

Hormone Environment

This is a measure of another host factor which until recently had been largely ignored. The use of the discriminant to predict the response to adrenalectomy or hypophysectomy has been mentioned previously (see p. 321) but it was not appreciated until 1962 (Bulbrook *et al.*, a and b) how the discriminant was distributed in the normal population and in patients with early breast cancer. It was then shown that almost all normal women had positive discriminants, although the values decreased with age and, in women over 65, were frequently negative. In

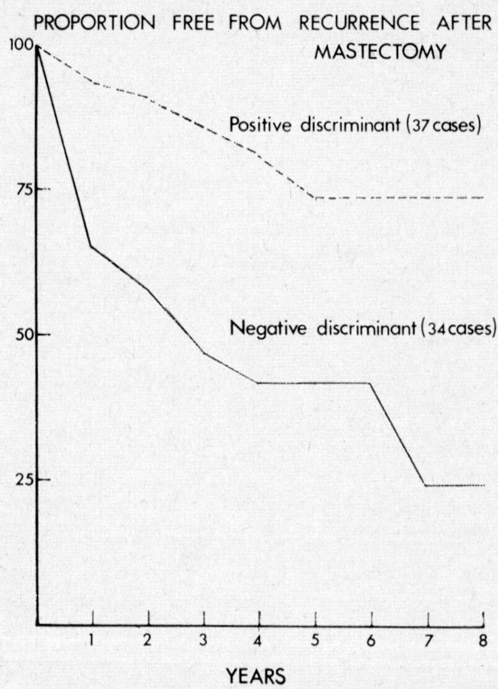

Fig. 18.6. Life table showing proportions free from recurrence after mastectomy.

patients with early breast cancer this regression with age did not occur and the distribution was almost identical with the pattern in patients with advanced disease i.e. about 50 per cent of patients of all ages had negative discriminants. In a subsequent report (Bulbrook, Hayward and Thomas, 1964) it was shown that, in those patients with early breast cancer and negative discriminants, the disease recurred soon after mastectomy; also the patients with negative discriminants had a much lower survival rate when compared with the positives. The work has now been carried further and Fig. 18.6 shows a life table comparing the fate of those with negative discriminants and those with positives.

This appears to be another parameter which can be added to the Grade, Stage etc. to determine prognosis. When sufficient data are available to make use of all these factors, a highly accurate picture may be obtained of the likely fate of any individual patient.

The Future

In discussing the many topics included in this chapter it has become obvious that chronologically the disease is in an interim period. Policies for the treatment of early and advanced breast cancer, and ideas on aetiology and prognosis, are static. And yet the reason for this is not inactivity. We are at last in the healthy position where active and proper steps are being taken to throw light on problems which for so many years have been the subject of fruitless argument. Therapy is no longer dictated by the groundless suppositions of the few who have the ears of the medical profession. Surgeons now change their practice only when they have proof that the change is in the best interest of their patients, rather than on the recommendation of a famous name.

This is the era of the controlled clinical trial and we are awaiting the results of the many that are taking place. When these results are available, each surgeon and physician will have the opportunity of judging them for himself, and altering his thoughts and practice accordingly.

Trials are now taking place which should soon end the tedious debate on the proper approach to the early disease. More important still, investigations on more basic problems may soon throw light on aetiology and possible prevention. The next decade could be decisive in the long story of cancer of the breast.

References

American Joint Committee on Cancer Staging and End Result Reporting (1962). Clinical Staging System for Cancer of the Breast.

ATKINS, H. J. B. (1958). *Brit. Med. J.*, *i*, 187.

ATKINS, H. J. B. (1966). *Ann. R. C. S. Eng.*, **38**, 133.

ATKINS, H. J. B., FALCONER, M. A., HAYWARD, J. L., MacLEAN, K. S., SCHURR, P. H. and ARMITAGE, P. (1960). *Lancet, ii*, 1148.

ATKINS, H. J. B., FALCONER, M. A., HAYWARD, J. L., MacLEAN, K. S. and SCHURR, P. H. (1966). *Lancet, i*, 827.

ATKINS, H. J. B. and WOLFF, B. (1965). *Brit. J. Surg.*, **51**, 602.

BAILAR, J. C. (1963). *Cancer*, **16**, 842.

BEATSON, G. T. (1896). *Lancet, ii*, 104, 162.

BITTNER, J. J. (1937). *J. Hered.*, **28**, 363.

BLOOM, H. J. G. (1950). *Br. J. Cancer*, **4**, 259, 347.

BUELL, P. and DUNN, J. E. (1965). *Cancer*, **18**, 656.

BULBROOK, R. D., GREENWOOD, F. C. and HAYWARD, J. L. (1960). *Lancet, i*, 1154.

BULBROOK, R. D., HAMAGUCHI, E., MacDONALD, W. C., THOMAS, B. S. and UTSUNOMIYA, J. (1966). *Abs. Ninth Int. Canc. Congress.* p. 653.

BULBROOK, R. D., HAYWARD, J. L., SPICER, C. C. and THOMAS, B. S. (1962a). *Lancet, ii*, 1238.

BULBROOK, R. D., HAYWARD, J. L., SPICER, C. C. and THOMAS, B. S. (1962b). *Lancet, ii*, 1235.

BULBROOK, R. D., HAYWARD, J. L. and THOMAS, B. S. (1964). *Lancet, i*, 947.

BULBROOK, R. D., THOMAS, B. S. and UTSUNOMIYA, J. (1964). *Nature*, **201**, 189.

Chemotherapy Statistical Unit: "Surgical Adjuvant Breast Study—I". Progress Report, 1964. Buffalo, N.Y. Roswell Park Memorial Institute.

COLE, M. P. (1964). *Brit. J. Surg.*, **51**, 216.

CUTLER, S. J., BLACK, M. M. and GOLDENBERG, I. S. (1963). *Cancer*, **16**, 1589.

DENOIX, P. F. (1944). *Bull. Inst. Natn. Hyg.* (Paris), *i*, 69.

EISENBERG, H. S. and GOLDENBERG, I. S. (1966). In "Clinical Evaluation in Breast Cancer". (Editors J. L. Hayward and R. D. Bulbrook) p. 93. Academic Press, New York and London.

FORREST, A. P. M. and STEWART, H. J. (1967). In "Major Endocrine Surgery for the Treatment of Cancer of the Breast in Advanced Stages". (Editors M. Dargent and Cl. Romieu), p. 89, SIMEP Editions, Lyon.

FORREST, A. P. M. and PEEBLES BROWN, D. A. (1955). *Lancet, i*, 1054.

GROSS, L., McCARTY, K. S. and GESSLER, A. E. (1952). *Ann. N. Y. Acad. Sci.*, **54**, 1018.

HAAGENSEN, C. D. (1949). *Am. J. Roentg.*, **62**, 328.

HAYWARD, J. L. (1957). *Guy's Hospital Rep.*, **106**, 254.

HAYWARD, J. L. (1964). *Brit. J. Surg.*, **51**, 224.

HAYWARD, J. L. and BULBROOK, R. D. (1965). *Cancer Res.*, **25**, 1129.

HAYWARD, J. L. and BULBROOK, R. D. (1968). In "Prognostic Factors in Breast Cancer". (Editors A. P. M. Forrest and P. B. Kunkler). p. 383, Livingstone, Edinburgh.

HUGGINS, C. and BERGENSTAL, D. M. (1952). *Cancer Res.*, **12**, 134.

JURET, P., HAYEM, M. and FLEISLER, A. (1964). *J. Chir.* (Paris), **87**, 409.

KUMAOKA, S., ABE, O., SAKAUCHI, M., TAKATANI, O. and KUSAMA, M. (1966). *Abs. Ninth Int. Canc. Congress*, p. 653.

LANE-CLAYPON, J. E. (1926). Public Health and Medical Subjects No. 32 London: British Ministry of Health.

LEWISON, E. F. and ALLEN, L. W. (1953). *Ann. Surg.*, **138**, 39.

LILIENFELD, A. M. (1963). *Cancer Res.*, **23**, 1503.

LUFT, R. and OLIVECRONA, H. (1953). *J. Neurosurg.*, **10**, 301.

NISSEN-MEYER, R. (1955). *Nordisk Medicin*, **53**, 186.

NISSEN-MEYER, R. (1966). In "Clinical Evaluation in Breast Cancer". (Editors J. L. Hayward and R. D. Bulbrook), p. 175, Academic Press, New York and London.

PASSEY, R. D., DMOCHOWSKI, L., ASTBURY, W. T., REED, R. and EAVES, G. (1951). *Nature*, **167**, 643.

PATERSON, R. (1948). In "The Treatment of Malignant Disease by Radium and X-rays", p. 309, Arnold and Co., London.

PATEY, D. H. and NURICK, A. W. (1953). *Brit. Med. J.*, *i*, 15.

PELLER, S. (1940). *Surg. Gynec. Obstet.*, **71**, 1.

PRUDENTE, A. (1945). *Surg. Gynec. Obstet.*, **80**, 575.

RIDDELL, V. (1954). In "Progress in Clinical Surgery" (Editor Rodney Smith). p. 217, Churchill, London.

ROBBINS, G. F. and BERG, J. W. (1964). *Cancer*, **17**, 1501.

SCHINZINGER, A. (1889). *Centrabl. Chir.*, **16**, 55.

SEGI, M. (1957). "Cancer Mortality Statistics in Japan 1953–1955." Sendai, Japan. Department of Public Health, Tohoku University.

SHAPIRO, S., STRAX, P. and VENET, L. (1966). *J. Amer. Med. Ass.*, **195**, 731.

STEVENS, G. M. and WEIGEN, J. F. (1966). *Cancer*, **19**, 51.

UHLRICH, P. (1939). *Acta Union Internat. contre cancer*, **4**, 377.

WAINWRIGHT, J. H. (1931). *Am. J. Cancer.*, **15**, 2610.

WESTOVER, J. L., RAND, R. W. and GREENFIELD, M. A. (1960). *Radiology*, **74**, 86.

WOLFF, B. (1966). *Br. J. Cancer*, **20**, 36.

WYNDER, E. L., BROSS, I. J. and HIRAYAMA, T. (1960). *Cancer*, **13**, 180.

WYNDER, E. L., KAJITANI, T., KUNO, J., LUCAS, J. C., DE PALO, A. and FARROW, J. (1963). *Surg. Gynec. Obstet.*, **117**, 196.

CHAPTER 19

THE ZOLLINGER-ELLISON SYNDROME

RODNEY SMITH

This syndrome was first described by Zollinger and Ellison in 1955, their original paper calling attention to an association between the presence of a non-beta islet cell tumour in the pancreas and peptic ulceration of the jejunum. Since that date some 600 cases have been reported in the literature and it has become clear that the early definition of the syndrome requires some broadening.

In the majority of cases, for instance, the peptic ulceration is not situated in the jejunum, the common sites being the stomach or the

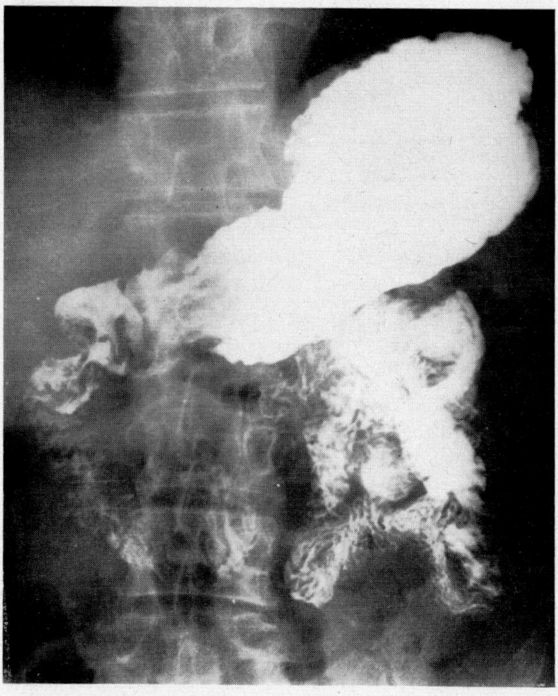

FIG. 19.1. In the Zollinger-Ellison Syndrome, the ulcer or ulcers are present in unusual sites in only a minority of cases. This X-ray shows a large ulcer in the first part of the duodenum, cured by removal of an islet cell carcinoma in the tail of the pancreas.

first part of the duodenum (Fig. 19.1). In fact, in only about 25 per cent of cases is the ulceration at an unusual site. In over 90 per cent of cases gastric hypersecretion is present and it can usually be shown that this is caused by a hormone identical with, or at least indistinguishable from, gastrin, secreted by the pancreatic tumour tissue. The tumour itself in the pancreas is composed of cells which are not beta cells but either alpha cells or agranular cells. Unlike the beta cell tumour producing hyperinsulinism, the non-beta cell tumour producing the Zollinger-

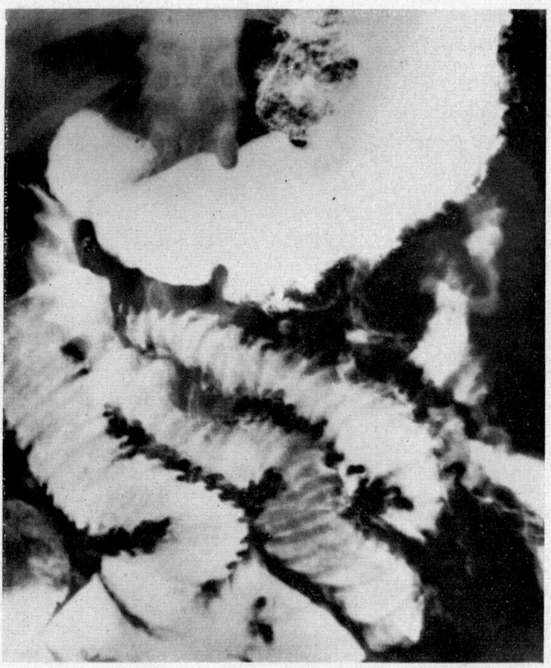

Fig. 19.2. Diarrhoea in the Zollinger-Ellison Syndrome is usually accounted for by the intense jejunitis produced by the gastric hypersecretion. The appearance of the jejunum is well shown in the X-ray above.

Ellison syndrome is in 60 per cent of cases a malignant tumour, and even when benign is quite likely to be present at more than one site in the pancreas. Many patients in addition to having severe peptic ulceration and gastric hypersecretion, also have diarrhoea as a symptom and this may be caused by the severe jejunitis consequent upon the gastric hypersecretion or by the direct effect upon the intestine of some additional hormone other than gastrin (Fig. 19.2). In a small proportion of cases, less than 10 per cent, severe diarrhoea is present without gastric hypersecretion or peptic ulceration.

Diagnosis

The possibility that a patient may be suffering from the Zollinger-Ellison syndrome should be suspected if peptic ulcers have been shown to be multiple in the stomach and duodenum, or to be in unusual sites, particularly the lower duodenum and the jejunum. The possibility should also be suspected in any patient who after surgery which would normally be regarded as adequate rapidly develops a recurrence of peptic ulceration.

Gastric hypersecretion is usually gross. The basal (resting) juice is often as much as 2 to 3 litres in 12 hr., and cases reaching an amount of 7 or 8 litres have been reported. The juice usually contains 80 to 100 mEq. of free hydrochloric acid per litre, and this figure is sometimes exceeded. The stomach is already putting out as much acid as the cells are capable of producing, so little or no alteration occurs after the administration of histamine, and this is a valuable diagnostic point. Estimation of pepsin in the serum and of uropepsin in the urine also gives very high levels. Another feature which may be identified is gross hypertrophy of the gastric and duodenal mucosa, which may be shown by x-rays or by gastroscopy. If diarrhoea is a major symptom considerable electrolyte imbalance may occur and in particular potassium deficiency.

In any patient strongly suspected of having a Zollinger-Ellison syndrome a search should be made for other endocrine lesions and enquiries should extend to relatives of the patient, for multiple endocrine lesions are far from uncommon and it is not uncommon to find that relatives of the patient have also presented troubles of an endocrine nature. As an example of this, one patient of the writer died of a malignant non-beta islet cell tumour producing gross gastric hypersecretion and peptic ulceration, eventually metastasizing widely in the thorax. Before death he had also developed hyper-parathyroidism, and his daughter had been successfully operated upon for the removal of a beta cell insulin-producing tumour in her pancreas.

Pancreatic Scanning—Patients suspected of having an islet cell tumour in the pancreas may be investigated by pancreatic scanning with alpha-selenomethionine-75 (Blau and Bender, 1962; Brown *et al.*, 1968). A clear definition of the pancreas using this method is not often obtained, and as islet cell tumours are often small the chances of successfully demonstrating a tumour are poor.

Selective angiography, contrast medium being introduced by the Seldinger technique into the coeliac or superior mesenteric artery or both, has a rather better chance of demonstrating an islet cell tumour, but even here the results so far reported are not impressive.

11*

Clinical Course

Most patients are in serious trouble with peptic ulceration and many have had unsuccessful surgery already which has failed to prevent recurrent ulceration. Although the tumour is often malignant it is usually slow growing, and study of the causes of death in those patients dying of the syndrome show clearly that they die of haemorrhage, perforation or peritonitis rather than of metastases in the liver, the lungs or elsewhere, even though such metastases are often present. This has a bearing upon treatment.

Treatment

Surgical treatment is usually essential, but an occasional case has been reported where the syndrome has been controlled by the use of the anticholinergic drug Poldine Methyl Methosulphate.

As regards the type of surgery to be undertaken there are two apparently opposing views which have been expressed. The first of these, which is accepted in most centres in the United States, insists that the only surgery to be contemplated is total gastrectomy. The arguments in favour of this view run as follows. The tumour more often than not is a malignant tumour and there may already be metastases in lymph nodes or in the liver which are functioning and producing gastrin. Even if the tumour is not malignant, benign adenomata may be present at multiple sites in the pancreas. Taking these two facts together it is often far from easy to be sure that all tumour tissue has been removed and if all tumour tissue is not removed the syndrome is bound to continue. Patients dying from the syndrome usually die of the complications of peptic ulceration rather than the tumour itself. Therefore, the argument goes, clearly the correct treatment is to assume that the syndrome is likely to continue as long as the stomach is present, and the initial surgical treatment should be total gastrectomy.

The opposing view is that the pancreas should first be explored in the hope that the tumour, or tumours, in it can be eradicated surgically, reserving total gastrectomy for those cases where this proves impossible, or where there are already functioning metastastic tumours.

The writer's experiences have led to the conclusion that the second of these two views is the more logical, but it is certainly true that inadequate pancreatic surgery is just as futile as inadequate gastric surgery in these very severe disorders.

Eight personal cases of the Zollinger-Ellison syndrome have been encountered. Of these, one presented with very severe diarrhoea without peptic ulceration or gastric hypersecretion and underwent a total pancreatectomy for a diffuse multicentric non-beta islet cell carcinoma

(Fig. 19.3). Three patients had already had multiple gastric operations for recurrent peptic ulceration. Their tumours were malignant and already beyond the stage where pancreatectomy could be considered. The other four cases are worth referring to in a little more detail.

One of these, a lady aged 38 in 1956, had a laparotomy for a huge duodenal ulcer and marked gastric hypersecretion (12 hr. gastric secretion was over 4 litres, containing 425 mEq. of hydrochloric acid). (Fig. 19.1.) At her operation a tumour in the distal pancreas was found and this was treated by distal pancreatectomy. The tumour was a malignant

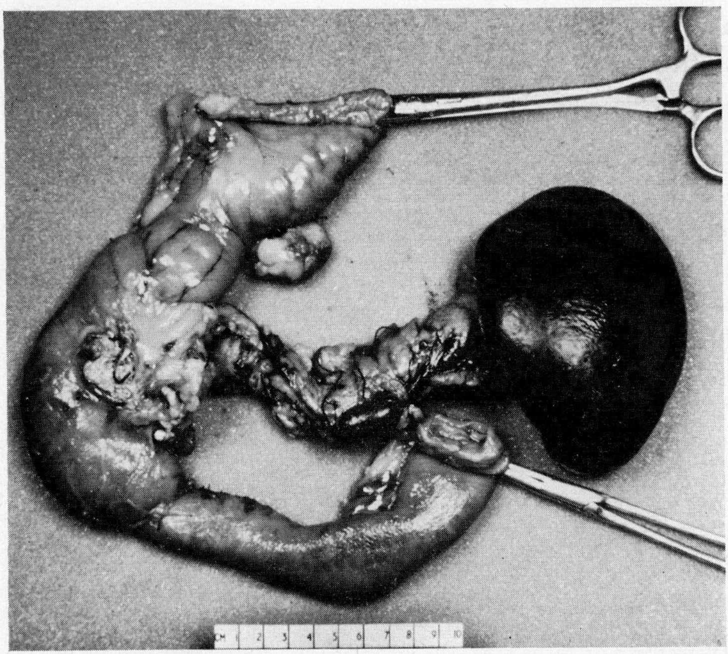

FIG. 19.3. Total pancreatectomy specimen. The entire pancreas was the site of a multi-centric non-beta cell carcinoma, presenting with intense diarrhoea but no gastric hypersecretion or peptic ulceration.

non-beta islet cell tumour with one lymph node in the hilum of the spleen containing metastastic tumour. The stomach was not removed nor was vagotomy performed. The patient, 12 years later, is well and free from recurrence of her syndrome.

A lady of 30 in 1957, was found to have multiple peptic ulcers extending from the subcardiac region through the stomach, duodenum and well down into the jejunum. She had severe gastric hypersecretion (12 hr. secretion was 7½ litres containing 750 mEq. of hydrochloric acid). At operation multiple adenomas were found in the pancreas for which she underwent a subtotal pancreatectomy. Later the demonstration of hyperparathyroidism led to the removal of three parathyroid adenomas. The stomach was not removed, vagotomy was not performed. Post-operatively all ulcers healed, all symptoms disappeared, gastric hypersecretion slowly returned to normal. The patient, 11 years later, remains in good health without signs of recurrence of her syndrome.

A lady of 35 in 1962 had had, at another hospital, a cholecystojejunostomy performed for obstructive jaundice caused by a tumour in the head of the pancreas. Epigastric pain had been a feature already and post-operatively although her jaundice cleared, pain had continued and repeated severe gastric haemorrhages had occurred. In 1963 she was referred to the writer and underwent a radical pancreatoduodenectomy together with removal of three-quarters of the stomach. The operation was difficult and involved opening the portal vein and removal of a long extension of the tumour, freely mobile in the lumen of the portal vein. Histologically the tumour was shown to be a non-beta islet cell carcinoma and the source of the bleeding had been a huge peptic ulcer of the duodenum. This lady died $3\frac{1}{2}$ years post-operatively from metastases of the tumour, but in spite of this there was no recurrence of the epigastric pain or haemorrhage.

A man of 27 in 1964 underwent an emergency gastrectomy for haemorrhage, the bleeding coming from a very large duodenal ulcer. Within six weeks two new ulcers had appeared,

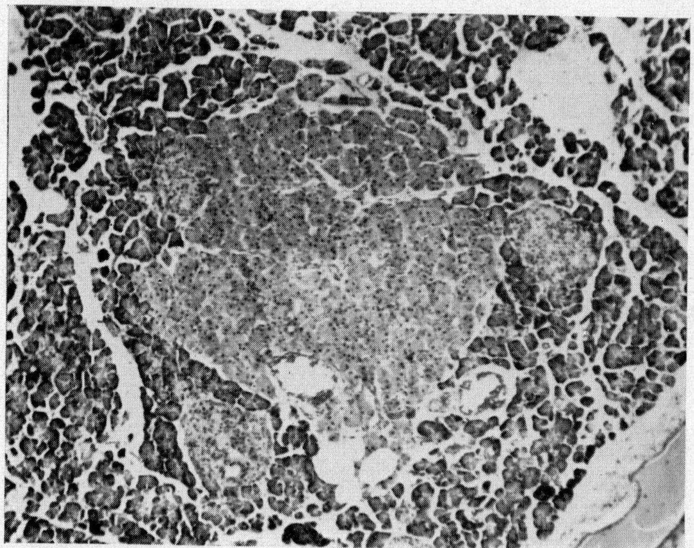

FIG. 19.4. Micro-adenosis producing the Zollinger-Ellison Syndrome. The distal pancreas contained a number of discrete micro-adenomata as shown above.

one above and one below the anastomosis. Exploration was undertaken with the diagnosis of a possible Zollinger-Ellison syndrome. The pancreas was grossly normal. Subtotal gastrectomy and vagotomy was carried out together with distal pancreatectomy. The histology of the pancreas showed clearly micro-adenosis of a non-beta cell pattern affecting particularly the tail of the pancreas (Fig. 19.4). The patient remains well and free from symptoms four years later.

It is possible to draw some conclusions at least from these four patients. The first two of them, both thin young women in their 30s, subjected to pancreatic surgery, one 12 years ago and one 11 years ago, both without recurrence of the syndrome, clearly had the right operation, for there would be few who would say that either patient would today be better off had a total gastrectomy been performed. The third patient appeared to have had an inadequate operation and it remains uncertain why, when metastases from the tumour appeared, the syndrome itself was not re-established with further severe peptic ulceration. In similar circumstances, in the light of the knowledge we have now, such a patient would probably be better treated by removal of the whole stomach as part of the excision, rather than three-quarters of the stomach as was practised in this case. The fourth patient, a young man of 27, on the face of it also appears to have had an inadequate operation in that the remaining pancreas was unlikely to be normal. Nevertheless, gastrectomy in his case was followed by recurrence of severe ulceration within a matter of weeks, whereas distal pancreatectomy has been followed by freedom from symptoms for four years. It is clearly right to continue to follow such a patient's progress and not advise further surgery unless recurrence of the syndrome occurs. Should the syndrome recur however in this patient, total gastrectomy would probably be the operation of choice.

Summary

It would seem logical to explore the abdomen of a patient with the Zollinger-Ellison syndrome with the primary intention of examining the pancreas. If it appears to be possible to remove all tumour tissue by enucleation or pancreatectomy, then this should be the procedure selected. However, post-operatively the patient should remain in hospital for further study. If the result of pancreatic surgery is that ulcers heal, symptoms disappear and gastric hypersecretion returns to normal (although this may take time) then total gastrectomy should not be performed. If however the result of pancreatic surgery is unsatisfactory and it appears likely that tumour tissue has been left behind, then re-operation should be advised and total gastrectomy performed. In those cases where from the outset it becomes apparent that total removal of all pancreatic tumour tissue is unlikely, total gastrectomy remains the procedure of choice. The two apparently opposing views about surgical treatment of the Zollinger-Ellison Syndrome have in fact much in common, for it must be accepted that both inadequate gastric surgery and inadequate pancreatic surgery can only lead to disaster.

References

Blau M. and Bender, M. A. (1962) *Radiology*, **78**: 974.

Brown P. W., Sircus W., Smith A. N., Donaldson A. A., Dymock I. W., Falcome C. W. A. and Small W. P. (1968) *Lancet*, **1**: 160.

Zollinger R. M. and Ellison E. H. (1955) *Ann. Suy.* **142**: 709.

Chapter 20

CHRONIC PANCREATITIS

Rodney Smith

Twenty or thirty years ago chronic pancreatitis was regarded as a rare condition. Today it is encountered more frequently and although this is probably due in part to better diagnosis there is some evidence that the disorder itself has become more common.

Origins

A great number of factors are possibly concerned with the aetiology of chronic pancreatitis. The two most common of these are alcohol and cholelithiasis. The place of other possible origins is less well defined— such as pathology in the blood supply to the pancreas, trauma, primary pancreatic duct obstruction, metabolic origins, virus or bacterial infections and so on. A recent survey at St. George's Hospital showed that the patients admitted with pancreatitis fell into three more or less equal groups as follows:

One third of patients had gallstones and an infected biliary tract.
One third of patients consumed a good deal more alcohol than was good for them.
One third of patients had neither alcohol nor biliary tract infection as a cause: some of these had other identifiable aetiological factors, but a fair proportion had perforce to be classified as "idiopathic" in origin.

The aetiological factors vary considerably from country to country, and in some areas clinical reports of chronic pancreatitis place the origins on an alcoholic basis in as high as 90 per cent of cases.

Pathology

In the relapsing subacute type of pancreatitis the gland passes recurrently through the changes characteristic of acute inflammation, and may between attacks return substantially to normal. These attacks may quite often be relatively minor ones during which the local changes do not progress beyond a generalized pancreatic oedema. If however, there has been actual necrosis, some subsequent replacement with fibrous tissue and permanent intrapancreatic scarring is inevitable. In

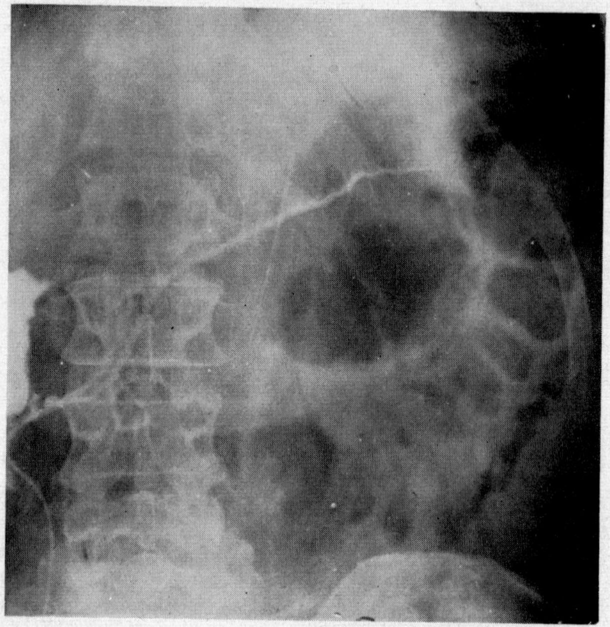

FIG. 20.1. Normal pancreatic duct as shown by ascending operative pancreatography.

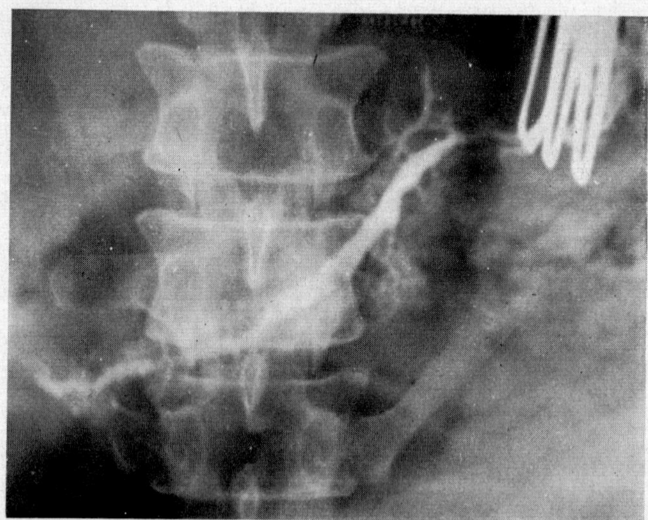

FIG. 20.2. Dilated roughened pancreatic duct characteristic of chronic pancreatitis as shown by ascending operative pancreatography.

chronic pancreatitis, with or without acute exacerbations, there is a progressive replacement of the gland by fibrous tissue affecting the exocrine tissue first and the islets of Langerhans much later. The pancreatic duct system may become secondarily obstructed and widely dilated, sometimes with multiple strictures dividing up the duct of Wirsung into a "chain of lakes" (Fig. 20.1-2-3). The pancreas may however become the site of a dense generalized sclerosis without dilatation of the duct system.

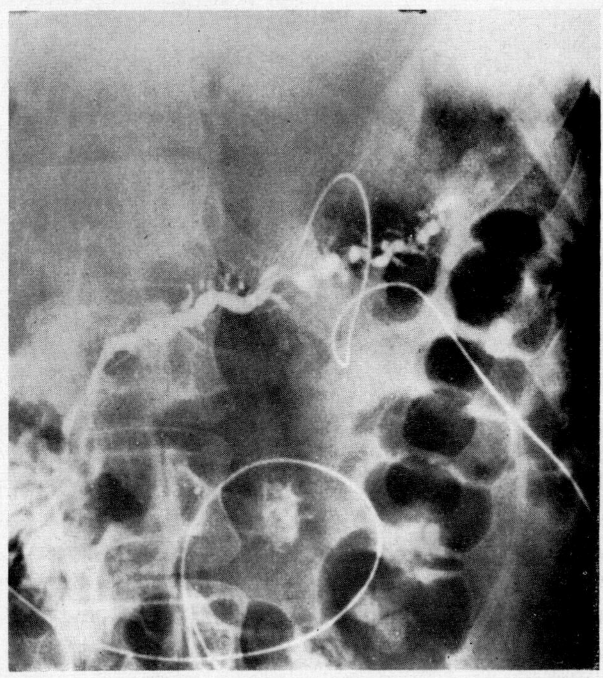

FIG. 20.3. Dilated pancreatic duct with multiple strictures producing the so-called "chain of lakes" appearance as shown by descending pancreatography.

Pancreatic calculi may form within the main and subsidiary ducts (Fig. 20.4) and occasionally calcification of the gland parenchyma has occurred. Important secondary pathological changes include pancreatic pseudocyst, abscess, fistula, portal vein obstruction, splenic vein obstruction, splenomegaly, duodenal obstruction.

Clinical Presentation:

Relapsing Sub-acute Pancreatitis. Patients in this group suffer from recurring attacks of upper abdominal pain with gastro-intestinal upsets, between which they are free from symptoms. In many instances

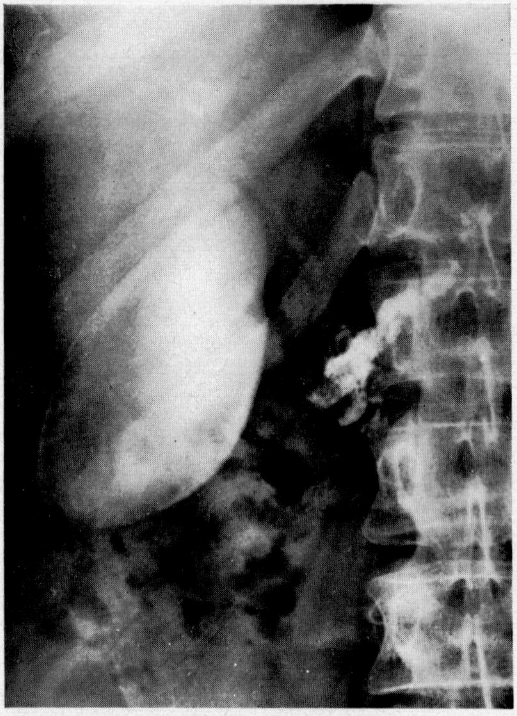

Fig. 20.4. Gross intraductal pancreatic stones demonstrated during intravenous cholangiogram series. The gallbladder is large but the common bile duct is slim and not dilated.

investigations have been carried out over several years without the cause being found. Clinical evidence that the correct diagnosis may be relapsing pancreatitis is provided by observing in some cases that:

(1) Pain is characteristically *pancreatic*. It is sited centrally in the epigastrium. It radiates through to the back, or to the right or left costal margin. It is a very constant pain, not colicky, not relieved by milk or alkalis (as is the pain of a duodenal ulcer), in fact sometimes made worse by milk.

(2) Nausea and anorexia are common—vomiting less so.

(3) Diarrhoea is a common accompaniment of the acute episodes.

(4) Each attack may last from 24 hr. to several days, and may be precipitated by alcohol or a large meal with an unusually high fat content.

(5) A mild pyrexia may accompany the attacks lasting for several days.

(6) Infrequently a history of mild transient jaundice is obtained during the attacks or an account that the urine has been very dark.

Chronic and Chronic Relapsing Pancreatitis.—Patients in this group differ from those of the preceding group in that some symptoms are present all the time.

(1) Pancreatic pain varies in intensity but remains as a constant background, never really leaving the patient who has learned to rely on a wide range of pain killers to get through the day, and has frequently discovered that pethidine is the only drug which will temporarily abolish the pain completely. Addiction to this drug is thus common in patients with chronic pancreatitis.

(2) Gastro-intestinal upsets of one kind or another are almost universal. Anorexia, nausea, vomiting and diarrhoea occur during exacerbations and in long-standing cases the nutritional state is poor.

(3) Clinical evidence of pancreatic insufficiency may be found, such as steatorrhoea and symptoms suggestive of diabetes mellitus.

(4) Physical examination may reveal merely tenderness in the epigastrium but in advanced cases there may be secondary pancreatic pathology such as a pseudocyst giving rise to an abdominal mass.

Radiological Investigations

(1) Plain films, including tomography, may demonstrate pancreatic calcification.

(2) A barium meal may provide evidence of gastric or duodenal mucosal oedema or pressure or distortion by an enlarged pancreas or a pseudocyst.

(3) Radiological studies of the biliary tract may show intrinsic pathology, or distortion of the common bile duct by pancreatic pathology.

(4) "Scanning" of the pancreas using alpha-selenomethionine-75 has been employed during the last few years in the study of various pancreatic lesions. Evidence of chronic pancreatitis may be obtained if the patchy reduced uptake of the isotope characteristic of this disorder is identified (Blau and Bender, 1962; Brown *et al.*, 1968).

(5) Coeliac artery angiography has similarly proved to be of some limited value in cases suspected of chronic pancreatitis.

In general it should be said that scanning of the pancreas and selective coeliac artery angiography have proved disappointing as diagnostic aids. Positive evidence is quite often obtained in advanced cases where the diagnosis is in little doubt but in the early doubtful case these methods of investigation are often unhelpful.

Laboratory Investigations

(1) *Serum amylase estimation* may be helpful during exacebations. In chronic pancreatitis estimation of serum amylase levels is likely to yield normal values.

(2) *Tests of pancreatic exocrine function*, the secretin-pancreozymin test, the Lundh test and others may provide evidence that there is a reduction in the production of pancreatic juice or that the pancreatic duct is occluded. In general such evidence is found when a clear cut diagnosis of chronic pancreatitis (or pancreatic carcinoma) can already be made without the use of such tests. They are not therefore usually helpful in relapsing acute pancreatitis or in the early doubtful case of chronic pancreatitis.

(3) *Glucose tolerance curve*. In chronic pancreatitis diabetes mellitus is not uncommon and some disturbance of carbohydrate metabolism is frequently found. The glucose tolerance curve is abnormal in a fairly high percentage of cases.

Diagnosis

The major factors leading to a diagnosis of chronic or relapsing pancreatitis are thus as follows:

(1) Presence of known aetiological factors, such as alcohol or biliary tract disease.

(2) Pain, probably the most pressing symptom, which appears to be "pancreatic" in character.

(3) Gastro-intestinal upsets such as loose stools which float, fat intolerance, alcohol intolerance.

(4) Complications diagnostic of a pancreatic origin such as pancreatic pseudocyst or a pancreatic fistula.

(5) Evidence of pancreatic insufficiency; steatorrhoea, frank diabetes or abnormal glucose tolerance curve, abnormal results to pancreatic function tests.

(6) Radiological evidence on plain films, barium studies, films of the biliary apparatus, angiograms or in a pancreatic scan.

In late cases the clinical picture may be complicated by severe malabsorption and by secondary compression of the portal vein or splenic vein with the production of oesophagogastric varices which bleed.

Treatment

The first essential in treatment is the elimination where possible of any obvious cause. Thus if alcohol is a factor it may well be found that if the patient takes no alcohol at all, some considerable improvement will follow. Merely to reduce the alcohol intake, however, seldom has any useful effect. If there are no obvious causes or if the patient is unable to give up alcohol it is no easy matter to improve the lot of the sufferer from chronic pancreatitis. Pancreatic insufficiency can clearly be treated medically. There is, however, no effective medical treatment for chronic or relapsing pancreatitis. The patient therefore has the choice of accepting his symptoms and possible potential dangers or accepting an operation in the hope of improvement.

Normally speaking surgery should be undertaken on one or more of the following indications:

(1) Intractable pain (far the most common indication for surgery).
(2) Frequent attacks of acute or sub-acute pancreatitis.
(3) Complications, such as a cyst, a fistula, or portal vein obstruction.
(4) A doubtful diagnosis and in particular the possibility of carcinoma of the pancreas.

The Scope of Surgery

The uncertainty of bringing about a cure by means of surgery is adequately demonstrated by the number of different procedures advocated. The most useful way of assessing these is perhaps to examine them one by one indicating the physiological object of each and hence the type of pancreatic pathology likely to be influenced.

Cholecystectomy; Cholecystogastrostomy; Cholecystojejunostomy

The removal of a pathological gallbladder containing stones may well eliminate a mild relapsing sub-acute pancreatitis. Here the surgery is logically treating the cause. Anastomosis, however, of a normal gallbladder to stomach or jejunum cannot on theoretical grounds be expected to help in chronic or relapsing pancreatitis, nor in practice will it do so.

Sphincterotomy.—Much argument centres around this operation. It was originally thought that attacks of pancreatitis were commonly produced by reflux of bile up the main pancreatic duct and that sphincterotomy would prevent this by laying open the common channel through which bile and pancreatic juice enter the duodenum. It is not now generally believed that reflux of bile into the pancreatic duct is of primary importance although reflux of infected bile into a damaged pancreatic duct system, particularly if there is stasis in addition, may be a contributing factor. When the operation of sphincterotomy is effective therefore the reason probably is that it eliminates a partial obstruction and prevents stasis in the pancreatic duct system.

The writer's personal experiences of this operation suggests the following conclusions:

(1) It is only of use in some cases of relapsing sub-acute pancreatitis and is totally ineffective in established chronic pancreatitis.

(2) It is particularly likely to succeed in those cases in which there is biliary tract pathology in addition.

(3) The clear demonstration at operation of a fibrous obstructive lesion at the level of the papilla of Vater the division of which releases pancreatic juice from a dilated pancreatic duct system, suggests a probable good outcome to the operation.

Biliary Diversion (e.g. Choledochoduodenostomy). This procedure grew out of the belief that sphincterotomy, if it succeeded, did so by diverting bile from the pancreatic duct and that therefore this might be more effectively achieved by anastomosis of the common bile duct to the duodenum. The theoretical basis is thus unsound and it seems probable that the only usefulness of procedures of this kind lies in the treatment of the occasional case of pancreatitis where the picture is complicated by a recurrent ascending cholangitis.

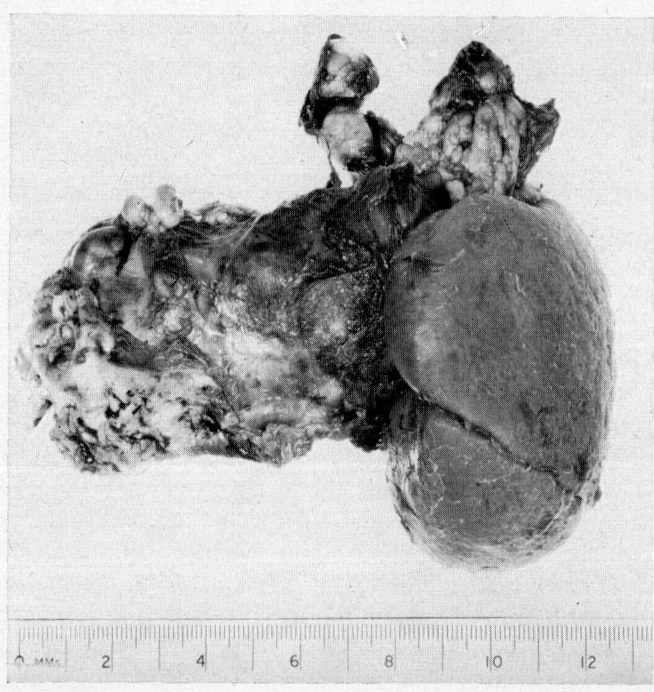

FIG. 20.5. Distal pancreatectomy specimen from a case of severe chronic pancreatitis.

Operations aimed at Providing Retrograde Drainage of the Pancreatic Duct

The state of the pancreatic duct system in chronic pancreatitis varies from case to case, but a dilated duct which is clearly obstructed may be decompressed in a number of ways and this is a reasonable approach to the problem. Professor Charles Puestow of Chicago advocates slitting up the pancreatic duct from the tail of the gland right up to the head

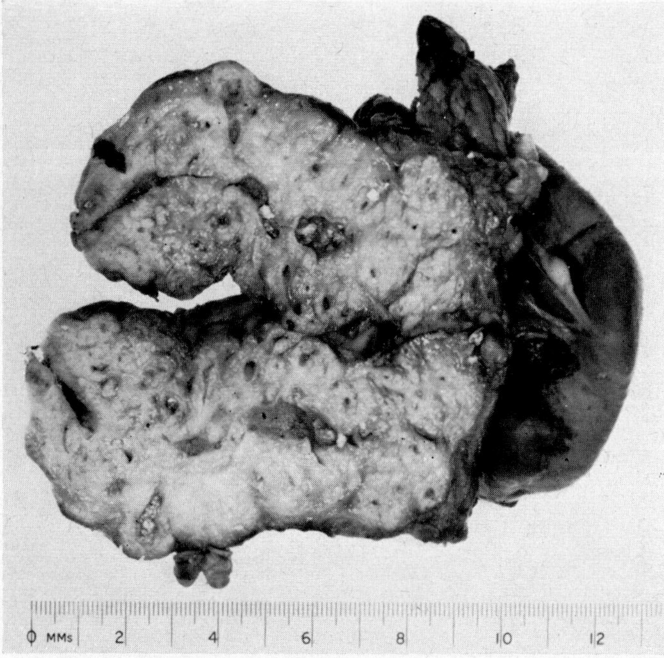

FIG. 20.6. Sub-total distal pancreatectomy specimen from a case of severe chronic pancreatitis with calcification.

after removal of the spleen and draining this widely opened duct into a long Roux loop of jejunum, arguing that this major procedure is necessary because obstruction is often due to multiple strictures with the duct system resembling "a chain of lakes" (Puestow, 1957). If this is indeed the pathology present, ductal decompression would require a Puestow operation if the pancreas is to be left behind. However, many surgeons, of whom the author is one, feel that a distal pancreatectomy is in many instances a safer operation than a Puestow operation, the whole of the pancreas up to the neck being removed and the duct remaining in the head and neck being drained retrogradely either into the stomach or into the jejunum (Fig. 20.5).

If investigation at operation of the pancreatic duct system shows that this duct is generally dilated from one end of the pancreas to the other, without strictures, then effective decompression may be secured by

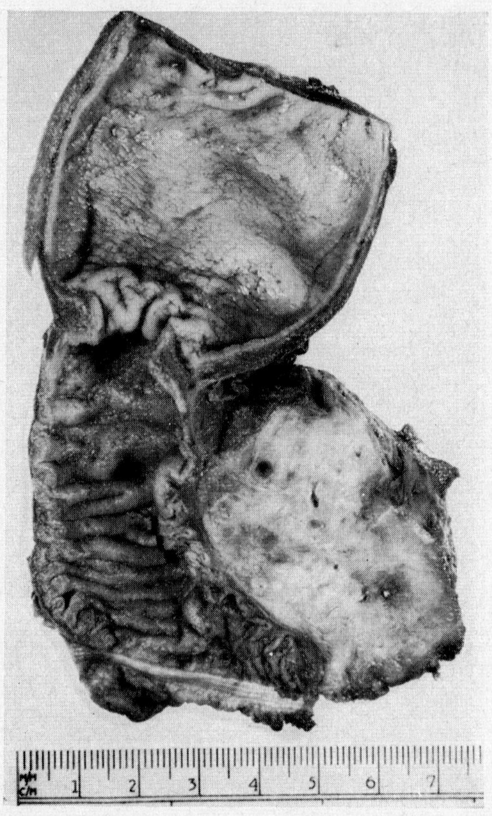

FIG. 20.7. Pancreatoduodenectomy specimen from a case of severe chronic pancreatitis the main feature of which was fibrosis and calcification in the head of the pancreas.

draining this duct into either the stomach or the jejunum without removal of any pancreatic substance at all.

Sub-total Distal Pancreatectomy (Fig. 20.6). Severe generalized chronic pancreatitis without duct dilatation may be treated by re-section of the whole of the gland except a thin crescentic fragment left in the concavity of the second part of the duodenum. After this procedure diabetes mellitus is likely to occur and the patient will need pancreatic extracts by mouth (both of these effects may of course occur without an operation).

Pancreatoduodenectomy (Fig. 20.7). Resection of the head of the gland with the duodenum, similar to the resection carried out for carcinoma of the head or periampullary region, is sometimes necessary if the head is grossly disorganized by disease and the symptoms sufficiently severe. Reconstruction includes anastomosis of the divided pancreatic

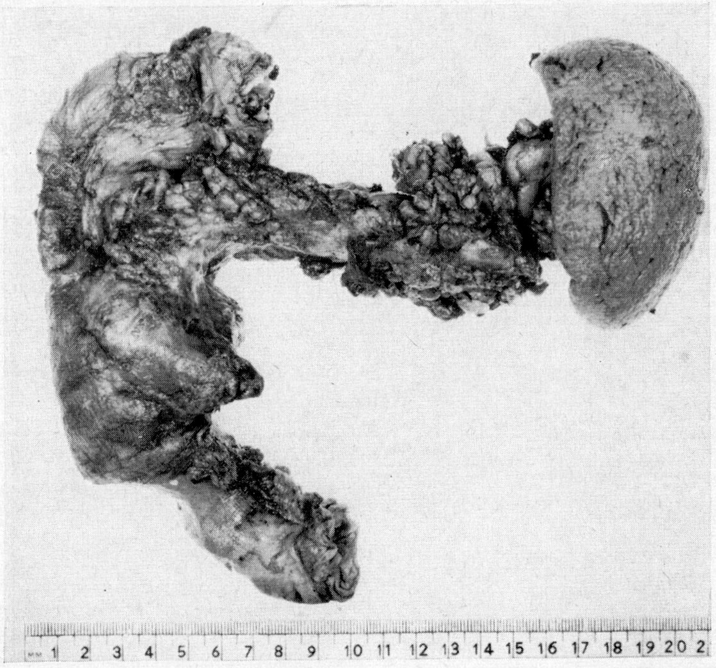

FIG. 20.8. Total pancreatectomy specimen from a case of severe generalized chronic pancreatitis.

duct to the jejunum. The operative hazard is relatively high but the results of this procedure are good.

Total Pancreatectomy (Fig. 20.8). Occasionally the pancreas is so extensively destroyed by inflammatory disease that it is not possible to retain any part of it with safety if surgery is to succeed. Another infrequent indication for total pancreatectomy is the combination of a pancreatic or ampullary carcinoma with extensive pancreatitis.

Splanchnicectomy.—Division of the autonomic nerve supply of the pancreas can reduce or even eliminate pancreatic pain and this has some part to play in the treatment of chronic pancreatitis. It is however a treatment for pancreatic *pain* and not of pancreatitis. Moreover its effect in relieving pain is unfortunately usually only a temporary one.

Results

The overall results of operative treatment of chronic pancreatitis are disappointing considered purely in terms of patients *cured*. Nevertheless some 75 to 80 per cent of patients can be improved, some of them so materially that they profess themselves cured, only admitting to symptoms on questioning, and are able to return to their employment and a normal enjoyment of life. This is an undoubted improvement on medical treatment, which can deal with pancreatic insufficiency, endocrine or exocrine, but is ineffective in controlling the symptoms of chronic pancreatitis, particularly pain.

Finally it must be emphasized that any doctor attempting to treat a patient with chronic pancreatitis must indeed remember that he is treating a patient and not a disease and often to treat the patient may be the more difficult problem. If, for instance, he will not give up alcohol and is also perhaps addicted to pethidine, the clinician (physician or surgeon) attempting to treat him is fighting a losing battle from the start.

References

Blau M. and Bender M. A. (1962) *Radiology*, **78**: 974.

Brown P. W., Sircus W., Smith A. N., Donaldson A. A., Dymock I. W., Falcome C. W. A. and Small W. P. (1968) *Lancet*, **1**: 160

Puestow C. B. (1957) "Surgery of the Biliary Tract, Pancreas and Spleen", Year Book Publishers, Chicago.

PRINTED IN GREAT BRITAIN BY THE WHITEFRIARS PRESS LTD.
LONDON AND TONBRIDGE